VOLUME NINETY THREE

VITAMINS AND HORMONES

Hormones and Breast Cancer

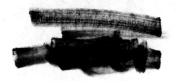

VOLUME NINETY THREE

VITAMINS AND HORMONES

Hormones and Breast Cancer

Editor-in-Chief

GERALD LITWACK, PhD

Toluca Lake, North Hollywood, California

ELSEVIER

AMSTERDAM • BOSTON • HEIDELBERG • LONDON
NEW YORK • OXFORD • PARIS • SAN DIEGO
SAN FRANCISCO • SINGAPORE • SYDNEY • TOKYO
Academic Press is an imprint of Elsevier

Cover photo credit:
Giulianelli S., Molinolo A. and Lanari C.
Targeting Progesterone Receptors in Breast Cancer
Vitamins and Hormones (2013) **93**, pp. 161–184.

Academic Press is an imprint of Elsevier
32 Jamestown Road, London, NW1 7BY, UK
The Boulevard, Langford Lane, Kidlington, Oxford, OX5 1GB, UK
Linacre House, Jordan Hill, Oxford OX2 8DP, UK
225 Wyman Street, Waltham, MA 02451, USA
525 B Street, Suite 1800, San Diego, CA 92101-4495, USA

First edition 2013

ISBN: 978-0-12-416673-8
ISSN: 0083-6729

For information on all Academic Press publications
visit our website at store.elsevier.com

Printed and bound in USA
13   14   15   16   11   10   9   8   7   6   5   4   3   2   1

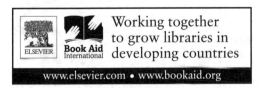

CONTENTS

CONTRIBUTORS

Jarlath C. Bolger
Endocrine Oncology Research, Royal College of Surgeons in Ireland, Dublin 2, Ireland

Ceshi Chen
Key Laboratory of Animal Models and Human Disease Mechanisms of Chinese Academy of Sciences & Yunnan Province, Kunming Institute of Zoology, Kunming, Yunnan, China

Nina D'Abreo
Oncology/Hematology Division, Winthrop University Hospital, Mineola, and SUNY Stony Brook School of Medicine, Stony Brook, New York, USA

Rawan Damouni
Diabetes and Metabolism Clinical Research Center of Excellence, Clinical Research Institute at Rambam (CRIR), Rambam Medical Center, P.O. Box 9602, Haifa, Israel

Jin-Tang Dong
Winship Cancer Institute, Emory University School of Medicine, Atlanta, Georgia, USA

Julia Dunn
School of Population and Public Health, University of British Columbia, Vancouver, British Columbia, Canada

Çağatay Erşahin
Department of Pathology, Loyola University Chicago Division of Health Sciences, Maywood, Illinois, USA

Rosalyn D. Ferguson
Division of Endocrinology, Diabetes and Bone Diseases, Samuel Bronfman Department of Medicine, Mount Sinai School of Medicine, P.O. Box 1055, New York, USA

Gilles Flouriot
Institut de Recherche en Santé-Environnement-Travail (IRSET), University of Rennes 1, INSERM U1085, Team TREC, Biosit, Rennes, France

Emily J. Gallagher
Division of Endocrinology, Diabetes and Bone Diseases, Samuel Bronfman Department of Medicine, Mount Sinai School of Medicine, P.O. Box 1055, New York, USA

Sebastián Giulianelli
Laboratory of Hormonal Carcinogenesis, Institute of Experimental Biology and Medicine (IBYME), Consejo Nacional de Investigaciones Científicas y Técnicas (CONICET), Buenos Aires, Argentina

Carolyn Gotay
School of Population and Public Health, University of British Columbia, Vancouver, British Columbia, Canada

Alexander A. Hindenburg
Oncology/Hematology Division, Winthrop University Hospital, Mineola, and SUNY
Stony Brook School of Medicine, Stony Brook, New York, USA

Kuniko Horie-Inoue
Division of Gene Regulation and Signal Transduction, Research Center for Genomic
Medicine, Saitama Medical University, Saitama, Japan

Kuo-Sheng Hsu
Department of Biochemistry, School of Medicine, Case Western Reserve University
(CWRU), The Comprehensive Cancer Center of CWRU, Cleveland, Ohio, USA

Nobuhiro Ijichi
Division of Gene Regulation and Signal Transduction, Research Center for Genomic
Medicine, Saitama Medical University, Saitama, Japan

Kazuhiro Ikeda
Division of Gene Regulation and Signal Transduction, Research Center for Genomic
Medicine, Saitama Medical University, Saitama, Japan

Satoshi Inoue
Division of Gene Regulation and Signal Transduction, Research Center for Genomic
Medicine, Saitama Medical University, Saitama; Department of Geriatric Medicine, and
Department of Anti-Aging Medicine, Graduate School of Medicine, The University of
Tokyo, Tokyo, Japan

V. Craig Jordan
Department of Oncology, Georgetown University, Lombardi Comprehensive Cancer
Center, Washington, District of Columbia, USA

Hung-Ying Kao
Department of Biochemistry, School of Medicine, Case Western Reserve University
(CWRU), The Comprehensive Cancer Center of CWRU, Cleveland, Ohio, USA

Gwenneg Kerdivel
Institut de Recherche en Santé-Environnement-Travail (IRSET), University of Rennes 1,
INSERM U1085, Team TREC, Biosit, Rennes, France

Todd P. Knutson
Department of Medicine, and Department of Pharmacology (Division of Hematology,
Oncology, and Transplantation), Masonic Cancer Center, University of Minnesota,
Minneapolis, Minnesota, USA

Claudia Lanari
Laboratory of Hormonal Carcinogenesis, Institute of Experimental Biology and Medicine
(IBYME), Consejo Nacional de Investigaciones Científicas y Técnicas (CONICET), Buenos
Aires, Argentina

Carol A. Lange
Department of Medicine, and Department of Pharmacology (Division of Hematology,
Oncology, and Transplantation), Masonic Cancer Center, University of Minnesota,
Minneapolis, Minnesota, USA

Derek LeRoith
Division of Endocrinology, Diabetes and Bone Diseases, Samuel Bronfman Department of Medicine, Mount Sinai School of Medicine, P.O. Box 1055, New York, USA, and Diabetes and Metabolism Clinical Research Center of Excellence, Clinical Research Institute at Rambam (CRIR), Rambam Medical Center, P.O. Box 9602, Haifa, Israel

Rong Liu
Key Laboratory of Animal Models and Human Disease Mechanisms of Chinese Academy of Sciences & Yunnan Province, Kunming Institute of Zoology, Kunming, Yunnan, China

Philipp Y. Maximov
Department of Oncology, Georgetown University, Lombardi Comprehensive Cancer Center, Washington, District of Columbia, USA

Russell E. McDaniel
Department of Oncology, Georgetown University, Lombardi Comprehensive Cancer Center, Washington, District of Columbia, USA

Alfredo Molinolo
Oral and Pharyngeal Cancer Branch, National Institute of Dental and Craniofacial Research, NIDCR, NIH, Bethesda, Maryland, USA

Clodia Osipo
Department of Pathology; Oncology Institute, and Department of Microbiology and Immunology, Loyola University Chicago Division of Health Sciences, Maywood, Illinois, USA

Farzad Pakdel
Institut de Recherche en Santé-Environnement-Travail (IRSET), University of Rennes 1, INSERM U1085, Team TREC, Biosit, Rennes, France

Sol Recouvreux
Área Investigación, Instituto de Oncología "Angel H. Roffo", Avda. San Martin 5481, Buenos Aires, Argentina

Rocio Sampayo
Área Investigación, Instituto de Oncología "Angel H. Roffo", Avda. San Martin 5481, Buenos Aires, Argentina

Dipak K. Sarkar
Endocrinology Program and Department of Animal Sciences, Rutgers, The State University of New Jersey, New Brunswick, New Jersey, USA

Eyal J. Scheinman
Diabetes and Metabolism Clinical Research Center of Excellence, Clinical Research Institute at Rambam (CRIR), Rambam Medical Center, P.O. Box 9602, Haifa, Israel

Marina Simian
Área Investigación, Instituto de Oncología "Angel H. Roffo", Avda. San Martin 5481, Buenos Aires, Argentina

Jodi J. Speiser
Department of Pathology, Loyola University Chicago Division of Health Sciences, Maywood, Illinois, USA

Leonie S. Young
Endocrine Oncology Research, Royal College of Surgeons in Ireland, Dublin 2, Ireland

Changqing Zhang
Endocrinology Program and Department of Animal Sciences, Rutgers, The State University
of New Jersey, New Brunswick, New Jersey, USA

PREFACE

Breast cancer has been a terrible disease and one where progress in therapy has been improving. The American Cancer Society estimated that, in 2011, there would be 230,480 new cases of breast cancer in females in the United States and 2140 new cases in males with an annual death rate of 39,520 of the involved women, a number of deaths not much different going back as far as 1998 although the percentage of deaths in 1998 was about 22% while in 2011 it was estimated to be about 17% of the existing cases. There definitely has been progress in treating this complex disease, but much more needs to be learned.

In this volume, many aspects of the disease are approached: the complex of sex hormone receptors involved and the nature of the cancer when one or more receptors are no longer being expressed, signifying a degree of dedifferentiation in the tumor cell; the relationship of other environmental factors, both external and internal, as they are related to the development of breast cancer; the many hormonal involvements that are primary factors in cancer development and the related drugs that are used to treat this disease; the many newly investigated genes whose expressions are related; and finally the behavior of the patient in terms of compliance with the drug treatments.

In the first chapter, a state-of-the-art review of the overall treatment of this disease is authored by R.E. McDaniel, P.Y. Maximov, and Y.C. Jordan entitled: "Estrogen-mediated mechanisms to control the growth and apoptosis of breast cancer cells: a translational research success story." In the chapter that follows, R.D. Ferguson, E.J. Gallagher, E. Scheinman, R. Damouni, and D. LeRoith present a comprehensive treatment of "The epidemiology and molecular mechanisms linking obesity, diabetes, and cancer." "Sex hormone receptors in breast cancer" is the title of the third contribution by N. D'Abreo and A.A. Hindenburg. Following this, G. Kerdivel, G. Flouriot, and F. Pakdel consider "Modulation of estrogen receptor alpha activity and expression during breast cancer progression." "Targeting progesterone receptors in breast cancer" is the topic of S. Giulianelli, A. Molinolo, and C. Lanari. The next report involves "The hyperplastic phenotype in PR-A and PR-B transgenic mice: lessons on the role of estrogen and progesterone receptors in the mouse mammary gland and breast cancer" by E. Sampayo, S. Recouvreux, and M. Simian.

In the next group of chapters, various genes and their products are the focus. N. Ijichi, K. Ikeda, K. Horie-Inoue, and S. Inoue discuss "FOXP1 and estrogen signaling in breast cancer." "The role of KLF5 in hormonal signaling and breast cancer development" is reported by R. Liu, J.-T. Dong, and C. Chen. T.P. Knutson and C.A. Lange focus on "Dynamic regulation of steroid hormone receptor transcriptional activity by reversible SUMOylation." D.K. Sarkar and C. Zhang target a role of the pituitary in "Beta-endorphin neuron regulates stress response and innate immunity to prevent breast cancer growth and progression." "The functional role of notch signaling in triple negative breast cancer" is the next chapter authored by J.J. Speiser, C. Ersahin, and C. Osipo. J.C. Bolger and L.S. Young proceed to discuss "ADAM22 as a prognostic and therapeutic drug target in the treatment of endocrine-resistant breast cancer." As a finale to this section, K.-S. Hsu and H.-Y. Kao review "Alpha-actinin 4 and tumorigenesis of breast cancer."

As the finale, J. Dunn and C. Gotay report on "Adherence rates and correlates in long-term hormonal therapy."

Collaborators in the assembly and processing of this volume are Helene Kabes and Mary Ann Zimmerman, of Elsevier, both stationed in the U.K.

The cover illustration is Figure 1 of Chapter 5 authored by S. Giulianelli, A. Molinolo, and C. Lanari.

GERALD LITWACK
North Hollywood, California
March 19, 2013

Estrogen-Mediated Mechanisms to Control the Growth and Apoptosis of Breast Cancer Cells: A Translational Research Success Story

Russell E. McDaniel, Philipp Y. Maximov, V. Craig Jordan[1]
Department of Oncology, Georgetown University, Lombardi Comprehensive Cancer Center, Washington, District of Columbia, USA
[1]Corresponding author: e-mail address: vcj2@georgetown.edu

Contents

Abstract

The treatment and prevention of solid tumors have proved to be a major challenge for medical science. The paradigms for success in the treatment of childhood leukemia, Hodgkin's disease, Burkett's lymphoma, and testicular carcinoma with cytotoxic chemotherapy did not translate to success in solid tumors—the majority of cancers that kill. In contrast, significant success has accrued for patients with breast cancer with antihormone treatments (tamoxifen or aromatase inhibitors) that are proved to enhance survivorship, and remarkably, there are now two approved prevention strategies using either tamoxifen or raloxifene. This was considered impossible 40 years ago. We describe the major clinical advances with nonsteroidal antiestrogens that evolved into selective estrogen receptor modulators (SERMs) which successfully exploited the ER

Vitamins and Hormones, Volume 93
ISSN 0083-6729
http://dx.doi.org/10.1016/B978-0-12-416673-8.00007-1

target selectively inside a woman's body. The standard paradigm that estrogen stimulates breast cancer growth has been successfully exploited for over 4 decades with therapeutic strategies that block (tamoxifen, raloxifene) or reduce (aromatase inhibitors) circulating estrogens in patients to stop breast tumor growth. But this did not explain why high-dose estrogen treatment that was the standard of care to treat postmenopausal breast cancer for 3 decades before tamoxifen caused tumor regression. This paradox was resolved with the discovery that breast cancer resistance to long-term estrogen deprivation causes tumor regression with physiologic estrogen through apoptosis. The new biology of estrogen action has been utilized to explain the findings in the Women's Health Initiative that conjugated equine estrogen alone given to postmenopausal women, average age 68, will produce a reduction of breast cancer incidence and mortality compared to no treatment. Estrogen is killing nascent breast cancer cells in the ducts of healthy postmenopausal women. The modulation of the ER using multifunctional medicines called SERMs has provided not only significant improvements in women's health and survivorship not anticipated 40 years ago but also has been the catalyst to enhance our knowledge of estrogen's apoptotic action that can be further exploited in the future.

1. INTRODUCTION

Translational research is a conversation between the laboratory and clinical practice. Pharmacology has always been by definition translational research. The goal in the laboratory is to discover a weakness in the disease that can be exploited selectively to kill the infection (or at least stop disease progression and the death of the host), but without injuring the normal tissue. The key word here is "selectively," as the proposed strategy for disease treatment leaves the safety of the laboratory to enter the uncertain world of treating patients.

At the outset, we will consider the disease to be controlled and the relentless threat to the patient the disease presents. Breast cancer is unique with its most important drug target, the estrogen receptor (ER). What is unique is the fact that the ER is not tumor specific. The ER is ubiquitous in one form or another (ERα or ERβ) within a woman's body. Nevertheless, the most progress during the past 40 years in patient survivorship has been made by targeting the ER in breast cancer. We will examine two ideas that have been essential to reduce the death rate from breast cancer: first, how do we develop drugs to treat disease? Second, how do we ensure selectivity, that is, kill the disease and not the patient. The story will advance rapidly through the twentieth century, but as with all journeys of discovery, surprises were in store along the way and dogma destroyed. These surprises are at the heart of our conversation with nature that is necessary for progress in medical science to save lives.

We will first describe the stages of breast cancer and its incidence in various countries. This is important not only to appreciate the extent of the disease worldwide but also to provide a basis to understand how fashions in treatment have evolved. The first fashion was to treat what could be seen, that is, metastatic breast cancer (stage IV) by endocrine ablative surgery or the empirical use of high-dose hormone therapy (Kennedy, 1965a). Endocrine therapy was palliative and no significant gains were anticipated. After the palliative use of endocrine approaches to treat stage IV breast cancer for 70 years, by the 1970s, nobody cared about palliative endocrine therapy. By the 1960s, combination cytotoxic chemotherapy was showing dramatic promise for the treatment of stage IV breast cancer so combination cytotoxic chemotherapy was used as an adjuvant to destroy micrometastases (stages I and II) that could not be seen but were predicted to grow and cause a recurrence of the disease. Regrettably, success was modest and cures elusive. However, the change in fashion to embrace long-term adjuvant therapy with antihormones saved millions of lives worldwide. The subsequent discovery and development of selective estrogen receptor modulators (SERMs) (Jordan, 2001) was the key step in developing a practical approach to reduce the incidence of breast cancer but, at the same time, maintained a hope to be able to reduce the morbidity produced by other diseases such as osteoporosis, coronary heart disease, strokes, and endometrial cancer. It has therefore been possible over the past 40 years to address effectively the targeted treatment of all stages of breast cancer and prevent the disease. As a result prognosis, survivorship has been enhanced and breast cancer incidence can now be reduced not only in the high-risk population but also in the general population.

2. CLINICAL PRESENTATION OF BREAST CANCER

Of the 275,370 American women that are estimated to die in 2012 from cancer, 39,510 of them (or approximately 14%) are projected to die from cancer of the breast (Howlader et al., 2009). Of the baby girls born today, 12.38% will be diagnosed with breast cancer at some point in their lifetime; 2.76% will die from breast cancer (Howlader et al., 2009). With the exception of skin cancers, breast cancer is the most common of all cancers in women, accounting for about one-third of all diagnoses in the United States (Breast Cancer Facts & Figures, 2011–2012). In recent years, 124.3 out of 100,000 women per year have been diagnosed with inva-sive breast cancer in the United States (31.4 out of 100,000 women per year have been diagnosed with *in situ* breast cancer; 23 out of 100,000 died (Howlander et al., 2009)). The District of Columbia has had the highest number of deaths due to invasive breast cancer in women with 27.96 out of 100,000 (Howlader et al., 2009). Louisiana, New Jersey, Ohio Missis-sippi, Missouri, Maryland, and Virginia all have relatively high death rates (above 24.18 per 100,000) (Howlader et al., 2009). While White American women have the highest rate of breast cancer diagnosis, African American women have an increased mortality rate from breast cancer, with 31.6 out of 100,000 dying (Howlader et al., 2009).

According to the American Cancer Society, 89% of women with breast cancer will still be living 5 years after their diagnosis (Breast Cancer Facts & Figures, 2011–2012). In fact, as of 2008, there were about 2.6 million women alive in America who had at one time been diagnosed with breast cancer (Breast Cancer Facts & Figures, 2011–2012).

Breast cancer also accounts for about 14% of cancer deaths among Canadian women, second only to lung cancer (Canadian Cancer Statistics, 2012). In Canada, in 2012, there will be an estimated 96 cases of breast cancer per 100,000 women or about 22,700 new diagnoses, with Ontario and Nova Scotia having the highest incidences. Five thousand one-hundred Canadian women will die in 2012 from breast cancer—out of 36,000 total female cancer deaths—with Prince Edward Island having the highest breast cancer mortality rate (Canadian Cancer Statistics, 2012).

In Brazil, in 2008, there were 49,400 new cases of breast cancer with 50.7 cases per 100,000 women (EISRCM, 2006) representing 28% of cancers in women (INCA, 2006). In 2006, there were 10,834 deaths due to breast can-cer (INCA, 2006). Malignant breast cancer is the seventh leading cause of death in Brazilian women (INCA, 2006). In the European Union, breast cancer represented about 30% of cancer incidences in women (Ferlay, Parkin, & Steliarova-Foucher, 2010), and about 16.6% of all female cancer deaths (Ferlay et al., 2010). In China, 168,013 new cases of breast cancer in women were estimated in 2005 (Yang, Parkin, Ferlay, Li, & Chen, 2005).

Breast cancer cases are divided into several stages, depending on the development of the disease. The population distribution of this relentlessly moving target, as it first occurs in the breast and subsequently breaks out, is illustrated in Fig. 1.1. Invasive breast cancer—or cancer cells from the breast that have overrun tissue beyond their origin, be it breast or other parts of the body—is divided into four stages. Potentially cancerous, abnormally

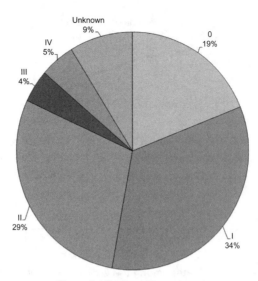

Stage distribution of breast cancer

Figure 1.1 Percentage of each stage of breast cancer as recorded by SEER between 2002 and 2008 (Howlader et al., 2009; Ries, Eisner, & Kosary, 2001). (See Color Insert.)

growing cells in the wall of the breast duct called ductal carcinoma *in situ*, or DCIS, is often referred to as stage 0 (Breast Cancer Survival Rates by Stage, 2011).

Stage I breast cancer is the first stage where the cancerous cells have spread into breast tissue away from the duct. This type of tumor is confined to the breast, and its diameter is no more than 2 cm. Stage II breast tumors have either spread to the lymph nodes under the arm or grown to be more than 2 cm in diameter (Breast Cancer Survival Rates by Stage, 2011).

Stage III breast cancer is known as "locally advanced cancer" and is divided into three subsections. Stage IIIA is when the tumor spreads to underarm lymph nodes that are attached to other bodily features (including other lymph nodes). Stage III also comprises tumors of greater than 5 cm diameter that have spread to isolated underarm lymph nodes. Stage IIIB is any breast tumor that has grown into the skin of the breast or into the chest wall. The size of the tumor is unimportant in stage IIIB classification. Stage IIIC tumors have either spread to the lymph nodes above or below the collarbone, or spread to the lymph nodes under the arm and behind the breastbone (Breast Cancer Survival Rates by Stage, 2011).

Metastatic breast cancer is known as stage IV. This cancer has spread from the breast to other organs. The brain, bones, and liver are frequent locations

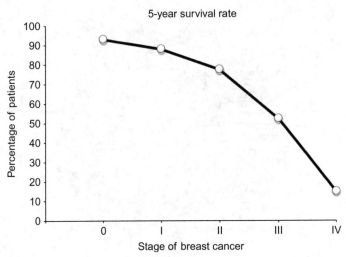

Figure 1.2 Five-year survival rates among the various stages of breast cancer (Breast Cancer Survival Rates by Stage, 2011).

for secondary breast cancers. Stage IV breast cancer has a poor prognosis with a 15% 5-year survival rate (Breast Cancer Survival Rates by Stage, 2011).

It is, therefore, important to stress that all "breast cancer" is not the same. We now know this from the molecular fingerprints from individual tumors that can be classified into subgroups (Hu et al., 2006; Perou et al., 2000; Sorlie et al., 2003). But personalized medicine has not yet arrived. Early detection and staging remain essential for survival (Fig. 1.2). Treatments with endocrine therapies have proved to be more successful the sooner they are deployed. But how did this happen?

3. TARGETED THERAPY

3.1. Foundations of chemical therapy

In 1908, Professor Paul Ehrlich was awarded the Nobel Prize for Medicine. In his Nobel Prize Lecture (Baumler, 1984), he described his work on antitoxins for diphtheria toxin and alluded to his side chain theory of receptors. However, he also alluded to his new studies on arsenicals (Baumler, 1984). He stated, "I want to show you that we are approaching the problem of obtaining an insight into the nature of the effects produced by drugs by following these points systematically, it will be easier than before to develop planned synthesis for pharmaceuticals targeted to requirements" (Baumler, 1984). He died of a heart attack and kidney failure on the afternoon of

August 20th, 1915, so he was not to receive his second Nobel Prize for his discovery that changed pharmacology and the treatment of disease forever. Based upon his early experience discovering dyes that stain bacteria but not human cells, he conceived of the idea that chemicals could be synthesized to kill the disease-causing bacteria specifically. Through his research, he created the process of synthesizing analogues of known toxic chemicals, testing the efficacy and safety of chemicals in appropriate animal models of human disease, and a suitable candidate could then be tested in clinical trial.

Sahachiro Hata, in Erlich's team, created the appropriate animal models of disease and ultimately discovered that chemical 606 was completely effective against laboratory models of syphilis. Ehrlich approached Hoescht to enter into mass production for clinical trials. These trials worked spectacularly to cure a fatal disease and Salvarsan became the first specific chemical therapy (or chemotherapy). Professor Ehrlich had created the roadmap for drug discovery by the pharmaceutical industry, but he also turned from the treatment of infections to cancer research. In 1909, the press announced, "The beginning of the end of the cancer problem is in sight," and an editorial in *Scientific American* in 1912 stated, "Unquestionably, their [Ehrlich and Wasseman's] investigations justify the hope of a cure for human cancer" (Schrek, 1960). However, in 1915, Ehrlich admitted defeat and stated, "I have wasted 15 years of my life in experimental cancer" (Schrek, 1960). So it would remain for the next 30 years, but this stagnation would change with the first successful use of a chemical therapy to treat metastatic breast cancer (stage IV) (Haddow, Watkinson, Paterson, & Koller, 1944).

3.2. The first chemical therapy to treat cancer

The link between estrogen and the growth of breast cancer is a fascinating tale. The interconnected research ventures in endocrinology and chemistry during the first 40 years of the twentieth century would create a new dimension in therapeutics, result in the use of high doses of synthetic estrogens to treat some metastatic breast cancers successfully, but also create a paradox. If ovarian estrogens fuel the growth of breast cancer, why does a high dose of estrogen kill breast cancer cells in postmenopausal women? This paradox has only recently been solved and we will use this chapter to illustrate how the twists and turns of endocrine therapy have both revolutionized patient care and exposed a new biology of estrogen action: estrogen-induced apoptosis.

In 1896, George Beatson reported the first case of oophorectomy as a treatment for breast cancer (Beatson, 1896). Although it is often said that he performed the operation empirically, he actually relied on his knowledge that farmers had discovered there was a link between the ovary and the lactating mammary gland. In 1900, Boyd (1900) collected all-known cases of oophorectomy from hospitals around Britain and discovered there was a 30% response rate. This is perhaps the first "clinical trial" and gave the medical community new knowledge that has stood the test of time. The response rate to any endocrine therapy is 30%. The work during the early decades of the twentieth century on laboratory mouse models of breast cancer by Lathrop and Loeb (1916) and Lacassagne (1933) would be valuable to advance knowledge about hormones and breast cancer growth. However, an understanding of why oophorectomy was beneficial to treat breast cancer and which tumor would be responsive would remain a mystery until the 1960s. The first clues that the ovaries contained a substance that causes responses in a target organ were reported by Allen and Doisey (1923). They named their substance in pig ovary estrogen. They determined the biological effect by ovariectomizing mice to stop the estrous cycles and discovered that the vaginal epithelium would undergo replication and cornification when pig ovarian extract was injected. The animal model in the mouse (referred to henceforth as the "Allen–Doisy test") would be the essential test system to discover synthetic estrogens a decade later during the 1930s.

The story of the discovery of potent nonsteroidal estrogens is remarkable (Jordan, Mittal, Gosden, Koch, & Lieberman, 1985). With only a few early clues that simple synthetic molecules could initiate mouse vaginal cornification, two major groups of potent estrogenic compounds were described in the 1930s: the stilbenes (Dodds, 1938; Dodds, Goldberg, Lawson, & Robinson, 1938) of which diethylstilbestrol (Fig. 1.3) would become a key compound and used clinically, and the longer acting triphenylethylenes (Robson, 1937; Robson & Schonberg, 1942; Robson, Schonberg, & Fahim, 1938; Thompson & Werner, 1953). These two classes of compounds would be the essential tools with which to change breast cancer therapy but most of the therapeutic advances over the decades between 1930 and 1980 would be almost by chance. Remarkably, the successful translational research would enhance survival from breast cancer and significantly improve women's health. Two practical facts emerged during this period: estrogens support mammary and breast tumorigenesis and growth; but, estrogen was used routinely to treat and cause regression of some metastatic breast cancers. This paradox would lie dormant until its rediscovery during the past decade.

Lacassagne (1936a, 1936b), Shimkin and Wyman (1945, 1946), and Shimkin, Wyman, and Andervont (1946) contributed evidence that estrogens could increase mouse mammary tumorigenesis. Lacassagne (1936b)

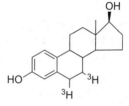

Diethylstilbestrol

Triphenylchlorethylene

Triphenylpropene

High-specific activity radiolabeled estrogens
to identify estrogen target tissues

[³H] Hexestrol

6,7 [³H] Estradiol

Figure 1.3 Compounds used by Haddow as the first "chemical therapy for cancer" (Haddow et al., 1944) and tritiated DES (hexestrol) and estradiol used in the first studies of retention of the estrogen in target tissues (Glascock & Hoekstra, 1959; Jensen & Jacobson, 1962).

went one step further at the Annual Meeting of the American Association of Cancer Research in Boston in 1936 by stating that

> If one accepts the consideration of adenocarcinoma of the breast as the consequence of a special hereditary sensibility to the proliferative actions of oestrone, one is led to imagine a therapeutic preventative for subjects predisposed by their heredity to this cancer. It would consist—perhaps in the very near future when the knowledge and use of hormones will be better understood—in the suitable use of a hormone antagonistic or excretory, to prevent the stagnation of oestrone in the ducts of the breast.

Unfortunately, there would be no "therapeutic antagonist" to use clinically until tamoxifen started its journey as an antiestrogen for the treatment of breast cancer (Jordan, 2003c, 2008b) some 40 years later!

In the first half of the twentieth century, breast cancer treatment was severe and unsuccessful. Radical mastectomy was the standard of care, radiation therapy was advancing from an art to a science, and nonspecific cytotoxic chemotherapy started to be introduced to treat cancer in general after the end of the Second World War. Prospects for the patient in general were abysmal and the examination of the state-of-the-art breast cancer treatment in 1977 (Stoll, 1977b) was not too much more hopeful. Nevertheless, with the wisdom of insight, one counterintuitive observation in the 1940s was to act as a catalyst for the eventual discovery of targeted cancer therapies. Alexander Haddow, conducting laboratory studies, discovered that carcinogenic polycyclic hydrocarbons actually caused tumor regression in animals but clearly one could not apply this "translational therapy" to patient care. However, he reasoned that the polycyclic synthetic estrogens had a similar sort of structure as the carcinogens (scary but true!), so following testing in the laboratory he compared and contrasted high-dose DES and triphenylethylenes (Fig. 1.3) as treatments for prostate cancer, breast cancer, and "other cancers." Prostate cancer responded as did metastatic breast cancer (stage IV) (30%) but none of the "other cancers" responded (Haddow et al., 1944). The application of high-dose estrogen therapy to provide palliative treatment for some postmenopausal women with metastatic breast cancer was the first chemical therapy to treat any cancer successfully. This approach became the standard of medical care in both the United Kingdom and the United States of America (Kennedy, 1965b; Kennedy & Nathanson, 1953) for the next 30 years until the resurrection of the triphenylethylene-based antiestrogen tamoxifen (Jordan, 2003c). In 1970, Sir Alexander Haddow FRS, during the inaugural Karnofsky (Haddow, 1970) lecture (the highest honor bestowed by the American Society for Clinical Oncology), stated his concerns for the future of specific and effective cancer therapy.

> In the first place, the fact that the cancer cell is but a modification of the normal somatic cell holds out little prospect of a chemotherapiaspecifica in Ehrlich's sense, whereby chemical substances which, on the one hand, are taken up by certain parasites and are able to kill them, are, on the other hand, tolerated well by the organism itself, or at any rate without too great damage.
>
> (Haddow, 1970)

In his Karnofsky lecture, Haddow also mentioned the importance of the few breast tumors that just melted away during high-dose estrogen therapy. However, he stated,

> ... the extraordinary extent of tumour regression observed in perhaps 1% of post-menopausal cases (with oestrogen) has always been regarded as of major theoretical importance, and it is a matter for some disappointment that so much of the underlying mechanisms continues to elude us ...
>
> (Haddow, 1970)

It is also important to stress that, at the time of Haddow's Karnofsky lecture in 1970, bacteria were routinely grown in the laboratory for testing antibiotic sensitivity; the right antibiotic could then be used appropriately to treat the right disease. No such tests existed for cancer. Practice was to give the drug and hope it might work. Therefore, the definition of the anticancer mechanism of DES in some breast tumors was the essential first step to determine which tumors will respond and which will not. What is the target for drug sensitivity or in Ehrlich's terms—the receptor? One study in 1949 by Walpole and Paterson (1949) declared defeat but the answer to the question "why" was to come ultimately from DES itself. The stilbene can be hydrogenated with tritium across the double bond to produce high-specific activity [^{3}H] hexestrol (Fig. 1.3). Hexestrol is a potent estrogen. Glascock and Hoekstra (1959) in fact showed the binding of [^{3}H] hexestrol in the estrogen target tissues of sheep and goats. The idea was subsequently translated to a clinical study in patients with metastatic breast cancer. Those patients whose breast tumor retained [^{3}H] hexestrol were more likely to respond to endocrine ablation (Folca, Glascock, & Irvine, 1961). These very preliminary findings were refined first by Jensen and Jacobson (1962) using [^{3}H] estradiol (Fig. 1.3) to describe the binding and retention of estradiol in the estrogen target tissues (uterus, vagina, pituitary gland) of the immature rat. Tritiated estradiol was bound initially, but not retained in tissues (muscle, lung) that were not targets of estrogen action. Gorski's group subsequently extracted and identified the soluble ER from the immature rat uterus (Toft & Gorski, 1966; Toft, Shyamala, & Gorski, 1967). These data were rapidly translated to identify the ER in breast tumors (Jordan, Wolf, Mirecki, Whitford, & Welshons, 1988) and there was a spectrum of none to a lot. Gorski's group discovered (Toft et al., 1967) that the extracted ER from target tissues could subsequently be liganded with [^{3}H] estradiol *in vitro*, so there was no need to inject radioactive estrogens into patients. The Jensen group went on to establish sucrose density gradient analysis as the method of choice to identify the breast tumor ER in the United States. In 1974 (McGuire, Carbone, & Vollmer, 1975), an NCI conference to consider the value of the ER assay to predict responsiveness of metastatic breast cancer to endocrine ablation or DES concluded that the absence of ER in a breast tumor predicted that the tumor would not respond to endocrine ablation or DES. If ER was present, there was about a 60% probability of an objective response. Thus, patients with ER-negative tumors should not be treated with endocrine ablation surgery; it would be worthless. At that time, in the mid-1970s, medical practice changed in America with a requirement that all patients with a diagnosis of breast cancer should have an ER assay on their tumor tissue. By the end of the 1970s, ER assay laboratories were springing up at most academic institutions (V.C.J. was involved in establishing one at the Worcester Foundation for Experimental Biology, Massachusetts in the early 1970s and was director of the steroid receptor laboratory at the Ludwig Unit in Bern, Switzerland (1979), organizing international quality control for the Ludwig clinical trials group, and the steroid receptor laboratory at the University of Wisconsin Clinical Cancer Center in the 1980s).

It should again be stressed that during the 1960s and 1970s the therapeutics of breast cancer was primitive. Only metastatic disease (stage IV) was addressed with therapy and this stage is fatal within a few years (Fig. 1.2). But the therapeutic options slowly evolved and this story again has its origins in the interest in synthetic estrogens. The synthetic estrogens, stilbenes or triphenylethylenes, used by Haddow in the 1940s (Haddow et al., 1944) (Fig. 1.3) were synthesized by Imperial Chemical Industries (ICI) Ltd. (now Astra Zeneca) but they were not alone in their interest in estrogens. Numerous pharmaceutical companies during the 1950s were interested in synthetic estrogens primarily because of the revolution in therapeutics that occurred with the development of the oral contraceptive that emanated from the vision of Gregory Pincus at the Worcester Foundation (Speroff, 2009). His chemical method stopped ovulation in the woman. No egg—no baby. It was reasoned by chemists in the pharmaceutical industry that if only another novel chemical method of contraception could be discovered, then the use of chemicals to prevent pregnancy, which was not a disease, could be expanded.

Leonard Lerner, a young scientist in the pharmaceutical industry in the 1950s, would take the next conceptual advance in reproduction research; that step would fail, but open the door for others to create the first targeted therapy for any cancer, the first endocrine therapy to save hundreds of thousands of women's lives, and the first chemical therapy approved to reduce the incidence of breast cancer in women of high risk for the disease. This did not occur because there was a specific plan by the pharmaceutical industry. The advance with tamoxifen would come from ICI Pharmaceuticals Division where their fertility control program would discover and then abandon ICI 46,474 to be resurrected and advanced by individuals with close friendships and who were in the right place at the right time and ready to exploit a unique opportunity.

3.3. Nonsteroidal antiestrogens

Leonard Lerner was tasked within the William S. Merrell Company to study nonsteroidal estrogens. At the time, the company marketed trianisylchlorethylene (TACE) (Fig. 1.4), but Lerner noticed a compound in the cardiovascular program was similar in structure—MER25 (Fig. 1.4) (Lerner, 1981). He tested the triphenylethanol and could detect no estrogenic activity in any species tested but it was a weak blocker of estrogen action (Lerner, Holthaus, & Thompson, 1958). However, what electrified the pharmaceutical industry was that MER25 and its successor clomiphene (Fig. 1.4) were postcoital antifertility agents in rats. Unfortunately, in clinical trial, the nonsteroidal antiestrogens were effective in inducing ovulation in subfertile women, so hopes of making a blockbuster drug disappeared. Clomiphene was tested as a breast cancer drug in metastatic disease (Hecker et al., 1974), as was nafoxidine (Legha, Slavik, & Carter, 1976), but development was abandoned because of concerns about toxic side effects (Fig. 1.4). No one was recommending careers in failed antifertility drugs or cancer therapy. Arthur Walpole was the head of the Fertility Control Program at ICI Pharmaceuticals Division in Alderley Park, Cheshire. He was interested in cancer research but was tasked to improve the toxicology profile of clomiphene that increased circulating desmosterol. Desmosterol was

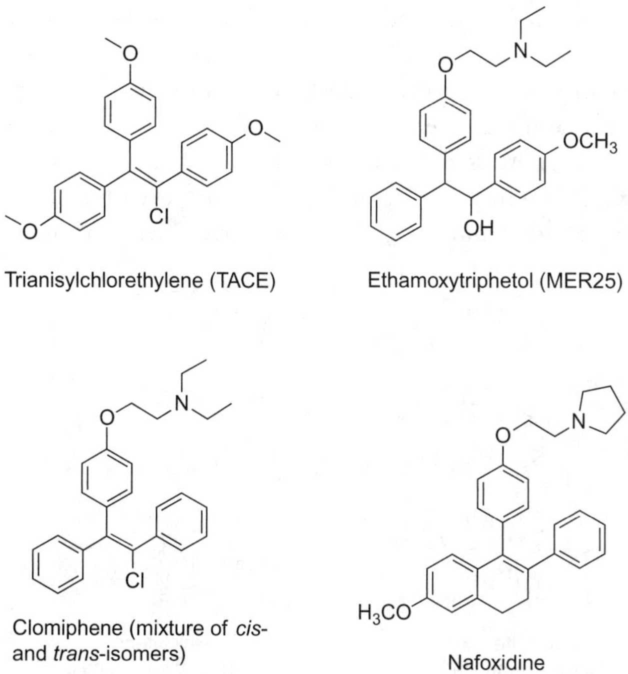

Trianisylchlorethylene (TACE)

Ethamoxytriphetol (MER25)

Clomiphene (mixture of *cis*-
and *trans*-isomers)

Nafoxidine

Figure 1.4 Structures of nonsteroidal estrogens and antiestrogens mentioned in the text.

associated with cataract formation in women (Laughlin & Carey, 1962). The result of the antifertility program at Alderley Park in the 1960s was ICI 46,474, the *trans*-isomer of a substituted triphenylethylene (Fig. 1.5) that was antiestrogenic with postcoital antifertility properties in the rat (Harper & Walpole, 1967a, 1967b). The patent application read,

> *The alkene derivatives of the invention are useful for the modification of the endocrine status in man and animals and they may be useful for the control of hormone-dependent tumours or for the management of the sexual cycle and aberrations thereof. They also have useful hypocholesterolaemic activity (Jordan, 2003c).*

Preliminary clinical studies demonstrated modest anticancer activity in metastatic breast cancer in postmenopausal women (Cole, Jones, & Todd, 1971) and the induction of ovulation in subfertile women (Klopper & Hall, 1971). However, after a review of all the data at Alderley Park in 1972, the Research Director decided to terminate clinical development—there was no financial future in ICI 46,474 (Jordan, 2006). However, Walpole reasoned that the company should put ICI 46,474 on the market as an orphan drug for the treatment of metastatic breast cancer and the induction of ovulation for subfertile women and "outsource" work to discover a strategy for the clinical use of tamoxifen. Walpole had recently met and examined the Ph.D. thesis of a young graduate student, Craig Jordan, in the Department of Pharmacology at the University of Leeds. Jordan was now spending 2 years as a visiting scientist as the Worcester foundation. Why not sponsor his research with an unrestricted grant? Let Jordan develop a clinical strategy for a nonsteroidal antiestrogen for the treatment of breast cancer.

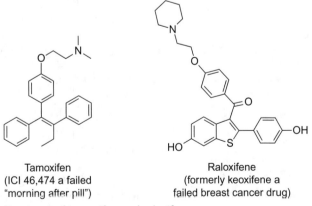

Tamoxifen
(ICI 46,474 a failed
"morning after pill")

Raloxifene
(formerly keoxifene a
failed breast cancer drug)

Figure 1.5 Structures of tamoxifen and raloxifene.

Scholarships were made available for Jordan students, technician's salaries were provided, and hundreds of laboratory rats were chauffeured from Alderley Park to the University of Leeds. This personal story has recently been told elsewhere (Poirot, 2011), but it is time now to focus on the pioneering medicine tamoxifen and how it not only changed breast cancer therapy but also acted as the catalyst to create new knowledge about the pharmacology of nonsteroidal antiestrogens that sequentially led to selective ER modulators, chemoprevention, the science of acquired drug resistance to antihormone therapy, and the new biology of estrogen–induced apoptosis.

4. TRANSITION TO TAMOXIFEN

Tamoxifen is unique in the annals of cancer therapeutics. While it is the first targeted therapy to treat cancer (a nonsteroidal antiestrogen targeted to the ER to stop estrogen-stimulated growth), the selective toxicity of tamoxifen was lucky. There are ERs all around the postmenopausal women's body, but as it turned out, these ERs do not appear to play a significant role in physiological homeostasis. Indeed, it was lucky that tamoxifen was also an antitumor agent in the premenopausal women without significant actions on normal physiology. Tamoxifen is approved by the FDA for the treatment of all stages of breast cancer, DCIS, male breast cancer, and for the reduction of breast cancer risk in both high-risk pre- and postmenopausal women. No other cancer therapy has such a spectrum of approved applications. At the outset of the translational research studies in the early years of the 1970s, it could not have been anticipated that a palliative medicine, FDA approved in December 1977 for the short-term (1–2 years) disease control of one in three postmenopausal patients with metastatic breast cancer, could so dramatically change the prognosis and survivorship for millions of women with ER–positive early breast cancer. During the 1970s, a laboratory strategy was put in place that would ultimately revolutionize thinking about the approach to treating breast cancer by targeting the tumor, killing the cancer cells not the patient, and treating earlier stages of the disease or even women only at risk for developing breast cancer (Jordan, 2008b). In the 1970s, the new fashion in therapeutics was combination cytotoxic chemotherapy that declared victory in childhood leukemia and was in the process of mopping up Hodgkin's disease (Stoll, 1977a). Justifiably, cytotoxic chemotherapy was king and only the appropriate acronym of drugs had now to be discovered to cure breast cancer. By contrast, no one in the pharmaceutical industry or clinical oncology was advocating a massive effort in endocrine therapy—or in fact any effort. Few cared.

The three publications that presaged the future clinical promise of tamoxifen as a pioneering medicine were all published in the *European Journal of Cancer* (Jordan, 2008b). The idea that tamoxifen blocked estrogen-stimulated breast cancer growth through blocking estradiol binding to the ER was controversial but was demonstrated both biochemically (Jordan & Koerner, 1975) and in cell culture (Lippman & Bolan, 1975). However, although these data were embraced in the United States, the same was not true for the United Kingdom where no clear clinical correlations between ER and tumor response could be demonstrated in clinical trial for the next 15 years (NATO, 1983; SCTO, 1987). Conceptually, this was important because the Europeans tended toward palliative applications with endocrine therapy, whereas in the United States, the goal was cure with combination cytotoxic chemotherapy. Simply stated, nobody cared about the mechanism of tamoxifen action but the good news was that in the United Kingdom everyone with breast cancer was to receive tamoxifen. This inadvertent policy was perhaps the correct decision for the wrong reason that ensured survivorship for tens of thousands of women in the United Kingdom.

The second conceptual advance was the finding that two sustained release subcutaneous injections of tamoxifen at the same time—as oral administration of dimethylbenzanthracene (DMBA) to 50–day-old female Sprague–Dawley rats, would prevent the initiation and growth of mammary carcinogenesis (Jordan, 1976). This observation was expanded (Jordan, Allen, & Dix, 1980; Jordan, Naylor, Dix, & Prestwich, 1980) and subsequently used as important laboratory evidence by Dr. Trevor Powles to explore the potential of tamoxifen to be used in the chemoprevention of breast cancer in high-risk women (Powles et al., 1989). The new dimension of the chemoprevention of breast cancer arrived in 1998 with the FDA approval of the pioneer tamoxifen for reducing the incidence of breast cancer in pre- and postmenopausal women at high risk (Fisher et al., 1998; Powles et al., 1998; Veronesi et al., 1998).

The third paper and advance that translated to clinical trial ultimately extended the survivorship of perhaps millions of women receiving long-term adjuvant tamoxifen therapy to prevent the recurrence of ER-positive breast cancer in patients with node-positive or node-negative breast cancer (stages I and II). In the early 1970s, the dilemma was when to use combination cytotoxic chemotherapy in the treatment plan for breast cancer. There was great enthusiasm that the use of combination cytotoxic chemotherapy would eventually lead to the cure of breast cancer. Very good results had been noted during the late 1960s (Cooper, 1969) and now a new strategy was considered: adjuvant therapy to destroy micro-metastatic disease that had spread systemically after the woman had a mastectomy and local radiation. The strategy seemed sound that combination cytotoxic would cure patients with a low tumor burden. Regrettably, early results were modest (Bonadonna et al., 1976; Fisher et al., 1975) with the best effect noted in premenopausal patients. However, subsequent work demonstrated that cytotoxic chemotherapy destroys the ovary so the treatment could reasonably be interpreted as an aggressive ovarian ablation (Jordan, 1998). With the slow development of the antiestrogen tamoxifen during the 1970s, attentions started to focus not on the palliative use of tamoxifen for metastatic breast cancer but on the idea that tamoxifen might have potential as an adjuvant therapy. In the laboratory, the DMBA rat mammary carcinoma model was considered to be "state of the art" for the study of the endocrine treatment of breast cancer. Huggins, Grand, and Brillantes (1961) first showed that a single oral administration of 20 mg DMBA to 50-day-old female Sprague–Dawley rats would produce multiple mammary carcinomas in all rats within 150 days after DMBA treatment. The development of tumors was endocrine dependent; the tumors contained ER and regressed in response to ovariectomy (Welsch, 1985). In the absence of any other experimental options, other than the DMBA model, to explore adjuvant therapy with tamoxifen, different durations of tamoxifen were used (or its potent metabolite 4-hydroxytamoxifen discovered around this time(Jordan, Collins, Rowsby, & Prestwich, 1977; Jordan, Dix, Naylor, Prestwich, & Rowsby, 1978) as tamoxifen actions was the sum of its antiestrogenic metabolites) to determine if a short course of the antiestrogen for a month (equivalent to a year in women as adjuvant therapy) would be cidal (Lippman & Bolan, 1975) or whether longer durations would be necessary to prevent tumor development. The idea was to destroy the early transformed cells, not unlike adjuvant therapy. The profound conclusion was that longer adjuvant therapy was going to be a better clinical strategy (Jordan, 1978; Jordan & Allen, 1980; Jordan, Allen, et al., 1980; Jordan, Dix, & Allen, 1979). The laboratory studies also derived another conclusion that was to have ramifications for the later use of polar nonsteroidal antiestrogen for the treatment of breast cancer. Tamoxifen was metabolically activated to 4-hydroxytamoxifen (Jordan et al., 1977, 1978). This was not a requirement for antiestrogenic activity but an advantage (Jordan & Allen, 1980). Polar nonsteroidal antiestrogens may be better at blocking estrogen actions at the ER but they had poor bioavailability and were rapidly excreted (Jordan & Allen, 1980). The subsequent idea that tamoxifen needed to be metabolically activated by hydroxylation of the primary metabolite N-desmethyltamoxifen to endoxifen was to preoccupy pharmacogenomics research on tamoxifen during the past decade with arguments both for and against the critical role of different CYP2D6 genotypes (Brauch et al., 2013; Dieudonne et al., 2009; Kiyotani et al., 2010; Lammers et al., 2010; Lash et al., 2011; Madlensky et al., 2011; Rae et al., 2012; Regan et al., 2012; Schroth et al., 2009). Simply stated, if CYP2D6 was aberrant then there is low metabolism to endoxifen and a lower probability of a response of the patients tumor to tamoxifen. Be that as it may, the fundamental issue in the 1970s was to select an appropriate duration of adjuvant tamoxifen therapy to test in breast cancer clinical trials.

The clinical community selected a 1-year course of adjuvant tamoxifen therapy in all early clinical trials (LBCSG, 1984; Rose et al., 1985). This was an obvious choice based on the limited effectiveness of tamoxifen to treat metastatic breast cancer. Tamoxifen is only effective for about 1 year (Ingle et al., 1981) so there was an understandable concern that longer adjuvant tamoxifen therapy would precipitate early drug resistance and recurrent disease that would now be fatal. But the studies with the DMBA rat mammary carcinoma model did not comply with clinical "predictions" based on the treatment of metastatic breast cancer. Short-term therapy (1 month equivalent to a year in a patient) was unable to control tumorigenesis in the rat but continuous therapy for six months (6 years in a patient) was 90% effective in controlling tumorigenesis (Jordan, Allen, et al., 1980). The DMBA rat model was to be proved to predict accurately subsequent clinical trials data. Five years of adjuvant tamoxifen therapy became the standard of care for the treatment of breast cancer for 20 years and remains so for the premenopausal patient.

There are several notable features of adjuvant tamoxifen therapy that were exposed during clinical trials and these data were enhanced and amplified by the regular review of ongoing adjuvant clinical trials through the Oxford Overview Analysis process. The survival advantage for these women taking long-term tamoxifen therapy is profound, whereas short term (1 year of treatment) is not of significance in premenopausal patients (Davies et al., 2011; EBCTCG, 1998, 2005). Most importantly, and we will examine this clinical observation in more detail during the discussions of acquired tamoxifen resistance, is the sustained decrease in mortality noted *after* 5 years of adjuvant tamoxifen. This was a surprising observation that now has a plausible scientific explanation. The science will be considered in Section 7.

The next step in the tamoxifen tale was the evaluation of its worth to prevent breast cancer in high-risk women. The evidence to support this decision to test the hypothesis in clinical trial was solid. The expanding database on tamoxifen as the endocrine adjuvant therapy of choice during 1980s and 1990s was reassuring for clinicians. Most important in this regard was the use of adjuvant tamoxifen therapy for the treatment of node-negative breast cancer because 80% of patients are cured by surgery and local radiotherapy, which meant that an increasing proportion of "cured" patients were already being treated with 5 years of adjuvant therapy (Fisher et al., 1989; SCTO, 1987). The fact that adjuvant tamoxifen reduced contralateral breast cancer (primary breast cancer) by 50% (Cuzick & Baum, 1985) was proof of principle: primary prevention would be successful and the earlier knowledge that tamoxifen prevented mammary tumorigenesis in rodents (Jordan, 1976) enhanced the opportunities for the clinical trials community.

Overall, the placebo-controlled clinical trials of chemoprevention demonstrated a significant decrease in the incidence of breast cancer following tamoxifen therapy that was sustained even when the drug treatment was terminated (Cuzick, Forbes, & Howell, 2006; Fisher et al., 2005, 1998; Powles, Ashley, Tidy, Smith, & Dowsett, 2007). However, the strategy was flawed as only a few women (2–5 per thousand per year) has their breast cancer prevented but hundreds of women per thousand would experience significant side effects such as menopausal symptoms and there would be an increased risk of deep vein thrombosis in postmenopausal women. Perhaps more serious was the finding in the laboratory that tamoxifen increased the growth of human endometrial cancer implanted in athymic mice but did block estrogen-stimulated growth of breast cancer completely in the same athymic mouse (Gottardis, Robinson, Satyaswaroop, & Jordan, 1988). These observations moved rapidly from the laboratory to clinical care within 3 years once the laboratory findings were confirmed in a placebo-controlled clinical trial (Fornander et al., 1989). Clinical findings demonstrated a three- to fivefold increase in the risk of developing endometrial cancer in postmenopausal women who now, as a treatment population, would have regular gynecological examinations when using tamoxifen. Although endometrial cancer was not significant for the treatment of breast cancer as the decreases in mortality were profound (EBCTCG, 2005), for the well women, this was a troubling side effect. It was said "one cancer was being substituted for another." In the prevention setting, this and the emerging new laboratory knowledge during the early 1990s that tamoxifen was a hepatocarcinogen in rats (Greaves, Goonetilleke, Nunn, Topham, & Orton, 1993; Hard et al., 1993) (this laboratory observation has never translated to patient populations—fortunately) mandated that a profoundly different strategy was essential, if chemoprevention was ever to be accepted as a reality in clinical practice.

5. SELECTIVE ESTROGEN RECEPTOR MODULATION

Up until the mid-1970s, the nonsteroidal antiestrogens were initially potential and then failed postcoital contraceptives. The antiestrogens became agents of interest to be exploited in gynecology. Both clomiphene and tamoxifen were successful for the induction of ovulation in subfertile women. A review by Lunan and Klopper (1975) focuses almost entirely on the potential applications in gynecology and there is only passing references to breast cancer treatment. By the mid-1980s, with tamoxifen FDA approved in December 1977 and adjuvant clinical trials well underway it was now time to consolidate all the information about the nonsteroidal antiestrogens as pharmacological agents (Jordan, 1984), so that further effective translational research could help patients. It was time also to review all that was known about tamoxifen (Furr & Jordan, 1984). After all, tamoxifen was, and is, the only nonsteroidal antiestrogen to be approved for the therapeutics of all stages of breast cancer and chemoprevention. It is, however, of interest to mention that tamoxifen had not been granted patent protection in the United States because of the perceived primacy of the earlier Merrel patents in the 1960s (Jordan, 2003c). That all changed in 1986 almost exactly at the time that long-term adjuvant tamoxifen therapy was the treatment strategy of choice for patients with ER-positive breast cancer (Consensus conference, Adjuvant chemotherapy for breast cancer, 1985). But it was the move toward using tamoxifen to prevent breast cancer in high-risk populations of women that now became the driving force behind understanding the "good, bad, and the ugly" of tamoxifen pharmacology. A surprise was in store.

It was reasoned at the time that, if estrogen was important to maintain bone density, then a nonsteroidal antiestrogen may prevent breast cancer in the few but create osteoporosis in the majority. The same argument was articulated about coronary heart disease and atherosclerosis, but it was already known in tamoxifen's patent (earlier described in Section 3.3) that circulating cholesterol was lowered by the drug (Harper & Walpole, 1967b).

The question of bone loss with nonsteroidal antiestrogen was addressed in the ovariectomized and intact rat using tamoxifen and the failed breast cancer drug keoxifene (Fig. 1.5), also a nonsteroidal antiestrogen (Black, Jones, & Falcone, 1983). Both nonsteroidal antiestrogens actually prevented bone loss from ovariectomy and a combination with estrogen further improved bone density (Jordan, Phelps, & Lindgren, 1987). These break-through data were confirmed (Turner, Evans, & Wakley, 1993; Turner, Wakley, Hannon, & Bell, 1987, 1988; Turner et al., 1998), but initially, these data in the refereed literature were ignored by the pharmaceutical industry. They did, however, act as preliminary data to initiate a prospective placebo-controlled clinical trial with tamoxifen in postmenopausal breast cancer patients with node-negative breast cancer. This trial was initiated at a time when node-negative breast cancer patients did not receive adjuvant therapy as a standard of care. The Wisconsin Tamoxifen Study demonstrated that tamoxifen lowered low-density lipoprotein (bad) cholesterol, did not substantially reduce high-density lipoprotein (good) cholesterol (Love et al., 1990, 1991), and improved bone density measured by dual photon absorptiometry (Love et al., 1992).Thus, not only did the animal studies unexpectedly translate to potential clinical benefit but also a new concept and vision was about to change medicine.

The laboratory studies with keoxifene and tamoxifen on bone density showed estrogen-like actions, but parallel studies at the same time demonstrated that tamoxifen and keoxifene could prevent rat mammary carcinogenesis (Gottardis & Jordan, 1987), an antiestrogenic effect. Thus, this class of compounds including clomiphene (Fig. 1.4), which was mixed isomers that are estrogenic or antiestrogenic (Beall et al., 1985), had all shown a similar effect on bone in the rat. So the potential new drug group had the potential to turn on and turn off sites around the body. At this time, it was already known that tamoxifen was more estrogenic in the rodent uterus (Harper & Walpole, 1967b) and human endometrial cancer would grow with tamoxifen (Gottardis et al., 1988) so this again illustrated the target site specific actions. The complex of the "antiestrogen" with the ER was being interpreted differently at different sites around the body (Jordan & Robinson, 1987). The endometrial cancer issue clearly was a "bad" for tamoxifen but others in the class, like keoxifene, were less estrogen-like in the uterus (Black et al., 1983), less likely to stimulate endometrial cancer in patients (Gottardis, Ricchio, Satyaswaroop, & Jordan, 1990), and were already known to maintain or build bone (Jordan et al., 1987). A road map for industry was proposed and simply stated (Lerner & Jordan, 1990):

Is this the end of the possible applications for antiestrogens? Certainly not. We have obtained valuable clinical information about this group of drugs that can be applied in other disease states. Research does not travel in straight lines and observations in one field of science often become major discoveries in another. Important clues have been garnered about the effects of tamoxifen on bone and lipids so it is possible that derivatives could find targeted applications to retard osteoporosis or atherosclerosis. The ubiquitous application of novel compounds to prevent diseases associated with the progressive changes after menopause may, as a side effect, significantly retard the development of breast cancer. The target population would be postmenopausal women in general, thereby avoiding the requirement to select a high risk group to prevent breast cancer.

In 1993, keoxifene was renamed raloxifene (Fig. 1.5) with patent protection to treat and prevent osteoporosis in postmenopausal women. The pivotal registration trial call Multiple Outcomes Relative to Evista was to demonstrate that raloxifene simultaneously could prevent fractures of the lumbar spine by about 50% (Ettinger et al., 1999) and reduce the incidence of ER-positive breast cancer by about 80% (Cummings et al., 1999) with no increase in endometrial cancer. Raloxifene became the first multifunctional medicine in women's health because of the positive results of the Study of Tamoxifen and Raloxifene (Vogel et al., 2006) where both drugs, now called selective ER modulators or SERMs, reduced breast cancer incidence in high-risk postmenopausal women by 50%. Two diseases, osteoporosis and breast cancer, were controlled by one drug. However, it was later shown (Vogel et al., 2010) that a 5-year course of raloxifene is not sufficient to maintain long-term benefit for the prevention of breast cancer-like tamoxifen. Raloxifene is approved by the FDA for indefinite administration for the prevention and treatment of osteoporosis, and breast cancer reduction is sustained during extended treatment (Martino et al., 2004). Again, the unanticipated merits of tamoxifen to sustain antitumor actions in chemoprevention (Powles et al., 2007) would raise the question why? A plausible answer would occur through serendipity and the examination of acquired drug resistance to SERMs in the laboratory.

6. ACQUIRED DRUG RESISTANCE AND THE SURPRISE OF SERMS

During the 1970s, the concept of acquired resistance to antihormone therapy was simple. Breast tumors were considered to be a mixture of cells: some were ER negative and some ER positive. The concentration of ER in a tumor was therefore an average of total tumor ER per unit protein, for example, 150 femtomoles ER per mg tumor protein. This was measured by extracting the unoccupied tumor ER, and following some competitive binding assay with tritiated estradiol plus/minus a massive excess of non-radioactive ligand, which was either an estrogen or an antiestrogen (Jordan et al., 1988), the total ER tumor concentrations was established. Based on the 1974 Conference in Bethesda (McGuire et al., 1975), it was decided that tumors would be classified as either ER positive (above 10 femtomoles/mg cytosol protein) or ER negative (below 10 femtomoles/mg cytosol protein). Tumors that were ER positive would most likely respond to endocrine ablation or high-dose estrogen therapy but ER-negative tumors were unlikely to respond (McGuire et al., 1975).

Failure of endocrine therapy (Ingle et al., 1981) usually occurs after about a year or two of treatment in metastatic breast cancer (stage IV). The received wisdom was that the ER-positive cells were dying and the tumor was being repopulated with ER-negative cells. However, this did not explain the fact that clinicians could identify an endocrine therapy responsive tumor that would respond and fail but then respond again to a different endocrine therapy. This could continue for several cycles and is referred to as the "endocrine cascade." Clearly some other mechanism of acquired resistance was occurring. The adaptations of the tumor to the environment during treatment were illustrated by the responses of some tumors to high-dose DES therapy. We noted earlier that Haddow observed that some tumors melted away, but during the 1960s and 1970s, Basil Stoll showed that some tumors would regress but they would regrow during DES therapy only to regress again once DES treatment was stopped (Stoll, 1977b). This was called a "withdrawal response." There was no explanation for all these events.

During the 1980s, with the general acceptance by the clinical community that clinical trials had to be started to test long-term adjuvant tamoxifen therapy, it became clear that there was a need for realistic laboratory models of acquired drug resistance to tamoxifen. These would be necessary to assess mechanisms of resistance and subvert the process, but more importantly, in the short term, to discover effective second-line therapies for patients that prematurely recur during adjuvant tamoxifen treatment.

Tamoxifen blocks estradiol-stimulated MCF-7 tumor growth when cells are inoculated into athymic mice (Osborne, Hobbs, & Clark, 1985). However, tamoxifen cannot control tumor growth indefinitely; eventually, MCF-7 tumors grow despite continuing tamoxifen treatment (Osborne, Coronado, & Robinson, 1987). This situation was examined from another perspective using serial transplantations of MCF-7 tumors with acquired tamoxifen resistance. Remarkably, the growth of tumors with acquired tamoxifen resistance is dependent upon tamoxifen (Gottardis & Jordan, 1988; Gottardis, Wagner, Borden, & Jordan, 1989) or indeed any SERM such as raloxifene or toremifene (O'Regan et al., 2002). Physiologic estrogen treatment also caused tumors to grow so the ER mechanism was reconfigured in the breast cancer cells to grow with either estrogen or tamoxifen as the binding ligand. No treatment or treatment with a pure steroidal antiestrogen ICI 164,384 (Gottardis, Jiang, Jeng, & Jordan, 1989) (the lead compound for the series that became the clinically approved drug fulvestrant) would therefore be predicted to be an appropriate clinical treatment strategy. These data in the laboratory presaged the subsequent clinical findings that either an aromatase inhibitor (no estrogen) or fulvestrant would be appropriate second-line therapies following treatment failure with tamoxifen (Howell et al., 2004; Osborne et al., 2002).

The issue of the development of acquired resistance to tamoxifen within a year or two when used for the treatment of metastatic breast cancer (stage IV) appeared to be replicated in the laboratory (Gottardis & Jordan, 1988), but the fact that adjuvant tamoxifen treatment could be continued for 5 years without rapid early treatment recurrences was not explained by the laboratory models developed in the 1980s. Again serendipity intervened with a chance observation that opened up the study of a new biology of estrogen-induced apoptosis.

7. ESTROGEN-INDUCED APOPTOSIS: BACK TO THE BEGINNING

The MCF-7 tumor model of acquired resistance to tamoxifen was a significant advance for the study of SERM resistance, but the tumor biology could only be retained *in vivo*, through repeated transplantation into generations of athymic mice every 4 or 5 months. Cell culture models of antihormone therapy were becoming available (Sweeney, McDaniel, Maximov, Fan, & Jordan, 2012) once it was realized that the MCF-7 cell line, that had actually been derived from a patient treated with high-dose DES, was subsequently grown and propagated *in vitro* in a media rich in an estrogen as a contaminant of the phenol red redox indicator (Berthois, Katzenellenbogen, & Katzenellenbogen, 1986; Bindal, Carlson, Katzenellenbogen, & Katzenellenbogen, 1988; Bindal & Katzenellenbogen, 1988). Studies removing all estrogens from media initially cause MCF-7 cells to die but remaining cells adapt and grow independent of estrogen but retain the ER (i.e., do not become ER negative) (Katzenellenbogen, Kendra, Norman, & Berthois, 1987; Welshons & Jordan, 1987). These early studies would replicate the action of aromatase inhibitor on the ER-positive tumor. During the next decade, numerous cell lines would be created (Herman & Katzenellenbogen, 1994; Jiang, Wolf, Yingling, Chang, & Jordan, 1992; Masamura, Santner, Heitjan, & Santen, 1995; Pink, Jiang, Fritsch, & Jordan, 1995; Shim et al., 2000) that would yield further insights into estrogen action in the twenty-first century. However, the breakthrough in the understanding of the evolution of acquired resistance to tamoxifen was to come from the years of retransplantation of MCF-7 tumors into tamoxifen-treated athymic mice. Continuous retransplantation into tamoxifen-treated mice over a 5-year period changes the tumor cell response to physiological estrogen treatment from a survival signal to a trigger of apoptosis (Wolf & Jordan, 1993; Yao et al., 2000). Small tumors do not grow with physiologic estradiol treatment but melt away completely. Large tumors undergo dramatic regression but eventually start to regrow vigorously with continuing estradiol treatment. Retransplantation of the growing tumors into new athymic mice demonstrates growth is dependent upon estrogen treatment, no treatment results in no tumor growth, and tamoxifen again inhibits estradiol-stimulated growth (Fig. 1.6). The estrogen destroys cells with acquired resistance to tamoxifen with the remaining tumor tissue again responsive to tamoxifen treatment. These laboratory findings were reproducible and exhibited a cyclical pattern of sensitivity and resistance indicating a plasticity in the tumor cell population (Balaburski et al., 2010; Yao et al., 2000). They also suggested a mechanism to explain the sustained and enhanced antitumor effect of tamoxifen *after* a long duration of the SERM had been administered (at least 5 years). It was proposed that acquired drug resistance evolves through Phase I resistance where both estrogen and tamoxifen stimulate tumor growth and then the survival mechanisms are reconfigured so that, in Phase II that occurs before 5 years, only tamoxifen supports the survival of micrometastases; physiologic estrogen causes tumor cell death (Fig. 1.6) (Jordan, 2004). The use of adjuvant tamoxifen for 5 years prepares the micrometastatic disease to be destroyed by the woman's own estrogen once the tamoxifen is stopped (Wolf & Jordan, 1993). Mortality continues to decrease as micrometastatic disease is eradicated (EBCTCG, 2005). The same events would explain the sustained effects of long-term tamoxifen treatment in the chemoprevention setting (Cuzick et al., 2006; Fisher et al., 2005; Powles et al., 2007).

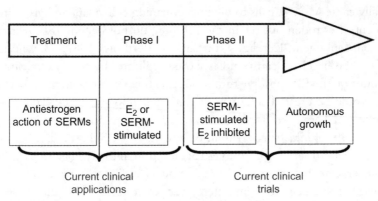

Figure 1.6 The evolution of drug resistance (Jordan, 2004). (See Color Insert.)

Table 1.1 Response rates to high-dose DES treatment of breast cancer patients in Lonning et al. (2001)
Response

Complete	Partial	Stable disease
4[a]/32	6/32	2/32

[a]One patient remains disease-free 10 years and 6 months after commencing DES treatment.

These laboratory data (Wolf & Jordan, 1993; Yao et al., 2000) also proposed the potential use of high- or low-dose estrogen treatment as a salvage therapy for patients who had received exhaustive (i.e., the endocrine cascade) antihormone therapy. This strategy has been evaluated clinically. Lonning et al. (2001) noted an overall 30% response rate to high-dose DES (15 mg daily) (Table 1.1) and one patient had a remarkable response continuing to last now for over 10 years.

> One of the patients (AO) who achieved a complete response of a 16 × 16 mm cytological confirmed chest wall relapse, received DES treatment for five years, where after she been subject to regular follow-up without active treatment. To this day, she remains disease-free 10 years and six months after commencing DES treatment.
>
> (Lonning, 2009)

Recently, Ellis et al. (2009) have tested the "low-dose" estrogen therapy hypothesis (Yao et al., 2000) and noted a similar clinical benefit (~29%) for women receiving either 6 mg estradiol daily or 30 mg estradiol daily, after failing an aromatase inhibitor. Responses were not as profound in the Ellis study (Ellis et al., 2009) compared with the Lonning study

(Lonning et al., 2001) probably because the patients in the Ellis study were not treated "exhaustively" with antihormones and had therefore not evolved to Phase II endocrine resistance.

The "Phase II" tamoxifen resistance model also taught another interesting lesson. The pure antiestrogen fulvestrant produced tumoristasis, whereas physiologic estrogen causes profound tumor regression starting after about 1 week (Osipo, Gajdos, Liu, Chen, & Jordan, 2003). However, a combination of fulvestrant plus physiologic estrogen causes dramatic tumor growth (Osipo et al., 2003). These data imply that a combination of fulvestrant and aromatase inhibitor as endocrine therapy following failure of long-term tamoxifen treatment may produce better tumor control than fulvestrant alone (presupposing one does not use physiologic estrogen to treat patients alone first!) Although results are not exactly optimal, two large treatment trials have recently been published using similar dosage regimens. One shows significant PFS and survival advantages for the combination (Mehta et al., 2012), whereas the other does not (Bergh et al., 2012). However, neither trial uses optimal fulvestrant therapy, that is, 500 mg, or twice the recommended monthly dose of 250 mg (Di Leo et al., 2010).

With the relentless rise of interest in the development of an aromatase inhibitor to replace tamoxifen as the long-term adjuvant therapy of choice for postmenopausal women, studies of resistance moved naturally to study the effect of estrogen withdrawal on ER-positive cells *in vitro*. The experimental results (Song et al., 2001) were to dovetail nicely into results from prior studies with tamoxifen *in vivo* (Yao et al., 2000). Long-term estrogen-deprived (LTED) MCF-7 cells could initially gain a "supersensitivity" to estrogen in the environment once the main source of estrogen had been removed. In other words, the original studies (Katzenellenbogen et al., 1987; Welshons & Jordan, 1987) that demonstrated initial cell death when MCF-7 cells were exposed to an estrogen-free environment, but then a population of cells grew spontaneously. This "estrogen-free growth" was interpreted as the cells being selected that were "hypersensitive" to extremely low estrogen concentrations (Masamura et al., 1995; Shim et al., 2000). But further examinations of concentration response relationship showed that estrogen-induced apoptosis occurred in these cells (Song et al., 2001), but not just at high concentrations but at low concentrations as predicted by the MCF-7 tamoxifen-resistant model *in vivo* (Jordan, Liu, & Dardes, 2002). Specific clones of MCF-7 cells generated from populations of LTED MCF-7 cells (Jiang et al., 1992; Pink et al., 1995) can undergo immediate estrogen-induced apoptosis (MCF-7:5C)

(Lewis et al., 2005) or apoptosis induced by estrogen a week later (MCF-7:2A) (Ariazi et al., 2011).

Several facts are emerging to understand the new biology of estrogen-induced apoptosis. The molecular events to trigger apoptosis with physiologic estrogen initiate the mitochondrial or intrinsic pathway first and then for the final execution there is recruitment of the extrinsic pathway (Lewis et al., 2005). This process is fundamentally different to cytotoxic chemotherapy that immediately causes a G1 blockade with a commitment to program cell death within 12 h. Massive DNA disruption requires immediate action by the cell.

What then is the physiologic trigger for estrogen-induced apoptosis? Apoptosis caused by estrogen can be modulated and is dependent upon the shape of the ligand ER complex. Estrogens are classified (Jordan et al., 2001) into Class I or planar estrogens such as estradiol or DES and Class II or angular estrogens such as hydroxylated triphenylethylenes. Both classes of estrogen *cause* cell replication but only Class I estrogens, which permit the ligand to be sealed within the ligand-binding domain (Brzozowski et al., 1997; Shiau et al., 1998), can initiate immediate estrogen-induced apoptosis in the correctly configured estrogen-deprived breast cancer cell. Coactivators must bind to the ER complex for growth or apoptosis (Hu et al., 2011). By contrast, an estrogenic triphenylethylene in Class II alters the shape of the ER complex "so that it temporarily adapts to the shape of an antiestrogenic ER complex" (Maximov et al., 2011) which cannot adequately bind coactivators to delay estrogen-induced apoptosis. These data dramatically illustrate the promiscuous nature of cell replication and survival with almost any signal input that is minimally adequate to bind to the ER. The signal for death must be precise because it is final for the cell.

One obvious application for the discovery of the cellular mechanisms that *prevent* estrogen-induced apoptosis is to deploy a companion therapy to neutralize resistance to apoptosis and enhance responsiveness to estrogen. Looked at simply, it would be an advantage to enhance apoptosis and convert clinical responses of 30% for estrogen-treated patients following exhaustive antihormone therapy to over 50%. Two approaches have addressed the goal of enhancing response rates to physiologic estrogen-induced apoptosis. First, the MCF-7:2A cells have a delayed response to estrogen-induced apoptosis and also have an enhanced glutathione synthetic pathway (Ariazi et al., 2011). Glutathione protects against oxidative stress. The administration of buthioninesulphoximine that blocks the synthesis of glutathione causes rapid estrogen-induced apoptosis (Lewis-Wambi, Swaby, Kim, & Jordan, 2009; Lewis-Wambi et al., 2008). Second, it was believed that blocking the cSrc oncogene, which is present in 70% of human breast cancer, would further enhance estrogen-induced apoptosis of the breast cancers treated exhaustively with antihormone therapy. In fact, blocking cSrc actually also blocked estrogen-induced apoptosis (Fan et al., 2012). This was not the anticipated result, but this is new knowledge that must, in the future, be considered when dissecting the trigger mechanism of estrogen-induced apoptosis. It could not have been predicted that cSrc was essential for estrogen-induced apoptosis. The discovery of the precise triggering mechanism for estrogen-induced apoptosis will, because it is biologically unique, provide additional approaches to discover new targeted therapies.

8. THE LEGACY OF TAMOXIFEN

In 1970, there was no tamoxifen, only ICI 46,474, a failed "morning after pill," that was abandoned by the pharmaceutical industry in 1972 (Jordan, 2003c, 2006). By a series of fortunate friendships and the key individuals being in the right place at the right time, the first target drug in breast cancer therapy, tamoxifen, was reinvented (Jordan, 2008b) to become a life-saving medicine, the first SERM, the first chemopreventive drug to reduce the risk of any cancer and the drug that would throw light on the "mechanism of estrogen-induced apoptosis" solving Haddow's paradox when he deployed the first chemical therapy, high-dose estrogen, to treat breast cancer successfully (Jordan, 2008a).

There are two additional therapeutic advances that tamoxifen catalyzed: the aromatase inhibitors and the development of the SERM principle as a multifunctional drug group.

Angela Brodie's dedicated and pioneering work (Brodie & Longcope, 1980; Brodie, Marsh, & Brodie, 1979; Brodie, Schwarzel, Shaikh, & Brodie, 1977; Coombes, Goss, Dowsett, Gazet, & Brodie, 1984) was essential as proof of principle that a selective aromatase inhibitor could be discovered with clinical efficacy. The problem with her discovery, 4-hydroxyandrostenedione, was that it was an injectable rather than a more convenient oral preparation. However, the fact that the failed "morning after pill" ICI 46,474 was transformed successfully into the "gold standard" tamoxifen for the adjuvant treatment of breast cancer provided a new target (the aromatase enzyme) to improve antihormonal therapy in breast cancer. With profits expanding from sales of tamoxifen in the United States after 1990, the key issue for the successful drug development of an aromatase inhibitor would be satisfied: profits. The patent from tamoxifen would run out in America, and aromatase inhibitors be substituted. Three orally active third-generation aromatase inhibitors were subsequently successfully developed for adjuvant therapy: anastrazole, letrozole, and exemestane. Each was demonstrated to have a small but consistent improvement over 5 years of tamoxifen alone whether given instead of tamoxifen in postmenopausal patients, after 5 years of tamoxifen or switching after a couple of years of tamoxifen (Baum et al., 2002; Boccardo et al., 2005; Coates et al., 2007; Coombes et al., 2004; Goss et al., 2003, 2005; Howell et al., 2005; Thurlimann et al., 2005). There has even been a successful trial of exemestane as a preventive in postmenopausal high-risk women (Goss et al., 2011). However, it is hard to see how this approach would be superior to a sophisticated third-generation SERM functioning as a multifunctional medicine in women's health.

The advantages of aromatase inhibitors for postmenopausal patients are clear in large population trials and for health-care systems. Patents for aromatase inhibitors are running out or have run out and cheap generics are becoming available. (The aromatase inhibitors were initially priced extremely high compared to tamoxifen to compensate for each only securing about one-third of the original tamoxifen market.) A disease-free survival advantage is noted for adding an aromatase inhibitor to the treatment plan compared to tamoxifen alone (Dowsett et al., 2010) and concerns about endometrial cancer and blood clots are diminished. Current clinical studies to improve endocrine response rates seek to exploit emerging knowledge about the molecular mechanisms of antihormone resistance to aromatase inhibitors (Roop & Ma, 2012). Combinations of letrozole and lapatinib, an inhibitor of the HER2 pathway, show some advantages over letrozole alone in ER-positive and HER-positive metastatic breast cancer (Riemsma et al., 2012). A similar improvement in responsiveness to aromatase inhibitors is noted with a combination with the mTor inhibitor everolimus (Bachelot et al., 2012; Baselga et al., 2012, 2009).

The second major advance in therapeutics catalyzed by tamoxifen is the SERM group of medicines. The cluster of laboratory findings in the 1980s that described the fact that the "nonsteroidal antiestrogens" were actually targeted estrogens and antiestrogens in select estrogen target tissues (Jordan, 2001) prompted a significant effort by the pharmaceutical industry to exploit the concept with new SERMs (Jordan, 2003a, 2003b). This, in large measure, was because both tamoxifen and raloxifene were so successful economically. The osteoporosis market is much bigger than the endocrine treatment of breast cancer.

Today considerable scientific success has been achieved with new SERMs, but it remains a challenge to create a drug with absolute safety guarantees for all women. The bar is now very high by necessity as prevention of multiple diseases implies that subjects who are the target population are in fact currently well. We will comment briefly on three compounds: lasofoxifene, basedoxifene, and ospemifene, but first it is worth mentioning that the molecules each have a "history" (Fig. 1.7). Lasofoxifene started its

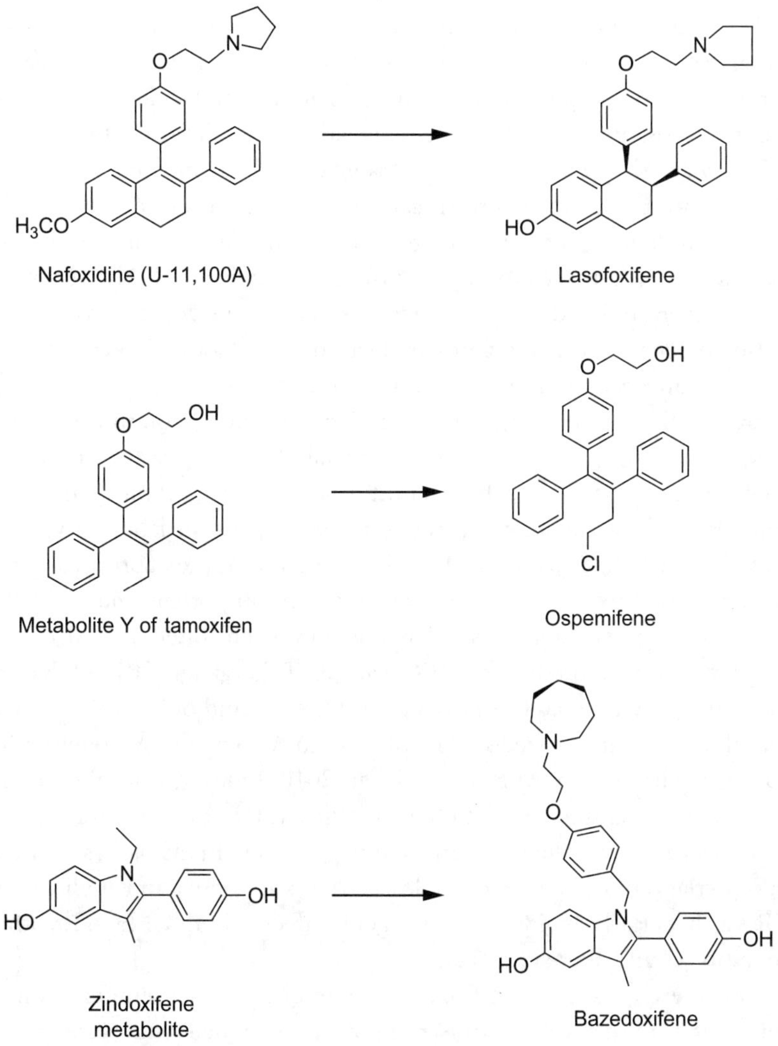

Figure 1.7 The historical origins of the new SERMs.

molecular odyssey from its origins in the fertility control program at Upjohn in Kalamazoo in the early 1960s (Lednicer, Emmert, Duncan, & Lyster, 1967; Lednicer, Lyster, & Duncan, 1967). The antiestrogen/postcoital contraceptive, U11,100A, was initially discovered by the fertility control program. But U11,100A was reinvented to become nafoxidine for the treatment of breast cancer (Legha et al., 1976). Unfortunately, this program was abandoned because of the severe side effect of photophobia. Lasofoxifene is a very potent SERM with an effective dose of 0.5 mg daily being recommended for the treatment and prevention of osteoporosis (Cummings et al., 2010). This is 1/100th the recommended daily dose of raloxifene (60 mg daily). Medicinal chemists discovered that the levorotatory enantiomer is resistant to glucuronidation so that the molecule is not readily excreted (Rosati et al., 1998). The registration trial of postmenopausal evaluation and risk-reduction with lasofoxifene documented significant decreases in ER-positive breast cancer, coronary heart disease, strokes, and endometrial cancer (Cummings et al., 2010). Basically, all that the original roadmap (Lerner & Jordan, 1990) predicted for a SERM to prevent breast cancer (and endometrial cancer) as beneficial side effect for the prevention of osteoporosis and coronary heart disease. Lasofoxifene is approved in the European Union, but not in the United States.

Bazedoxifene (Fig. 1.7) (Gruber & Gruber, 2004; Komm et al., 2005; Miller et al., 2001), evolved from the metabolite of an earlier compound, zindoxifene, that failed to have antitumor activity in clinical trial (Stein et al., 1990), actually showed estrogen-like activity in laboratory studies (Robinson, Koch, & Jordan, 1988). Introduction of the appropriate phenylalkylaminoethoxy side chain created an important new SERM. Bazedoxifene is of interest as it has not only been tested as a SERM for the prevention of osteoporosis (Kawate & Takayanagi, 2011; Silverman et al., 2012) but also has been evaluated as a new kind of hormone replacement therapy, that is, bazedoxifene plus conjugated equine estrogens (CEE) (Kagan, Williams, Pan, Mirkin, & Pickar, 2010; Lindsay, Gallagher, Kagan, Pickar, & Constantine, 2009; Pinkerton, Pickar, Racketa, & Mirkin, 2012). There is an additive effect on bone density, but the SERM blocks breast and endometrial actions of estrogen. Clearly, this is an innovation application of SERMs that clearly avoids the tumorigenic effect of both CEE and synthetic progestin (Crandall et al., 2012).

Last, there is ospemifene (Fig. 1.7). The history of ospemifene is interesting as it has also evolved from a previously researched predecessor. A new metabolite of tamoxifen (metabolite Y) was reported in 1982–1983 and was shown to have weak antiestrogenic properties (Bain & Jordan, 1983; Jordan, Bain, Brown, Gosden, & Santos, 1983). Later, a similar metabolite was found for another antiestrogen toremifene, and this metabolite is now known as ospemifene. Originally, ospemifene was developed to treat vaginal atrophy in postmenopausal women, but it also can be useful for the prevention and treatment of osteoporosis. In clinical trials, ospemifene was shown to be well tolerated and have a safe toxicity profile (DeGregorio et al., 2000; Rutanen et al., 2003; Voipio et al., 2002). However, there is still not enough data from the trials to assess the effectiveness of ospemifine in regard with osteoporosis or breast cancer prevention.

However, with all the SERMs, the principal issue can be the quality of life for the patient. Hormone replacement therapy solves the menopausal symptom of hot flashes and night sweats. This is an important issue for those with severe symptoms. The SERMs, at present, are known to exacerbate rather than resolve this issue. However, prompted by potential markets, pharmaceutical chemists are attempting to decipher the complexities of this important SERM side effect to allow therapeutic compliance with SERMs to become optimal (Jain et al., 2006, 2009; Wallace et al., 2006; Watanabe et al., 2003).

So how far can the SERM concept go? Already medicinal chemists have created selective agonist/antagonist for all members of the nuclear receptor superfamily (Fan & Jordan, 2013), and there is the promise of the further understanding of selective ERα/ERβ modulators (Sengupta & Jordan, 2013). The products, should they find applications in the clinic, hold the promise of treating diseases selectively that could never have been imagined 40 years ago.

But all is not resolved with SERMs and one discovery in the early 1980s remains a work in progress. The availability of [^{3}H] tamoxifen allowed the identification of an "antiestrogen-binding protein" by Sutherland et al. (1980). It was hypothesized that it could be linked with antiestrogen action, but in recent years, compelling evidence has been presented that it plays a role in cholesterol metabolism (Payre et al., 2008) and is identified in mice as membranous epoxide hydrolase. The biology is complex but there are suggestions that this may be a mechanism for tumoricidal action (Delarue et al., 1999; Payre et al., 2008).

In coming to the end of our story, we return to the beginning of chemical therapy for cancer. Sir Alexander Haddow FRS, it is fair to state, actually became the catalyst for change in the chemical treatment of cancer. In 1970, there were no tests to establish the sensitivity of a tumor to chemical therapy.

It was empirical medicine of trial and error in patients based on often suspect clinical experience rather than rigorously controlled clinical trials. Haddow advanced clinical certainty during his career from individual experience by organizing a small clinical trial to obtain preliminary data (Haddow et al., 1944), with a subsequent large multicentered trial to ensure a valid result was being promoted to improve clinical practice. To prove the validity and reproducibility of these preliminary data, a collaborative clinical trial was organized with a dozen centers throughout the United Kingdom organized by the Royal Society of Medicine (Haddow was the President of the Section of Oncology at the Royal Society of Medicine). He stated his discovery during his 1970 Karnofsky lecture:

> When the various reports were assembled at the end of that time, it was fascinating to discover that rather general impression, not sufficiently strong from the relatively small numbers in any single group, became reinforced to the point of certainty; namely, the beneficial responses were three times more frequent in women over the age of 60 years than in those under that age; that oestrogens may, on the contrary, accelerate the course of mammary cancer in younger women, and that their therapeutic use should be restricted to cases 5 years beyond the menopause. Here was an early and satisfying example of the advantages which may accrue from cooperative clinical trial.
>
> (Haddow, 1970)

A similar conclusion was noted by Stoll (1977b) through a review of his lifetime experience with 407 postmenopausal patients with stage IV breast cancer treated with high-dose estrogen (Table 1.2). It is clear a prolonged period of estrogen deprivation after the menopause is needed for the optimal apoptotic activity of estrogen to develop.

These early data have relevance to solve a current paradox in women's health that has major significance. The Women's Health Initiative (WHI) Study of combination CEE and the synthetic progestin medroxy-progesterone acetate (HRT) (to prevent endometrial cancer) was initiated to assess the effects of HRT on improving women's health, that is, preventing fractures, coronary heart disease, and Alzheimer's, and balancing

Table 1.2 Objective response rates in postmenopausal women with metastatic breast cancer using high-dose estrogen therapy

Age since menopause	Patient #	Regression (%)
Postmenopausal 0–5 years	63	9
Postmenopausal >5 years	344	35

The 407 patients are divided in relation to menopause (Stoll, 1977b).

this with the known side effects of increasing the incidence of breast cancer and thromboembolic disorders. The study did show a decrease in osteoporotic fractures but no benefit for coronary heart disease or for Alzheimer's disease (Rossouw et al., 2002). Breast cancer incidence was increased (Chlebowski et al., 2003; Shumaker et al., 2003). However, the examination of the second WHI trial of CEE alone versus placebo in hysterectomized postmenopausal women showed an initial decrease in breast cancer incidence (Anderson et al., 2004; Prentice et al., 2008), and then a further decrease that was sustained for 5 years after CEE treatment was terminated (LaCroix et al., 2011). A recent analysis demonstrates rather remarkably not only a sustained decrease in breast cancer incidence but also all cancers and a significant decrease in mortality (Anderson et al., 2012). The population of women were aged an average of 68 years, that is, following a long period of estrogen deprivation CEE causes a tumoricidal action which fits nicely with the Haddow/Stoll explanation of needing an "estrogen holiday" to create the correct antitumor sensitivity to estrogen. In other words, estrogen should not be given alone straight after menopause as an ERT. These data obtained in the modern era close the circle on our current understanding of estrogen action in the life and death of breast cancer cells (Jordan, 2008a). The saga of SERMs not only advanced women's health, dramatically improving survivorship and preventing both breast cancer and osteoporosis but also created the opportunity to discover the new biology of estrogen-induced apoptosis. This natural mechanism is programmed in a completely different way than the cellular response to cytotoxic therapy. Our ability to decipher the actual trigger of estrogen-induced apoptosis may open up new opportunities in targeted cancer therapeutics.

ACKNOWLEDGMENTS

This work (V. C. J.) was supported by the Department of Defense Breast Program under Award number W81XWH-06-1-0590 Center of Excellence, subcontract under the SU2C (AACR) Grant number SU2C-AACR-DT0409, the Susan G. Komen for the Cure Foundation under Award number SAC100009, and the Lombardi Comprehensive Cancer 1095 Center Support Grant (CCSG) Core Grant NIH P30 CA051008. The views and opinions of the author(s) do not reflect those of the U.S. Army or the Department of Defense.

REFERENCES

Allen, E., & Doisey, E. A. (1923). An ovarian hormone: Preliminary reports on its localization, extraction and partial purification and action in test animals. *Journal of the American Medical Association*, *81*(10), 819–821.

Anderson, G. L., Chlebowski, R. T., Aragaki, A. K., Kuller, L. H., Manson, J. E., Gass, M., et al. (2012). Conjugated equine oestrogen and breast cancer incidence and mortality in postmenopausal women with hysterectomy: Extended follow-up of the Women's Health Initiative randomised placebo-controlled trial. *The Lancet Oncology, 13*(5), 476–486.

Anderson, G. L., Limacher, M., Assaf, A. R., Bassford, T., Beresford, S. A., Black, H., et al. (2004). Effects of conjugated equine estrogen in postmenopausal women with hysterectomy: The Women's Health Initiative randomized controlled trial. *Journal of the American Medical Association, 291*(14), 1701–1712.

Ariazi, E. A., Cunliffe, H. E., Lewis-Wambi, J. S., Slifker, M. J., Willis, A. L., Ramos, P., et al. (2011). Estrogen induces apoptosis in estrogen deprivation-resistant breast cancer through stress responses as identified by global gene expression across time. *Proceedings of the National Academy of Sciences of the United States of America, 108*(47), 18879–18886.

Bachelot, T., Bourgier, C., Cropet, C., Ray-Coquard, I., Ferrero, J. M., Freyer, G., et al. (2012). Randomized phase II trial of everolimus in combination with tamoxifen in patients with hormone receptor-positive, human epidermal growth factor receptor 2-negative metastatic breast cancer with prior exposure to aromatase inhibitors: A GINECO study. *Journal of Clinical Oncology, 30*(22), 2718–2724.

Bain, R. R., & Jordan, V. C. (1983). Identification of a new metabolite of tamoxifen in patient serum during breast cancer therapy. *Biochemical Pharmacology, 32*(2), 373–375.

Balaburski, G. M., Dardes, R. C., Johnson, M., Haddad, B., Zhu, F., Ross, E. A., et al. (2010). Raloxifene-stimulated experimental breast cancer with the paradoxical actions of estrogen to promote or prevent tumor growth: A unifying concept in anti-hormone resistance. *International Journal of Oncology, 37*(2), 387–398.

Baselga, J., Campone, M., Piccart, M., Burris, H. A., 3rd., Rugo, H. S., Sahmoud, T., et al. (2012). Everolimus in postmenopausal hormone-receptor-positive advanced breast cancer. *The New England Journal of Medicine, 366*(6), 520–529.

Baselga, J., Semiglazov, V., van Dam, P., Manikhas, A., Bellet, M., Mayordomo, J., et al. (2009). Phase II randomized study of neoadjuvant everolimus plus letrozole compared with placebo plus letrozole in patients with estrogen receptor-positive breast cancer. *Journal of Clinical Oncology, 27*(16), 2630–2637.

Baum, M., Budzar, A. U., Cuzick, J., Forbes, J., Houghton, J. H., Klijn, J. G., et al. (2002). Anastrozole alone or in combination with tamoxifen versus tamoxifen alone for adjuvant treatment of postmenopausal women with early breast cancer: First results of the ATAC randomised trial. *The Lancet, 359*(9324), 2131–2139.

Baumler, E. (1984). *Paul Ehrlich: Scientist for life.* (1st ed.). New York: Holmes & Meier Publishers.

Beall, P. T., Misra, K. L., Young, R. L., Spjut, H. J., Evan, H. J., & LeBlanc, A. (1985). Clomiphene protects against osteoporosis in the mature ovariectomized rat. *Calcified Tissue International, 36*, 123–125.

Beatson, G. T. (1896). On the treatment of inoperable cases of carcinoma of the mamma: Suggestions for a new method of treatment, with illustrative cases. *The Lancet, 148*, 104–107.

Bergh, J., Jonsson, P. E., Lidbrink, E. K., Trudeau, M., Eiermann, W., Brattstrom, D., et al. (2012). FACT: An open-label randomized phase III study of fulvestrant and anastrozole in combination compared with anastrozole alone as first-line therapy for patients with receptor-positive postmenopausal breast cancer. *Journal of Clinical Oncology, 30*(16), 1919–1925.

Berthois, Y., Katzenellenbogen, J. A., & Katzenellenbogen, B. S. (1986). Phenol red in tissue culture media is a weak estrogen: Implications concerning the study of estrogen-responsive cells in culture. *Proceedings of the National Academy of Sciences of the United States of America, 83*(8), 2496–2500.

Bindal, R. D., Carlson, K. E., Katzenellenbogen, B. S., & Katzenellenbogen, J. A. (1988). Lipophilic impurities, not phenolsulfonaphthalein, account for the estrogenic activity in commercial preparations of phenol red. *Journal of Steroid Biochemistry, 31*(3), 287–293.

Bindal, R. D., & Katzenellenbogen, J. A. (1988). Bis(4-hydroxyphenyl)[2-(phenoxysulfonyl) phenyl]methane: Isolation and structure elucidation of a novel estrogen from commercial preparations of phenol red (phenolsulfonphthalein). *Journal of Medicinal Chemistry*, *31*(10), 1978–1983.

Black, L. J., Jones, C. D., & Falcone, J. F. (1983). Antagonism of estrogen action with a new benzothiophene derived antiestrogen. *Life Sciences*, *32*(9), 1031–1036.

Boccardo, F., Rubagotti, A., Puntoni, M., Guglielmini, P., Amoroso, D., Fini, A., et al. (2005). Switching to anastrozole versus continued tamoxifen treatment of early breast cancer: Preliminary results of the Italian Tamoxifen Anastrozole Trial. *Journal of Clinical Oncology*, *23*(22), 5138–5147.

Bonadonna, G., Brusamolino, E., Valagussa, P., Rossi, A., Brugnatelli, L., Brambilla, C., et al. (1976). Combination chemotherapy as an adjuvant treatment in operable breast cancer. *The New England Journal of Medicine*, *294*(8), 405–410.

Boyd, S. (1900). On oophorectomy in cancer of the breast. *British Medical Journal*, *2*, 1161–1167.

Brauch, H., Schroth, W., Goetz, M. P., Mürdter, T. E., Winter, S., Ingle, J. N., et al. (2013). Tamoxifen use in postmenopausal breast cancer: CYP2D6 matters. *Journal of Clinical Oncology*, *31*, 176–180.

Breast Cancer Facts and Figures (2011–2012). Atlanta, American Cancer Society: American Cancer Society, Inc.

Breast Cancer Survival Rates by Stage (2011). American Cancer Society.

Brodie, A. M., & Longcope, C. (1980). Inhibition of peripheral aromatization by aromatase inhibitors, 4-hydroxy- and 4-acetoxy-androstene-3,17-dione. *Endocrinology*, *106*(1), 19–21.

Brodie, A. M., Marsh, D., & Brodie, H. J. (1979). Aromatase inhibitors. IV. Regression of hormone-dependent, mammary tumors in the rat with 4-acetoxy-4-androstene-3,17-dione. *Journal of Steroid Biochemistry*, *10*(4), 423–429.

Brodie, A. M., Schwarzel, W. C., Shaikh, A. A., & Brodie, H. J. (1977). The effect of an aromatase inhibitor, 4-hydroxy-4-androstene-3,17-dione, on estrogen-dependent processes in reproduction and breast cancer. *Endocrinology*, *100*(6), 1684–1695.

Brzozowski, A. M., Pike, A. C., Dauter, Z., Hubbard, R. E., Bonn, T., Engstrom, O., et al. (1997). Molecular basis of agonism and antagonism in the oestrogen receptor. *Nature*, *389*(6652), 753–758.

Canadian Cancer Statistics (2012). Canadian Cancer Society.

Chlebowski, R. T., Hendrix, S. L., Langer, R. D., Stefanick, M. L., Gass, M., Lane, D., et al. (2003). Influence of estrogen plus progestin on breast cancer and mammography in healthy postmenopausal women: The Women's Health Initiative Randomized Trial. *Journal of the American Medical Association*, *289*(24), 3243–3253.

Coates, A. S., Keshaviah, A., Thurlimann, B., Mouridsen, H., Mauriac, L., Forbes, J. F., et al. (2007). Five years of letrozole compared with tamoxifen as initial adjuvant therapy for postmenopausal women with endocrine-responsive early breast cancer: Update of study BIG 1-98. *Journal of Clinical Oncology*, *25*(5), 486–492.

Cole, M. P., Jones, C. T., & Todd, I. D. (1971). A new anti-oestrogenic agent in late breast cancer. An early clinical appraisal of ICI46474. *British Journal of Cancer*, *25*(2), 270–275.

Consensus conference (1985). Adjuvant chemotherapy for breast cancer. *Journal of the American Medical Association*, *254*(24), 3461–3463.

Coombes, R. C., Goss, P., Dowsett, M., Gazet, J. C., & Brodie, A. (1984). 4-Hydroxyandrostenedione in treatment of postmenopausal patients with advanced breast cancer. *The Lancet*, *2*(8414), 1237–1239.

Coombes, R. C., Hall, E., Gibson, L. J., Paridaens, R., Jassem, J., Delozier, T., et al. (2004). A randomized trial of exemestane after two to three years of tamoxifen therapy in postmenopausal women with primary breast cancer. *The New England Journal of Medicine,* *350*(11), 1081–1092.

Cooper, R. G. (1969). Combination chemotherapy in hormone resistant breast cancer. *Proceeding of the American Association for Cancer Research,* *10,* 15.

Crandall, C. J., Aragaki, A. K., Cauley, J. A., McTiernan, A., Manson, J. E., Anderson, G., et al. (2012). Breast tenderness and breast cancer risk in the estrogen plus progestin and estrogen-alone women's health initiative clinical trials. *Breast Cancer Research and Treatment,* *132*(1), 275–285.

Cummings, S. R., Eckert, S., Krueger, K. A., Grady, D., Powles, T. J., Cauley, J. A., et al. (1999). The effect of raloxifene on risk of breast cancer in postmenopausal women: Results from the MORE randomized trial. Multiple Outcomes of Raloxifene Evaluation. *Journal of the American Medical Association,* *281*(23), 2189–2197.

Cummings, S. R., Ensrud, K., Delmas, P. D., LaCroix, A. Z., Vukicevic, S., Reid, D. M., et al. (2010). Lasofoxifene in postmenopausal women with osteoporosis. *The New England Journal of Medicine,* *362*(8), 686–696.

Cuzick, J., & Baum, M. (1985). Tamoxifen and contralateral breast cancer. *The Lancet,* *2*(8449), 282.

Cuzick, J., Forbes, J. F., & Howell, A. (2006). Re: Tamoxifen for the prevention of breast cancer: Current status of the National Surgical Adjuvant Breast and Bowel Project P-1 study. *Journal of the National Cancer Institute,* *98*(9), 643, author reply 643–644.

Davies, C., Godwin, J., Gray, R., Clarke, M., Cutter, D., Darby, S., et al. (2011). Relevance of breast cancer hormone receptors and other factors to the efficacy of adjuvant tamoxifen: Patient-level meta-analysis of randomised trials. *The Lancet,* *378*(9793), 771–784.

DeGregorio, M. W., Wurz, G. T., Taras, T. L., Erkkola, R. U., Halonen, K. H., & Huupponen, R. K. (2000). Pharmacokinetics of (deaminohydroxy)toremifene in humans: A new, selective estrogen-receptor modulator. *European Journal of Clinical Pharmacology,* *56*(6–7), 469–475.

Delarue, F., Kedjouar, B., Mesange, F., Bayard, F., Faye, J. C., & Poirot, M. (1999). Modifications of benzylphenoxy ethanamine antiestrogen molecules: Influence affinity for antiestrogen binding site (AEBS) and cell cytotoxicity. *Biochemical Pharmacology,* *57*(6), 657–661.

Di Leo, A., Jerusalem, G., Petruzelka, L., Torres, R., Bondarenko, I. N., Khasanov, R., et al. (2010). Results of the CONFIRM phase III trial comparing fulvestrant 250 mg with fulvestrant 500 mg in postmenopausal women with estrogen receptor-positive advanced breast cancer. *Journal of Clinical Oncology,* *28*(30), 4594–4600.

Dieudonne, A. S., Lambrechts, D., Claes, B., Vandorpe, T., Wildiers, H., Timmerman, D., et al. (2009). Prevalent breast cancer patients with a homozygous mutant status for CYP2D6*4: Response and biomarkers in tamoxifen users. *Breast Cancer Research and Treatment,* *118*(3), 531–538.

Dodds, E. (1938). Biological effects of the synthetic oestrogenic substance 4:4'-dihydroxy-alpha:beta-diethylstilbene. *The Lancet,* *232*(6015), 1389–1391.

Dodds, E. C., Goldberg, L., Lawson, W., & Robinson, R. (1938). Oestrogenic activity of esters of diethyl stilboestrol. *Nature,* *142*(3587), 211–212.

Dowsett, M., Cuzick, J., Ingle, J., Coates, A., Forbes, J., Bliss, J., et al. (2010). Meta-analysis of breast cancer outcomes in adjuvant trials of aromatase inhibitors versus tamoxifen. *Journal of Clinical Oncology,* *28*(3), 509–518.

EBCTCG, (1998). Tamoxifen for early breast cancer: An overview of the randomised trials. Early Breast Cancer Trialists' Collaborative Group. *The Lancet,* *351*(9114), 1451–1467.

EBCTCG, (2005). Effects of chemotherapy and hormonal therapy for early breast cancer on recurrence and 15-year survival: An overview of the randomised trials. *The Lancet,* *365*(9472), 1687–1717.

EISRCM, (2006). *O Câncer de Mama no Brasil Situacão epidemiológica e rastreamento*. Rio de Janeiro: Encontro Internacional Sobre Rastreamento de Cancer de Mama.

Ellis, M. J., Gao, F., Dehdashti, F., Jeffe, D. B., Marcom, P. K., Carey, L. A., et al. (2009). Lower-dose vs. high-dose oral estradiol therapy of hormone receptor-positive, aromatase inhibitor-resistant advanced breast cancer: A phase 2 randomized study. *Journal of the American Medical Association, 302*(7), 774–780.

Ettinger, B., Black, D. M., Mitlak, B. H., Knickerbocker, R. K., Nickelsen, T., Genant, H. K., et al. (1999). Reduction of vertebral fracture risk in postmenopausal women with osteoporosis treated with raloxifene: Results from a 3-year randomized clinical trial. Multiple Outcomes of Raloxifene Evaluation (MORE) Investigators. *Journal of the American Medical Association, 282*(7), 637–645.

Fan, P., & Jordan, V. C. (2013). An emerging principle: Selective nuclear receptor modulators. In V. C. Jordan (Ed.), *Estrogen actions, SERMs, and women's health*. London: Imperial College Press.

Fan, P., McDaniel, R. E., Kim, H. R., Clagett, D., Haddad, B., & Jordan, V. C. (2012). Modulating therapeutic effects of the c-Src inhibitor via oestrogen receptor and human epidermal growth factor receptor 2 in breast cancer cell lines. *European Journal of Cancer, 48*, 3488–3498.

Ferlay, J., Parkin, D. M., & Steliarova-Foucher, E. (2010). Estimates of cancer incidence and mortality in Europe in 2008. *European Journal of Cancer, 46*, 765–781.

Fisher, B., Carbone, P., Economou, S. G., Frelick, R., Glass, A., Lerner, H., et al. (1975). 1-Phenylalanine mustard (L-PAM) in the management of primary breast cancer. A report of early findings. *The New England Journal of Medicine, 292*(3), 117–122.

Fisher, B., Costantino, J., Redmond, C., Poisson, R., Bowman, D., Couture, J., et al. (1989). A randomized clinical trial evaluating tamoxifen in the treatment of patients with node-negative breast cancer who have estrogen-receptor-positive tumors. *The New England Journal of Medicine, 320*(8), 479–484.

Fisher, B., Costantino, J. P., Wickerham, D. L., Cecchini, R. S., Cronin, W. M., Robidoux, A., et al. (2005). Tamoxifen for the prevention of breast cancer: Current status of the National Surgical Adjuvant Breast and Bowel Project P-1 study. *Journal of the National Cancer Institute, 97*(22), 1652–1662.

Fisher, B., Costantino, J. P., Wickerham, D. L., Redmond, C. K., Kavanah, M., Cronin, W. M., et al. (1998). Tamoxifen for prevention of breast cancer: Report of the National Surgical Adjuvant Breast and Bowel Project P-1 Study. *Journal of the National Cancer Institute, 90*(18), 1371–1388.

Folca, P. J., Glascock, R. F., & Irvine, W. T. (1961). Studies with tritium-labelled hexoestrol in advanced breast cancer. Comparison of tissue accumulation of hexoestrol with response to bilateral adrenalectomy and oophorectomy. *The Lancet, 2*(7206), 796–798.

Fornander, T., Rutqvist, L. E., Cedermark, B., Glas, U., Mattsson, A., Silfversward, C., et al. (1989). Adjuvant tamoxifen in early breast cancer: Occurrence of new primary cancers. *The Lancet, 1*(8630), 117–120.

Furr, B. J., & Jordan, V. C. (1984). The pharmacology and clinical uses of tamoxifen. *Pharmacology and Therapeutics, 25*(2), 127–205.

Glascock, R. F., & Hoekstra, W. G. (1959). Selective accumulation of tritium-labelled hexoestrol by the reproductive organs of immature female goats and sheep. *The Biochemical Journal, 72*, 673–682.

Goss, P. E., Ingle, J. N., Ales-Martinez, J. E., Cheung, A. M., Chlebowski, R. T., Wactawski-Wende, J., et al. (2011). Exemestane for breast-cancer prevention in postmenopausal women. *The New England Journal of Medicine, 364*(25), 2381–2391.

Goss, P. E., Ingle, J. N., Martino, S., Robert, N. J., Muss, H. B., Piccart, M. J., et al. (2003). A randomized trial of letrozole in postmenopausal women after five years of tamoxifen therapy for early-stage breast cancer. *The New England Journal of Medicine*, *349*(19), 1793–1802.

Goss, P. E., Ingle, J. N., Martino, S., Robert, N. J., Muss, H. B., Piccart, M. J., et al. (2005). Randomized trial of letrozole following tamoxifen as extended adjuvant therapy in receptor-positive breast cancer: Updated findings from NCIC CTG MA.17. *Journal of the National Cancer Institute*, *97*(17), 1262–1271.

Gottardis, M. M., Jiang, S. Y., Jeng, M. H., & Jordan, V. C. (1989). Inhibition of tamoxifen-stimulated growth of an MCF-7 tumor variant in athymic mice by novel steroidal anti-estrogens. *Cancer Research*, *49*(15), 4090–4093.

Gottardis, M. M., & Jordan, V. C. (1987). Antitumor actions of keoxifene and tamoxifen in the N-nitrosomethylurea-induced rat mammary carcinoma model. *Cancer Research*, *47*(15), 4020–4024.

Gottardis, M. M., & Jordan, V. C. (1988). Development of tamoxifen-stimulated growth of MCF-7 tumors in athymic mice after long-term antiestrogen administration. *Cancer Research*, *48*(18), 5183–5187.

Gottardis, M. M., Ricchio, M. E., Satyaswaroop, P. G., & Jordan, V. C. (1990). Effect of steroidal and nonsteroidal antiestrogens on the growth of a tamoxifen-stimulated human endometrial carcinoma (EnCa101) in athymic mice. *Cancer Research*, *50*(11), 3189–3192.

Gottardis, M. M., Robinson, S. P., Satyaswaroop, P. G., & Jordan, V. C. (1988). Contrasting actions of tamoxifen on endometrial and breast tumor growth in the athymic mouse. *Cancer Research*, *48*(4), 812–815.

Gottardis, M. M., Wagner, R. J., Borden, E. C., & Jordan, V. C. (1989). Differential ability of antiestrogens to stimulate breast cancer cell (MCF-7) growth in vivo and in vitro. *Cancer Research*, *49*(17), 4765–4769.

Greaves, P., Goonetilleke, R., Nunn, G., Topham, J., & Orton, T. (1993). Two-year carcinogenicity study of tamoxifen in Alderley Park Wistar-derived rats. *Cancer Research*, *53*(17), 3919–3924.

Gruber, C., & Gruber, D. (2004). Bazedoxifene (Wyeth). *Current Opinion in Investigational Drugs*, *5*(10), 1086–1093.

Haddow, A. (1970). David A. Karnofsky memorial lecture. Thoughts on chemical therapy. *Cancer*, *26*(4), 737–754.

Haddow, A., Watkinson, J. M., Paterson, E., & Koller, P. C. (1944). Influence of synthetic oestrogens on advanced malignant disease. *British Medical Journal*, *2*(4368), 393–398.

Hard, G. C., Latropoulos, M. J., Jordan, K., Radi, L., Kaltenberg, O. P., Imondi, A. R., et al. (1993). Major difference in the hepatocarcinogenicity and DNA adduct forming ability between toremifene and tamoxifen in female Crl:CD(BR) rats. *Cancer Research*, *53*(19), 4534–4541.

Harper, M. J., & Walpole, A. L. (1967a). Mode of action of I.C.I. 46,474 in preventing implantation in rats. *The Journal of Endocrinology*, *37*(1), 83–92.

Harper, M. J., & Walpole, A. L. (1967b). A new derivative of triphenylethylene: Effect on implantation and mode of action in rats. *Journal of Reproduction and Fertility*, *13*(1), 101–119.

Hecker, E., Vegh, I., Levy, C. M., Magin, C. A., Martinez, J. C., Loureiro, J., et al. (1974). Clinical trial of clomiphene in advanced breast cancer. *European Journal of Cancer*, *10*(11), 747–749.

Herman, M. E., & Katzenellenbogen, B. S. (1994). Alterations in transforming growth factor-alpha and -beta production and cell responsiveness during the progression of MCF-7 human breast cancer cells to estrogen-autonomous growth. *Cancer Research*, *54*(22), 5867–5874.

Howell, A., Cuzick, J., Baum, M., Buzdar, A., Dowsett, M., Forbes, J. F., et al. (2005). Results of the ATAC (Arimidex, Tamoxifen, Alone or in Combination) trial after completion of 5 years' adjuvant treatment for breast cancer. *The Lancet*, *365*(9453), 60–62.

Howell, A., Robertson, J. F., Abram, P., Lichinitser, M. R., Elledge, R., Bajetta, E., et al. (2004). Comparison of fulvestrant versus tamoxifen for the treatment of advanced breast cancer in postmenopausal women previously untreated with endocrine therapy: A multinational, double-blind, randomized trial. *Journal of Clinical Oncology, 22*(9), 1605–1613.

Howlader, N., Noone, A. M., Krapcho, M., Neyman, N., Aminou, R., Altekruse, S. F., et al. (2009). *SEER cancer statistics review, 1975–2009 (Vintage 2009 populations)*. Bethesda, MD: National Cancer Institute. *http://seer.cancer.gov/csr/1975_2009_pops09/*.

Hu, Z., Fan, C., Oh, D. S., Marron, J. S., He, X., Qaqish, B. F., et al. (2006). The molecular portraits of breast tumors are conserved across microarray platforms. *BMC Genomics, 7*, 96.

Hu, Z. Z., Kagan, B. L., Ariazi, E. A., Rosenthal, D. S., Zhang, L., Li, J. V., et al. (2011). Proteomic analysis of pathways involved in estrogen-induced growth and apoptosis of breast cancer cells. *PLoS One, 6*(6), e20410.

Huggins, C., Grand, L. C., & Brillantes, F. P. (1961). Mammary cancer induced by a single feeding of polymucular hydrocarbons, and its suppression. *Nature, 189*, 204–207.

INCA (2006). *A Situacao do Cancer no Brasil*. Rio de Janeiro: Instituto Nacional de Cancer.

Ingle, J. N., Ahmann, D. L., Green, S. J., Edmonson, J. H., Bisel, H. F., Kvols, L. K., et al. (1981). Randomized clinical trial of diethylstilbestrol versus tamoxifen in postmenopausal women with advanced breast cancer. *The New England Journal of Medicine, 304*(1), 16–21.

Jain, N., Kanojia, R. M., Xu, J., Jian-Zhong, G., Pacia, E., Lai, M. T., et al. (2006). Novel chromene-derived selective estrogen receptor modulators useful for alleviating hot flushes and vaginal dryness. *Journal of Medicinal Chemistry, 49*(11), 3056–3059.

Jain, N., Xu, J., Kanojia, R. M., Du, F., Jian-Zhong, G., Pacia, E., et al. (2009). Identification and structure-activity relationships of chromene-derived selective estrogen receptor modulators for treatment of postmenopausal symptoms. *Journal of Medicinal Chemistry, 52*(23), 7544–7569.

Jensen, E. V., & Jacobson, H. I. (1962). Basic guides to the mechanism of estrogen action. *Recent Progress in Hormone Resistence, 18*, 387–414.

Jiang, S. Y., Wolf, D. M., Yingling, J. M., Chang, C., & Jordan, V. C. (1992). An estrogen receptor positive MCF-7 clone that is resistant to antiestrogens and estradiol. *Molecular and Cellular Endocrinology, 90*(1), 77–86.

Jordan, V. C. (1976). Effect of tamoxifen (ICI 46,474) on initiation and growth of DMBA-induced rat mammary carcinomata. *European Journal of Cancer, 12*(6), 419–424.

Jordan, V. C. (1978). Use of the DMBA-induced rat mammary carcinoma system for the evaluation of tamoxifen treatment as a potential adjuvant therapy. *Reviews on Endocrine-Related Cancer*, (October Suppl.), 49–55.

Jordan, V. C. (1984). Biochemical pharmacology of antiestrogen action. *Pharmacological Reviews, 36*(4), 245–276.

Jordan, V. C. (1998). Chemotherapy is antihormonal therapy-how much proof doOncologists need? *European Journal of Cancer, 34*(5), 606–608.

Jordan, V. C. (2001). Selective estrogen receptor modulation: A personal perspective. *Cancer Research, 61*(15), 5683–5687.

Jordan, V. C. (2003a). Antiestrogens and selective estrogen receptor modulators as multifunctional medicines. 1. Receptor interactions. *Journal of Medicinal Chemistry, 46*(6), 883–908.

Jordan, V. C. (2003b). Antiestrogens and selective estrogen receptor modulators as multifunctional medicines. 2. Clinical considerations and new agents. *Journal of Medicinal Chemistry, 46*(7), 1081–1111.

Jordan, V. C. (2003c). Tamoxifen: A most unlikely pioneering medicine. *Nature Reviews. Drug Discovery, 2*(3), 205–213.

Jordan, V. C. (2004). Selective estrogen receptor modulation: Concept and consequences in cancer. *Cancer Cell*, *5*(3), 207–213.

Jordan, V. C. (2006). Tamoxifen (ICI46,474) as a targeted therapy to treat and prevent breast cancer. *British Journal of Pharmacology*, *147*(Suppl. 1), S269–S276.

Jordan, V. C. (2008a). The 38th David A. Karnofsky lecture: The paradoxical actions of estrogen in breast cancer—Survival or death? *Journal of Clinical Oncology*, *26*(18), 3073–3082.

Jordan, V. C. (2008b). Tamoxifen: Catalyst for the change to targeted therapy. *European Journal of Cancer*, *44*(1), 30–38.

Jordan, V. C., & Allen, K. E. (1980). Evaluation of the antitumour activity of the non-steroidal antioestrogen monohydroxytamoxifen in the DMBA-induced rat mammary carcinoma model. *European Journal of Cancer*, *16*(2), 239–251.

Jordan, V. C., Allen, K. E., & Dix, C. J. (1980). Pharmacology of tamoxifen in laboratory animals. *Cancer Treatment Reports*, *64*(6–7), 745–759.

Jordan, V. C., Bain, R. R., Brown, R. R., Gosden, B., & Santos, M. A. (1983). Determination and pharmacology of a new hydroxylated metabolite of tamoxifen observed in patient sera during therapy for advanced breast cancer. *Cancer Research*, *43*(3), 1446–1450.

Jordan, V. C., Collins, M. M., Rowsby, L., & Prestwich, G. (1977). A monohydroxylated metabolite of tamoxifen with potent antioestrogenic activity. *The Journal of Endocrinology*, *75*(2), 305–316.

Jordan, V. C., Dix, C. J., & Allen, K. E. (1979). The effectiveness of longterm treatment in a laboratory model for adjuvant hormone therapy of breast cancer. In S. E. Salmone & S. E. Jones (Eds.), *Adjuvant therapy of cancer II* (pp. 19–26). New York: Grune and Stratton.

Jordan, V. C., Dix, C. J., Naylor, K. E., Prestwich, G., & Rowsby, L. (1978). Nonsteroidal antiestrogens: Their biological effects and potential mechanisms of action. *Journal of Toxicology and Environmental Health*, *4*(2–3), 363–390.

Jordan, V. C., & Koerner, S. (1975). Tamoxifen (ICI 46,474) and the human carcinoma 8S oestrogen receptor. *European Journal of Cancer*, *11*(3), 205–206.

Jordan, V. C., Liu, H., & Dardes, R. (2002). Re: Effect of long-term estrogen deprivation on apoptotic responses of breast cancer cells to 17 beta-estradiol and the two faces of Janus: Sex steroids as mediators of both cell proliferation and cell death. *Journal of the National Cancer Institute*, *94*(15), 1173, author reply 1173–1175.

Jordan, V. C., Mittal, S., Gosden, B., Koch, R., & Lieberman, M. E. (1985). Structure-activity relationships of estrogens. *Environmental Health Perspectives*, *61*, 97–110.

Jordan, V. C., Naylor, K. E., Dix, C. J., & Prestwich, G. (1980). Anti-oestrogen action in experimental breast cancer. *Recent Results in Cancer Research*, *71*, 30–44.

Jordan, V. C., Phelps, E., & Lindgren, J. U. (1987). Effects of anti-estrogens on bone in castrated and intact female rats. *Breast Cancer Research and Treatment*, *10*(1), 31–35.

Jordan, V. C., & Robinson, S. P. (1987). Species-specific pharmacology of antiestrogens: Role of metabolism. *Federation Proceedings*, *46*(5), 1870–1874.

Jordan, V. C., Schafer, J. M., Levenson, A. S., Liu, H., Pease, K. M., Simons, L. A., et al. (2001). Molecular classification of estrogens. *Cancer Research*, *61*(18), 6619–6623.

Jordan, V. C., Wolf, M., Mirecki, D. M., Whitford, D., & Welshons, W. V. (1988). Hormone receptor assays: Clinical usefulness in the management of carcinoma of the breast. *CRC Critical Reviews in Clinical Laboratory Sciences*, *26*, 97–152.

Kagan, R., Williams, R. S., Pan, K., Mirkin, S., & Pickar, J. H. (2010). A randomized, placebo- and active-controlled trial of bazedoxifene/conjugated estrogens for treatment of moderate to severe vulvar/vaginal atrophy in postmenopausal women. *Menopause*, *17*(2), 281–289.

Katzenellenbogen, B. S., Kendra, K. L., Norman, M. J., & Berthois, Y. (1987). Proliferation, hormonal responsiveness, and estrogen receptor content of MCF-7 human breast cancer cells grown in the short-term and long-term absence of estrogens. *Cancer Research*, *47*(16), 4355–4360.

Kawate, H., & Takayanagi, R. (2011). Efficacy and safety of bazedoxifene for postmenopausal osteoporosis. *Clinical Interventions in Aging*, *6*, 151–160.

Kennedy, B. J. (1965a). Hormone therapy for advanced breast cancer. *Cancer*, *18*(12), 1551–1557.

Kennedy, B. J. (1965b). Systemic effects of androgenic and estrogenic hormones in advanced breast cancer. *Journal of the American Geriatrics Society*, *13*, 230–235.

Kennedy, B. J., & Nathanson, I. T. (1953). Effect of intensive sex steroid hormone therapy in advanced breast cancer. *Journal of the American Medical Association*, *152*, 1135–1141.

Kiyotani, K., Mushiroda, T., Imamura, C. K., Hosono, N., Tsunoda, T., Kubo, M., et al. (2010). Significant effect of polymorphisms in CYP2D6 and ABCC2 on clinical outcomes of adjuvant tamoxifen therapy for breast cancer patients. *Journal of Clinical Oncology*, *28*(8), 1287–1293.

Klopper, A., & Hall, M. (1971). New synthetic agent for the induction of ovulation: Preliminary trials in women. *British Medical Journal*, *1*(5741), 152–154.

Komm, B. S., Kharode, Y. P., Bodine, P. V., Harris, H. A., Miller, C. P., & Lyttle, C. R. (2005). Bazedoxifene acetate: A selective estrogen receptor modulator with improved selectivity. *Endocrinology*, *146*(9), 3999–4008.

Lacassagne, A. (1933). Influence d'un facteur familial dans la production par la folliculine, de cancers mammaires chez la souris male. *Comptes Rendus des Seances de la Societe de Biologie et des ses Filiales (Paris)*, *114*, 427–429.

Lacassagne, A. (1936a). A comparative study of the carcinogenic action of certain oestrogenic hormones. *American Journal of Cancer*, *28*, 735–740.

Lacassagne, A. (1936b). Hormonal pathogenesis of adenocarcinoma of the breast. *American Journal of Cancer*, *27*(2), 217–228.

LaCroix, A. Z., Chlebowski, R. T., Manson, J. E., Aragaki, A. K., Johnson, K. C., Martin, L., et al. (2011). Health outcomes after stopping conjugated equine estrogens among postmenopausal women with prior hysterectomy: A randomized controlled trial. *Journal of the American Medical Association*, *305*(13), 1305–1314.

Lammers, L. A., Mathijssen, R. H., van Gelder, T., Bijl, M. J., de Graan, A. J., Seynaeve, C., et al. (2010). The impact of CYP2D6-predicted phenotype on tamoxifen treatment outcome in patients with metastatic breast cancer. *British Journal of Cancer*, *103*(6), 765–771.

Lash, T. L., Cronin-Fenton, D., Ahern, T. P., Rosenberg, C. L., Lunetta, K. L., Silliman, R. A., et al. (2011). CYP2D6 inhibition and breast cancer recurrence in a population-based study in Denmark. *Journal of the National Cancer Institute*, *103*(6), 489–500.

Lathrop, A. E., & Loeb, L. (1916). Further investigations on the origin of tumors in mice. III. On the part played by internal secretion in the spontaneous development of tumors. *Journal of Cancer Research*, *1*(1), 1–19.

Laughlin, R. C., & Carey, T. F. (1962). Cataracts in patients treated with triparanol. *Journal of the American Medical Association*, *181*, 369–370.

LBCSG (1984). Randomised trial of chemo-endocrine therapy, endocrine therapy, and mastectomy alone in postmenopausal patients with operable breast cancer and axillary node metastasis. *The Lancet*, *1*(8384), 1256–1260.

Lednicer, D., Emmert, D. E., Duncan, G. W., & Lyster, S. C. (1967). Mammalian antifertility agents. V. 5,6-Diarylhodronaphtalenes. *Journal of Medicinal Chemistry*, *10*(6), 1051–1054.

Lednicer, D., Lyster, S. C., & Duncan, G. W. (1967). Mammalian antifertility agents. IV. Basic 3,4-dihydronaphthalenes and 1,2,3,4-tetrahydro-1-naphthols. *Journal of Medicinal Chemistry*, *10*(1), 78–84.

Legha, S. S., Slavik, M., & Carter, S. K. (1976). Nafoxidine—An antiestrogen for the treatment of breast cancer. *Cancer, 38*(4), 1535–1541.

Lerner, L. J. (1981). The first nonsteroidal antiestrogen—MER25. In R. L. Sutherland & V. C. Jordan (Eds.), *Nonsteroidal antiestrogens, molecular pharmacology and antitumor activity* (pp. 1–16). Sydney: Academic Press.

Lerner, L. J., Holthaus, F. J., Jr., & Thompson, C. R. (1958). A non-steroidal estrogen antiagonist 1-(p-2-diethylaminoethoxyphenyl)-1-phenyl-2-p-methoxyphenyl ethanol. *Endocrinology, 63*(3), 295–318.

Lerner, L. J., & Jordan, V. C. (1990). Development of antiestrogens and their use in breast cancer: Eighth Cain memorial award lecture. *Cancer Research, 50*(14), 4177–4189.

Lewis, J. S., Meeke, K., Osipo, C., Ross, E. A., Kidawi, N., Li, T., et al. (2005). Intrinsic mechanism of estradiol-induced apoptosis in breast cancer cells resistant to estrogen deprivation. *Journal of the National Cancer Institute, 97*(23), 1746–1759.

Lewis-Wambi, J. S., Kim, H. R., Wambi, C., Patel, R., Pyle, J. R., Klein-Szanto, A. J., et al. (2008). Buthionine sulfoximine sensitizes antihormone-resistant human breast cancer cells to estrogen-induced apoptosis. *Breast Cancer Research, 10*(6), R104.

Lewis-Wambi, J. S., Swaby, R., Kim, H., & Jordan, V. C. (2009). Potential of l-buthionine sulfoximine to enhance the apoptotic action of estradiol to reverse acquired antihormonal resistance in metastatic breast cancer. *The Journal of Steroid Biochemistry and Molecular Biology, 114*(1–2), 33–39.

Lindsay, R., Gallagher, J. C., Kagan, R., Pickar, J. H., & Constantine, G. (2009). Efficacy of tissue-selective estrogen complex of bazedoxifene/conjugated estrogens for osteoporosis prevention in at-risk postmenopausal women. *Fertility and Sterility, 92*(3), 1045–1052.

Lippman, M. E., & Bolan, G. (1975). Oestrogen-responsive human breast cancer in long term tissue culture. *Nature, 256*(5518), 592–593.

Lonning, P. E. (2009). Additive endocrine therapy for advanced breast cancer—Back to the future. *Acta Oncologica, 48*(8), 1092–1101.

Lonning, P. E., Taylor, P. D., Anker, G., Iddon, J., Wie, L., Jorgensen, L. M., et al. (2001). High-dose estrogen treatment in postmenopausal breast cancer patients heavily exposed to endocrine therapy. *Breast Cancer Research and Treatment, 67*(2), 111–116.

Love, R. R., Mazess, R. B., Barden, H. S., Epstein, S., Newcomb, P. A., Jordan, V. C., et al. (1992). Effects of tamoxifen on bone mineral density in postmenopausal women with breast cancer. *The New England Journal of Medicine, 326*(13), 852–856.

Love, R. R., Newcomb, P. A., Wiebe, D. A., Surawicz, T. S., Jordan, V. C., Carbone, P. P., et al. (1990). Effects of tamoxifen therapy on lipid and lipoprotein levels in postmenopausal patients with node-negative breast cancer. *Journal of the National Cancer Institute, 82*(16), 1327–1332.

Love, R. R., Wiebe, D. A., Newcomb, P. A., Cameron, L., Leventhal, H., Jordan, V. C., et al. (1991). Effects of tamoxifen on cardiovascular risk factors in postmenopausal women. *Annals of Internal Medicine, 115*(11), 860–864.

Lunan, C. B., & Klopper, A. (1975). Antioestrogens. A review. *Clinical Endocrinology, 4*(5), 551–572.

Madlensky, L., Natarajan, L., Tchu, S., Pu, M., Mortimer, J., Flatt, S. W., et al. (2011). Tamoxifen metabolite concentrations, CYP2D6 genotype, and breast cancer outcomes. *Clinical Pharmacology and Therapeutics, 89*(5), 718–725.

Martino, S., Cauley, J. A., Barrett-Connor, E., Powles, T. J., Mershon, J., Disch, D., et al. (2004). Continuing outcomes relevant to Evista: Breast cancer incidence in postmenopausal osteoporotic women in a randomized trial of raloxifene. *Journal of the National Cancer Institute, 96*(23), 1751–1761.

Masamura, S., Santner, S. J., Heitjan, D. F., & Santen, R. J. (1995). Estrogen deprivation causes estradiol hypersensitivity in human breast cancer cells. *The Journal of Clinical Endocrinology and Metabolism, 80*(10), 2918–2925.

Maximov, P., Sengupta, S., Lewis-Wambi, J. S., Kim, H. R., Curpan, R. F., & Jordan, V. C. (2011). The conformation of the estrogen receptor directs estrogen-induced apoptosis in breast cancer: A hypothesis. *Hormonal Molecular Biology and Clinical Investigation, 5*(1), 27–34.

McGuire, W. L., Carbone, P. P., & Vollmer, E. P. (Eds.), (1975). *Estrogen receptors in human breast cancer.* New York: Raven Press.

Mehta, R. S., Barlow, W. E., Albain, K. S., Vandenberg, T. A., Dakhil, S. R., Tirumali, N. R., et al. (2012). Combination anastrozole and fulvestrant in metastatic breast cancer. *The New England Journal of Medicine, 367*(5), 435–444.

Miller, C. P., Collini, M. D., Tran, B. D., Harris, H. A., Kharode, Y. P., Marzolf, J. T., et al. (2001). Design, synthesis, and preclinical characterization of novel, highly selective indole estrogens. *Journal of Medicinal Chemistry, 44*(11), 1654–1657.

NATO (1983). Controlled trial of tamoxifen as adjuvant agent in management of early breast cancer. Interim analysis at four years by Nolvadex Adjuvant Trial Organisation. *The Lancet, 1*(8319), 257–261.

O'Regan, R. M., Gajdos, C., Dardes, R. C., De Los Reyes, A., Park, W., Rademaker, A. W., et al. (2002). Effects of raloxifene after tamoxifen on breast and endometrial tumor growth in athymic mice. *Journal of the National Cancer Institute, 94*(4), 274–283.

Osborne, C. K., Coronado, E. B., & Robinson, J. P. (1987). Human breast cancer in the athymic nude mouse: Cytostatic effects of long-term antiestrogen therapy. *European Journal of Cancer & Clinical Oncology, 23*(8), 1189–1196.

Osborne, C. K., Hobbs, K., & Clark, G. M. (1985). Effect of estrogens and antiestrogens on growth of human breast cancer cells in athymic nude mice. *Cancer Research, 45*(2), 584–590.

Osborne, C. K., Pippen, J., Jones, S. E., Parker, L. M., Ellis, M., Come, S., et al. (2002). Double-blind, randomized trial comparing the efficacy and tolerability of fulvestrant versus anastrozole in postmenopausal women with advanced breast cancer progressing on prior endocrine therapy: Results of a North American trial. *Journal of Clinical Oncology, 20*(16), 3386–3395.

Osipo, C., Gajdos, C., Liu, H., Chen, B., & Jordan, V. C. (2003). Paradoxical action of fulvestrant in estradiol-induced regression of tamoxifen-stimulated breast cancer. *Journal of the National Cancer Institute, 95*(21), 1597–1608.

Payre, B., de Medina, P., Boubekeur, N., Mhamdi, L., Bertrand-Michel, J., Terce, F., et al. (2008). Microsomal antiestrogen-binding site ligands induce growth control and differentiation of human breast cancer cells through the modulation of cholesterol metabolism. *Molecular Cancer Therapeutics, 7*(12), 3707–3718.

Perou, C. M., Sorlie, T., Eisen, M. B., van de Rijn, M., Jeffrey, S. S., Rees, C. A., et al. (2000). Molecular portraits of human breast tumours. *Nature, 406*(6797), 747–752.

Pink, J. J., Jiang, S. Y., Fritsch, M., & Jordan, V. C. (1995). An estrogen-independent MCF-7 breast cancer cell line which contains a novel 80-kilodalton estrogen receptor-related protein. *Cancer Research, 55*(12), 2583–2590.

Pinkerton, J. V., Pickar, J. H., Racketa, J., & Mirkin, S. (2012). Bazedoxifene/conjugated estrogens for menopausal symptom treatment and osteoporosis prevention. *Climacteric, 15*(5), 411–418.

Poirot, M. (2011). Four decades of discovery in breast cancer research and treatment—An interview with V. Craig Jordan. *The International Journal of Developmental Biology, 55*, 703–712.

Powles, T. J., Ashley, S., Tidy, A., Smith, I. E., & Dowsett, M. (2007). Twenty-year follow-up of the Royal Marsden randomized, double-blinded tamoxifen breast cancer prevention trial. *Journal of the National Cancer Institute, 99*(4), 283–290.

Powles, T., Eeles, R., Ashley, S., Easton, D., Chang, J., Dowsett, M., et al. (1998). Interim analysis of the incidence of breast cancer in the Royal Marsden Hospital tamoxifen randomised chemoprevention trial. *The Lancet, 352*(9122), 98–101.

Powles, T. J., Hardy, J. R., Ashley, S. E., Farrington, G. M., Cosgrove, D., Davey, J. B., et al. (1989). A pilot trial to evaluate the acute toxicity and feasibility of tamoxifen for prevention of breast cancer. *British Journal of Cancer, 60*(1), 126–131.

Prentice, R. L., Chlebowski, R. T., Stefanick, M. L., Manson, J. E., Langer, R. D., Pettinger, M., et al. (2008). Conjugated equine estrogens and breast cancer risk in the Women's Health Initiative clinical trial and observational study. *American Journal of Epidemiology, 167*(12), 1407–1415.

Rae, J. M., Drury, S., Hayes, D. F., Stearns, V., Thibert, J. N., Haynes, B. P., et al. (2012). CYP2D6 and UGT2B7 genotype and risk of recurrence in tamoxifen-treated breast cancer patients. *Journal of the National Cancer Institute, 104*(6), 452–460.

Regan, M. M., Leyland-Jones, B., Bouzyk, M., Pagani, O., Tang, W., Kammler, R., et al. (2012). CYP2D6 genotype and tamoxifen response in postmenopausal women with endocrine-responsive breast cancer: The breast international group 1-98 trial. *Journal of the National Cancer Institute, 104*(6), 441–451.

Riemsma, R., Forbes, C. A., Amonkar, M. M., Lykopoulos, K., Diaz, J. R., Kleijnen, J., et al. (2012). Systematic review of lapatinib in combination with letrozole compared with other first-line treatments for hormone receptor positive (HR+) and HER2+ advanced or metastatic breast cancer (MBC). *Current Medical Research and Opinion, 28*(8), 1263–1279.

Ries, L. A. G., Eisner, M. P., & Kosary, C. L. (2001). *SEER cancer statistics review, 1973–1998.* Bethesda, Maryland: National Cancer Institute.

Robinson, S. P., Koch, R., & Jordan, V. C. (1988). In vitro estrogenic actions in rat and human cells of hydroxylated derivatives of D16726 (zindoxifene), an agent with known antimammary cancer activity in vivo. *Cancer Research, 48*(4), 784–787.

Robson, J. M. (1937). Oestrous reactions, including mating, produced by triphenyl ethylene. *Nature, 140*(3535), 196.

Robson, J. M., Schonberg, A., & Fahim, H. A. (1938). Duration of action of natural and synthetic oestrogens. *Nature, 142*, 292–293.

Robson, J. M., & Schonberg, A. (1942). A new synthetic oestrogen with prolonged action when given orally. *Nature, 150*(3792), 22–23.

Roop, R. P., & Ma, C. X. (2012). Endocrine resistance in breast cancer: Molecular pathways and rational development of targeted therapies. *Future Oncology, 8*(3), 273–292.

Rosati, R. L., Da Silva Jardine, P., Cameron, K. O., Thompson, D. D., Ke, H. Z., Toler, S. M., et al. (1998). Discovery and preclinical pharmacology of a novel, potent, nonsteroidal estrogen receptor agonist/antagonist, CP-336156, a diaryltetrahydronaphthalene. *Journal of Medicinal Chemistry, 41*(16), 2928–2931.

Rose, C., Thorpe, S. M., Andersen, K. W., Pedersen, B. V., Mouridsen, H. T., Blichert-Toft, M., et al. (1985). Beneficial effect of adjuvant tamoxifen therapy in primary breast cancer patients with high oestrogen receptor values. *The Lancet, 1*(8419), 16–19.

Rossouw, J. E., Anderson, G. L., Prentice, R. L., LaCroix, A. Z., Kooperberg, C., Stefanick, M. L., et al. (2002). Risks and benefits of estrogen plus progestin in healthy postmenopausal women: Principal results from the Women's Health Initiative randomized controlled trial. *Journal of the American Medical Association, 288*(3), 321–333.

Rutanen, E. M., Heikkinen, J., Halonen, K., Komi, J., Lammintausta, R., & Ylikorkala, O. (2003). Effects of ospemifene, a novel SERM, on hormones, genital tract, climacteric symptoms, and quality of life in postmenopausal women: A double-blind, randomized trial. *Menopause, 10*(5), 433–439.

Schrek, R. (1960). Fashions in cancer research. In W. B. Wartman (Ed.), *1959–1960 Year book* (pp. 26–39). Chicago: The Year Book Publishers.

Schroth, W., Goetz, M. P., Hamann, U., Fasching, P. A., Schmidt, M., Winter, S., et al. (2009). Association between CYP2D6 polymorphisms and outcomes among women with early stage breast cancer treated with tamoxifen. *Journal of the American Medical Association, 302*(13), 1429–1436.

SCTO (1987). Adjuvant tamoxifen in the management of operable cancer: The Scottish Trial. Report from the Breast Cancer Trials Committee, Scottish Cancer Trials Office (MRC), Edinburgh. *The Lancet, 2*(8852), 171–175.

Sengupta, S., & Jordan, V. C. (2013). Novel selective estrogen receptor modulators. In V. C. Jordan (Ed.), *Estrogen actions, SERMs, and women's health.* London: Imperial College Press.

Shiau, A. K., Barstad, D., Loria, P. M., Cheng, L., Kushner, P. J., Agard, D. A., et al. (1998). The structural basis of estrogen receptor/coactivator recognition and the antagonism of this interaction by tamoxifen. *Cell, 95*(7), 927–937.

Shim, W. S., Conaway, M., Masamura, S., Yue, W., Wang, J. P., Kmar, R., et al. (2000). Estradiol hypersensitivity and mitogen-activated protein kinase expression in long-term estrogen deprived human breast cancer cells in vivo. *Endocrinology, 141*(1), 396–405.

Shimkin, M. B., & Wyman, R. S. (1945). Effect of adrenalectomy and ovariectomy on mammary carcinogenesis in strain C3H mice. *Journal of the National Cancer Institute, 6,* 187–189.

Shimkin, M. B., & Wyman, R. S. (1946). Mammary tumors in male mice implanted with estrogen-cholesterol pellets. *Journal of the National Cancer Institute, 7*(2), 71–75.

Shimkin, M. B., Wyman, R. S., & Andervont, H. B. (1946). Mammary tumors in mice following transplantation of mammary tissue. *Journal of the National Cancer Institute, 7*(2), 77.

Shumaker, S. A., Legault, C., Rapp, S. R., Thal, L., Wallace, R. B., Ockene, J. K., et al. (2003). Estrogen plus progestin and the incidence of dementia and mild cognitive impairment in postmenopausal women: The Women's Health Initiative Memory Study: A randomized controlled trial. *Journal of the American Medical Association, 289*(20), 2651–2662.

Silverman, S. L., Chines, A. A., Kendler, D. L., Kung, A. W., Teglbjaerg, C. S., Felsenberg, D., et al. (2012). Sustained efficacy and safety of bazedoxifene in preventing fractures in postmenopausal women with osteoporosis: Results of a 5-year, randomized, placebo-controlled study. *Osteoporosis International, 23*(1), 351–363.

Song, R. X., Mor, G., Naftolin, F., McPherson, R. A., Song, J., Zhang, Z., et al. (2001). Effect of long-term estrogen deprivation on apoptotic responses of breast cancer cells to 17beta-estradiol. *Journal of the National Cancer Institute, 93*(22), 1714–1723.

Sorlie, T., Tibshirani, R., Parker, J., Hastie, T., Marron, J. S., Nobel, A., et al. (2003). Repeated observation of breast tumor subtypes in independent gene expression data sets. *Proceedings of the National Academy of Sciences of the United States of America, 100*(14), 8418–8423.

Speroff, L. (2009). *A good man, Gregory Goodwin Pincus: The man, his story, the birth control pill.* Portland, Oregon: Arnica Publishing.

Stein, R. C., Dowsett, M., Cunningham, D. C., Davenport, J., Ford, H. T., Gazet, J. C., et al. (1990). Phase I/II study of the anti-oestrogen zindoxifene (D16726) in the treatment of advanced breast cancer. A Cancer Research Campaign Phase I/II Clinical Trials Committee study. *British Journal of Cancer, 61*(3), 451–453.

Stoll, B. (1977a). *Breast cancer management early and late.* London: William Herman Medical Books Ltd.

Stoll, B. A. (1977b). Palliation by castration or by hormone administration. In B. A. Stoll (Ed.), *Breast cancer management early and late* (pp. 133–146). London: W. Heinemann Medical Books Ltd.

Sutherland, R. L., Murphy, L. C., San Foo, M., Green, M. D., Whybourne, A. M., & Krozowski, Z. S. (1980). High-affinity anti-oestrogen binding site distinct from the oestrogen receptor. *Nature, 288*(5788), 273–275.

Sweeney, E. E., McDaniel, R. E., Maximov, P. Y., Fan, P., & Jordan, V. C. (2012). Models and mechanisms of acquired antihormone resistance in breast cancer: Significant clinical progress despite limitations. *Hormonal Molecular Biology and Clinical Investigation*, *9*(2), 143–163.

Thompson, C. R., & Werner, H. W. (1953). Fat storage of an estrogen in women following orally administered tri-p-anisyl chloroethylene. *Proceedings of the Society for Experimental Biology and Medicine*, *84*, 491–492.

Thurlimann, B., Keshaviah, A., Coates, A. S., Mouridsen, H., Mauriac, L., Forbes, J. F., et al. (2005). A comparison of letrozole and tamoxifen in postmenopausal women with early breast cancer. *The New England Journal of Medicine*, *353*(26), 2747–2757.

Toft, D., & Gorski, J. (1966). A receptor molecule for estrogens: Isolation from the rat uterus and preliminary characterization. *PNAS*, *55*(6), 1574–1581.

Toft, D., Shyamala, G., & Gorski, J. (1967). A receptor molecule for estrogens: Studies using a cell-free system. *Proceedings of the National Academy of Sciences of the United States of America*, *57*(6), 1740–1743.

Turner, R. T., Evans, G. L., Sluka, J. P., Adrian, M. D., Bryant, H. U., Turner, C. H., et al. (1998). Differential responses of estrogen target tissues in rats including bone to clomiphene, enclomiphene, and zuclomiphene. *Endocrinology*, *139*(9), 3712–3720.

Turner, R. T., Evans, G. L., & Wakley, G. K. (1993). Mechanism of action of estrogen on cancellous bone balance in tibiae of ovariectomized growing rats: Inhibition of indices of formation and resorption. *Journal of Bone and Mineral Research*, *8*(3), 359–366.

Turner, R. T., Wakley, G. K., Hannon, K. S., & Bell, N. H. (1987). Tamoxifen prevents the skeletal effects of ovarian hormone deficiency in rats. *Journal of Bone and Mineral Research*, *2*(5), 449–456.

Turner, R. T., Wakley, G. K., Hannon, K. S., & Bell, N. H. (1988). Tamoxifen inhibits osteoclast-mediated resorption of trabecular bone in ovarian hormone-deficient rats. *Endocrinology*, *122*(3), 1146–1150.

Veronesi, U., Maisonneuve, P., Costa, A., Sacchini, V., Maltoni, C., Robertson, C., et al. (1998). Prevention of breast cancer with tamoxifen: Preliminary findings from the Italian randomised trial among hysterectomised women. Italian Tamoxifen Prevention Study. *The Lancet*, *352*(9122), 93–97.

Vogel, V. G., Costantino, J. P., Wickerham, D. L., Cronin, W. M., Cecchini, R. S., Atkins, J. N., et al. (2006). Effects of tamoxifen vs. raloxifene on the risk of developing invasive breast cancer and other disease outcomes: The NSABP Study of Tamoxifen and Raloxifene (STAR) P-2 trial. *Journal of the American Medical Association*, *295*(23), 2727–2741.

Vogel, V. G., Costantino, J. P., Wickerham, D. L., Cronin, W. M., Cecchini, R. S., Atkins, J. N., et al. (2010). Update of the national surgical adjuvant breast and bowel project study of tamoxifen and raloxifene (STAR) P-2 trial: Preventing breast cancer. *Cancer Prevention Research (Philadelphia, Pa.)*, *3*(6), 696–706.

Voipio, S. K., Komi, J., Kangas, L., Halonen, K., DeGregorio, M. W., & Erkkola, R. U. (2002). Effects of ospemifene (FC-1271a) on uterine endometrium, vaginal maturation index, and hormonal status in healthy postmenopausal women. *Maturitas*, *43*(3), 207–214.

Wallace, O. B., Lauwers, K. S., Dodge, J. A., May, S. A., Calvin, J. R., Hinklin, R., et al. (2006). A selective estrogen receptor modulator for the treatment of hot flushes. *Journal of Medicinal Chemistry*, *49*(3), 843–846.

Walpole, A. L., & Paterson, E. (1949). Synthetic oestrogens in mammary cancer. *The Lancet*, *2*(6583), 783–786.

Watanabe, N., Ikeno, A., Minato, H., Nakagawa, H., Kohayakawa, C., & Tsuji, J. (2003). Discovery and preclinical characterization of (+)-3-[4-(1-piperidinoethoxy)phenyl] spiro[indene-1,1'-indane]-5,5'-diol hydrochloride: A promising nonsteroidal estrogen receptor agonist for hot flush. *Journal of Medicinal Chemistry*, *46*(19), 3961–3964.

Welsch, C. W. (1985). Host factors affecting the growth of carcinogen-induced rat mammary carcinomas: A review and tribute to Charles Brenton Huggins. *Cancer Research*, *45*(8), 3415–3443.

Welshons, W. V., & Jordan, V. C. (1987). Adaptation of estrogen-dependent MCF-7 cells to low estrogen (phenol red-free) culture. *European Journal of Cancer & Clinical Oncology*, *23*(12), 1935–1939.

Wolf, D. M., & Jordan, V. C. (1993). A laboratory model to explain the survival advantage observed in patients taking adjuvant tamoxifen therapy. *Recent Results in Cancer Research*, *127*, 23–33.

Yang, L., Parkin, D., Ferlay, J., Li, L., & Chen, Y. (2005). Estimates of cancer incidence in China for 2000 and projections for 2005. *Cancer Epidemiology, Biomarkers & Prevention*, *14*(1), 243–249.

Yao, K., Lee, E. S., Bentrem, D. J., England, G., Schafer, J. I., O'Regan, R. M., et al. (2000). Antitumor action of physiological estradiol on tamoxifen-stimulated breast tumors grown in athymic mice. *Clinical Cancer Research*, *6*(5), 2028–2036.

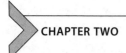

CHAPTER TWO

The Epidemiology and Molecular Mechanisms Linking Obesity, Diabetes, and Cancer

Rosalyn D. Ferguson[*], **Emily J. Gallagher**[*], **Eyal J. Scheinman**[†], **Rawan Damouni**[†], **Derek LeRoith**[*,†,1]

[*]Division of Endocrinology, Diabetes and Bone Diseases, Samuel Bronfman Department of Medicine, Mount Sinai School of Medicine, P.O. Box 1055, New York, USA
[†]Diabetes and Metabolism Clinical Research Center of Excellence, Clinical Research Institute at Rambam (CRIR), Rambam Medical Center, P.O. Box 9602, Haifa, Israel
[1]Corresponding author: e-mail address: derek.leroith@mssm.edu

Contents

Abstract

The worldwide epidemic of obesity is associated with increasing rates of the metabolic syndrome and type 2 diabetes. Epidemiological studies have reported that these conditions are linked to increased rates of cancer incidence and mortality. Obesity, particularly abdominal obesity, is associated with insulin resistance and the development of dyslipidemia, hyperglycemia, and ultimately type 2 diabetes. Although many

51

metabolic abnormalities occur with obesity and type 2 diabetes, insulin resistance and hyperinsulinemia appear to be central to these conditions and may contribute to dyslipidemia and altered levels of circulating estrogens and androgens. In this review, we will discuss the epidemiological and molecular links between obesity, type 2 diabetes, and cancer, and how hyperinsulinemia and dyslipidemia may contribute to cancer development. We will discuss how these metabolic abnormalities may interact with estrogen signaling in breast cancer growth. Finally, we will discuss the effects of type 2 diabetes medications on cancer risk.

1. INTRODUCTION

The worldwide epidemic of obesity is associated with rapidly increasing rates of the metabolic syndrome and type 2 diabetes. All three conditions are associated with increased rates of cancer risk and mortality. Obesity, particularly abdominal obesity, is associated with insulin resistance and the development of dyslipidemia, hyperglycemia, and ultimately type 2 diabetes. Although many metabolic abnormalities occur with obesity and type 2 diabetes, insulin resistance and hyperinsulinemia appear to be central to these conditions and may contribute to the dyslipidemia and altered levels of circulating estrogens. In this review, we will discuss how the hyperinsulinemia and dyslipidemia associated with these conditions may be contributing to cancer risk. We will discuss how these metabolic abnormalities may contribute to the estrogenic effects on breast cancer growth. Finally, we will discuss the effects of type 2 diabetes medications on cancer risk.

2. TYPE 2 DIABETES AND BREAST CANCER

2.1. Epidemiology

2.1.1 Type 2 diabetes and cancer

A connection between type 2 diabetes and breast cancer incidence, recurrence, and mortality in women of varying ages has been the subject of several epidemiological studies. The most recent of these have reported positive associations, such as in the Long Island Breast Cancer Specific Survival Project, where breast cancer risk was significantly elevated in Caucasian diabetic women over 65 [odds ratio (OR) = 1.35, 95% confidence interval (CI) = 0.99–1.85], while in nonwhite women, this OR rose to 3.89 (95% CI = 1.66–9.11) (Cleveland et al., 2012). An excess risk (OR = 1.76, 95%

CI = 1.34–2.32) of breast cancer specifically in postmenopausal women with preexisting type 2 diabetes has also been found during the analysis of a series of case–control studies in Italy and Switzerland (Bosetti et al., 2012). In a study in Asia, a lower breast cancer-specific survival rate (adjusted hazards ratio (HR) = 1.53, 95% CI = 1.14–2.05) has been reported for diabetic versus nondiabetic women over 40 years of age at both 2 and 5 years postsurgery (Chen et al., 2012). Similarly, another study has reported a modest association [HR = 1.31 (CI = 0.92–1.86)] between type 2 diabetes and breast cancer in postmenopausal women but no association in premenopausal women (Bowker, Richardson, Marra, & Johnson, 2011). A shorter disease-free survival period (36 months vs. 81 months, $P < 0.001$) for breast cancer has also been reported in type 2 diabetics versus nondiabetics in a Turkish study along with increased risk of tumor recurrence after surgery and overall poor prognosis (Kaplan et al., 2012). However, a recent study on Danish diabetic patients has found no association between diabetes and breast cancer in women of all ages (Carstensen, Witte, & Friis, 2012).

Many other epidemiological studies have examined the association between type 2 diabetes and breast cancer and these have been subject to various meta-analyses. The most recent of these eight evaluated studies performed between 1985 and 2002 revealed a 49% increased risk of all-cause mortality in women with breast cancer and preexisting type 2 diabetes, independent of possible confounding variables. Breast cancer-specific mortality in diabetics was, however, not evident (Peairs et al., 2011). In 2007, a meta-analysis of 20 studies revealed an elevated risk of breast cancer incidence [relative risk (RR) = 1.20, 95% CI = 1.12–1.28] in diabetics and, in an assessment of a further five studies, an increased risk [RR = 1.24 (95% CI = 0.95–1.62)] also existed for breast cancer mortality in women with type 2 diabetes (Larsson, Mantzoros, & Wolk, 2007). In the same year, a meta-analysis on how both type 2 diabetes and metabolic syndrome are related to breast cancer showed that in eight of nine case–control studies, patients with breast cancer were more likely to have had a history of diabetes; in four of these studies, the increase in odds became statistically significant. In 5 of 11 cohort studies, a significantly elevated risk of breast cancer was apparent in women with a history of type 2 diabetes (Xue & Michels, 2007). An earlier meta-analysis in 2005 gathered data from six cohort studies and four case–control studies and found that in both groups there was a moderate (10–20%) increase in the risk of breast cancer incidence (Wolf, Sadetzki, Catane, Karasik, & Kaufman, 2005).

2.1.2 Hyperinsulinemia and breast cancer

Insulin resistance and hyperinsulinemia are central to the pathogenesis of type 2 diabetes, and several epidemiological studies have focused specifically on these aspects with regard to breast cancer development. One such case–control study involved postmenopausal women initially recruited for the Women's Health Initiative Observational Study (WHI-OS). Of the 100,000 recruited, 800 individuals newly diagnosed with breast cancer and 800 cancer-free individuals were selected. Neither group included diagnosed diabetics. Analysis of blood samples from each group revealed that hyperinsulinemia, independent of body mass index (BMI), physical activity, age, ethnicity, parity, and other confounding factors, was a significant factor for incident breast cancer [highest ($\geq$9.5 µIU/ml) vs. lowest (<3.6 µIU/ml) hyperinsulinemia quartile (HR = 1.46, P = 0.02)] (Gunter et al., 2009).

In 2008, a meta-analysis on studies exploring hyperinsulinemia and all cancers included four prospective and five case–control breast cancer studies carried out between 1992 and 2007. Overall, the risk of breast cancer was 26% higher (RR = 1.26, 95% CI = 1.06–1.48) in the highest quintile of circulating C-peptide (a marker of circulating insulin). In all but one study, RRs were adjusted for BMI (Pisani, 2008). Another study in 2002 (not included in the above meta-analysis) measured fasting blood insulin between 1 and 3 months after surgical resection of early-stage breast cancer in women with no prior diagnosis of diabetes. Patients were then followed up for a median time of 50 months and metastatic events or breast cancer-associated deaths were recorded. Overall, the study found that plasma insulin levels were significantly associated with both metastasis (HR for upper vs. lower insulin quartile = 1.9, 95% CI = 1.2–3.2) and death (HR for upper vs. lower insulin quartile = 3.0, 95% CI = 1.6–5.7). Insulin levels were also significantly related to tumor stage and tumor grade (Goodwin et al., 2002).

The National Cancer Institute's Health, Eating, Activity, and Lifestyle (HEAL) study was a prospective, multiethnic cohort study of around 1200 women presenting with early-stage breast cancer. Its aim was to examine the associations of hormones, physical activity, eating habits, and weight patterns as prognostic factors for breast cancer recurrence after tumor resection. Fasting C-peptide levels were evaluated in around 600 women 3 years after breast cancer diagnosis and surgery. Individuals were then followed for a median period of 5 years or until death occurred. It was found that as little as a 1 ng/ml increase in C-peptide level was associated with a 31% increased risk (HR = 1.31, 95% CI = 1.06–1.63) of overall death and a 35% increased risk (HR = 1.35, 95% CI = 1.02–1.87) of breast cancer-specific death which was independent of variables such as disease stage, initial treatment, BMI, race, age, and estrogen receptor (ER) status. The association of C-peptide with mortality was particularly marked among women in the cohort with type 2 diabetes ($n = 58$) (Irwin et al., 2011). In an additional analysis on the same cohort of women (but excluding diabetics), Duggan and colleagues evaluated insulin resistance using the Homeostatic Model Assessment (HOMA) score whereby insulin resistance is directly related to HOMA score. It was found that higher HOMA scores were directly correlated with overall mortality (HR = 1.12, 95% CI = 1.05–1.20) and breast cancer-specific death (HR = 1.09, 95% CI = 1.02–1.15), suggesting the clinical relevance of insulin resistance in breast cancer (Duggan et al., 2011). A meta-analysis of these two studies and one other which investigated a link between hyperinsulinemia and breast cancer recurrence after tumor resection indicated that high levels of insulin were associated with a 57% increase in the risk of breast cancer recurrence (OR = 1.573, 95% CI = 1.009–2.453) (Formica, Tesauro, Cardillo, & Roselli, 2012).

A recent study has acknowledged the complex interaction between hyperinsulinemia, obesity, and breast cancer. In this analysis, both pre- and postmenopausal women who received surgical resection of breast tumors between 1989 and 1996 provided a blood sample between 5 and 9 weeks after surgery. Patients were then followed up for a median period of 12 years and then observed prospectively for local and distant recurrence, new primary cancers, and death. Evaluation of the study shows that insulin was associated with adverse prognosis only during the first 5 years of the study, whereas obesity-related variables exerted an adverse influence on prognosis that was constant throughout the period of follow-up (Goodwin et al., 2012).

2.2. Insulin and insulin receptor signaling in cancer

2.2.1 The dual role of insulin

The peptide hormone insulin is best known for its role as a homeostatic regulator of blood glucose, gluconeogenesis, and fatty acid metabolism in "metabolically active" tissues such as the liver, skeletal muscle, and adipose tissue. However, analysis of other physiological effects of insulin also suggests a highly developed and conserved role of this hormone as an important regulator of protein synthesis, cell growth, and proliferation. Widespread expression of the insulin receptor (IR) occurs in most classically "nonmetabolic" tissues such as breast, heart, brain, kidney, pancreas, and lung and in fibroblasts, monocytes, granulocytes, and erythrocytes (Kaplan, 1984). Insulin is involved in stimulating cell proliferation in embryonic mice

(Spaventi, Antica, & Pavelic, 1990), and IR-null mice have around 25% decreased body weight compared to controls (Accili et al., 1996). This growth-promoting ability of insulin under particular conditions is believed to be the primary mechanism behind the increased incidence and mortality of breast cancer in women with prolonged elevated circulating insulin, as is common in the etiology of type 2 diabetes.

2.2.2 Insulin as a metabolic regulator

Insulin binds the IR, a heterotetrameric protein consisting of two extracellular insulin-docking α-chains attached to two transmembrane β-chains which, upon ligand binding to the extracellular domain, result in tyrosine phosphorylation, thereby initiating the orderly recruitment and phosphorylation of downstream signaling proteins such as the insulin receptor substrate (IRS) proteins 1–4, the APS/Cbl complex, and adaptor proteins Shc and Grb2 (Saltiel & Pessin, 2002).

Of the IRS family members, IRS1 and IRS2 are the most important for insulin signaling pathways. Tyrosine phosphorylation of IRS1 and IRS2 generates docking sites for the p85 regulatory subunit and subsequent activation of the p110 catalytic subunit of phosphatidylinositol 3-kinase (PI3K), which leads to the conversion of PI (4,5)-bisphosphate (PIP$_2$) to PI (3,4,5)-trisphosphate (PIP$_3$). Formation of PIP$_3$ recruits pleckstrin homology domain-containing proteins such as the serine-threonine kinases, 3-phosphoinositide-dependent protein kinase-1 (PDK-1), and Akt (protein kinase B) that exist as three isoforms. Akt1 is involved principally in mediating cell growth and proliferation while Akt2 mediates mostly metabolic effects (Gonzalez & McGraw, 2009) and Akt3 is involved primarily in brain development (Gonzalez & McGraw, 2009). Akt is activated by PDK-1 (Alessi et al., 1997) and then functions as a core signaling molecule, directing the activation of multiple downstream pathways involved in metabolic regulation.

Crucial metabolic functions of Akt include the translocation and targeting of glucose transporter 4 (GLUT4) storage vesicles (GSV) to the cell surface to facilitate glucose uptake. Akt also phosphorylates glycogen synthase kinase, thereby abolishing its inhibition of glycogen synthase and allowing glycogen synthesis to proceed (Salas et al., 2003). Additionally, Akt is involved in lipogenesis through its activation of cyclic nucleotide phosphodiesterase-3B (Kitamura et al., 1999) and its inhibitory phosphorylation of AMP kinase (Berggreen, Gormand, Omar,

Degerman, & Goransson, 2009). Further to its role in lipid metabolism, Akt also phosphorylates and deactivates the forkhead transcription factor Foxa2, thereby inhibiting fatty acid β-oxidation (Li, Monks, Ge, & Birnbaum, 2007).

2.2.3 Insulin as a mitogen

As a core mediator of IR-mediated cell signaling, PI3K-activated Akt also drives the principal mitogenic effects of insulin which promote protein synthesis and cell growth and, in conditions of hyperinsulinemia, possibly cell proliferation leading to tumor development. Akt activation by PI3K is opposed by PTEN, a lipid phosphatase tumor suppressor that dephosphorylates PIP_2 and PIP_3 (Maehama & Dixon, 1998; Weng, Brown, & Eng, 2001). Specifically, PTEN has been shown to elevate p27 levels through downregulation of cyclin D1, resulting in cell cycle arrest at the G1 phase (Mamillapalli et al., 2001; Weng, Smith, Brown, & Eng, 2001). In up to 50% of breast cancers, PTEN is mutated (Di Cristofano & Pandolfi, 2000), suggesting a role of Akt in promoting tumor cell survival and proliferation. Loss of PTEN in breast cancer cell line T47D resulted in prolonged phosphorylation of both the insulin-like growth factor receptor I (IGF-IR) and Akt after IGF-I stimulation suggesting that PTEN may also interact upstream of PI3K in regulating receptor tyrosine kinase signaling (Miller et al., 2009). In cases of hyperinsulinemia, it is therefore possible that excess insulin signaling through the IR could further drive proliferation of breast cancer cells bearing PTEN mutations. Activating mutations in Akt1 have also been linked to breast cancer (Gonzalez & McGraw, 2009) and provide another possible means by which insulin signaling could promote cancer progression.

Insulin-mediated activation of Akt results in phosphorylation and thus deactivation of the GTPase activating protein tuberous sclerosis complex (TSC) (composed of TSC1 and TSC1) which results in Rheb reaching its GTP-bound state (Tee, Manning, Roux, Cantley, & Blenis, 2003) and subsequently activating the mTOR complex 1 (mTORC1), an assembly of proteins including mTOR, regulatory-associated protein of mTOR (raptor), GβL, and Deptor which regulate the balance between protein synthesis and protein degradation in response to physiological triggers in the cell such as nutrient quality and quantity and energy availability (reviewed in Sarbassov, Ali, & Sabatini, 2005). Active mTOR phosphorylates 4E binding protein 1, permitting its dissociation from eIF4E (Hay & Sonenberg, 2004). The association of eIF4E with other eIF4 proteins forms a ribosomal initiation complex, which allows the translation of proteins that promote G1 to S cell cycle progression, such as cyclin D1 and c-Myc, which are both known to be frequently upregulated in breast cancer (Ormandy, Musgrove, Hui, Daly, & Sutherland, 2003; Xu, Chen, & Olopade, 2010). Interestingly, insulin infusions during ovine fetal development increased eIF4E activity in a PI3K-independent manner (Shen, Yang, Boyle, Lee, & Liechty, 2001). In breast cancer, eIF4E can become deregulated and promote malignant progression (Byrnes et al., 2006; Li, Liu, Dawson, & De Benedetti, 1997; Li, McDonald, Nassar, & De Benedetti, 1998). Phosphorylated eIF4E is known to upregulate hypoxia inducible factor (HIF)-1α, a transcription factor implicated in the expression of angiogenic and prosurvival proteins such as vascular endothelial growth factor (VEGF) and epidermal growth factor (EGF) (Hudson et al., 2002; Toschi, Lee, Gadir, Ohh, & Foster, 2008). In the breast cancer cell line LCC6, knockdown of IR by shRNA resulted in reduced HIF1α, VEGF-A, and VEGF-D expression (Zhang et al., 2010). In breast tumor tissue, higher expression levels of eIF4E were found to correlate with elevated VEGF expression and increased tumor microvessel density (Byrnes et al., 2006). Further, high expression of eIF4E in breast cancer was associated with a significantly worse clinical outcome (Zhou, Wang, Liu, & Zhou, 2006). mTOR also targets S6 kinase (S6K)-1 and -2 which then phosphorylate S6 ribosomal protein, thereby stimulating protein synthesis through activation of translational machinery (Gingras, Raught, & Sonenberg, 2001; Hou, He, & Qi, 2007). Most studies to date have focused on the function of S6K1, which has been shown to enhance breast cancer proliferation by increasing ER levels (Yamnik et al., 2009). However, targeting of S6K1 has proved less than effective, due to its involvement in the negative regulation of the PI3K/Akt/mTOR pathway through its inhibitory phosphorylation of IRS1 (Haruta et al., 2000). Recently, it has been shown that S6K2 phosphorylation results in Akt activation (by one of several possible mechanisms) and subsequent downregulation of the proapoptotic protein Bid, leading to cell survival. Thus, S6K2 may play an important role in breast cancer progression and further may be a more suitable target than S6K1 for targeted therapies (Sridharan & Basu, 2011). The mTOR complex 2 (mTORC2) assembly includes mTOR, rapamycin-insensitive companion of mTOR (rictor), GβL, Sin1, PRR5/Protor-1, and Deptor and acts to promote cell survival by phosphorylating Akt (Glidden et al., 2012). Additionally, mTORC2 plays an important role in regulating the dynamics of cytoskeletal rearrangements (Sarbassov et al., 2004).

2.2.4 IR isoforms, hybrids, and cancer

Functional regulation of the IR (i.e., metabolic vs. mitogenic role) is controlled by alternative splicing of its transcript to produce IR-A and IR-B isoforms, where isoform A differs structurally from isoform B in its lack of exon 11 (Moller, Yokota, Caro, & Flier, 1989; Seino & Bell, 1989). The ratio of IR-A:IR-B in any particular tissue is regulated in a highly specific manner (Moller et al., 1989) and may change according to the developmental stage and differentiation state of the tissues and cells involved (Moller et al., 1989; Mosthaf et al., 1990). In fetal cells and cancer tissue (particularly breast and colon), the IR-A predominates (Frasca et al., 1999), while in classically metabolic tissues including the liver, muscle, and adipose tissues, a consistently lower IR-A:IR-B ratio is observed (Benecke, Flier, & Moller, 1992) suggesting that IR-A facilitates insulin's mitogenic role while IR-B promotes its metabolic effects. The mechanisms involved in the differential expression or activation of the two isoforms are not precisely clear; however, one study has suggested that the different spatial arrangement of IR-A and IR-B in the plasma membrane alters availability of the specific adaptor proteins that mediate IR downstream signal pathways (Uhles, Moede, Leibiger, Berggren, & Leibiger, 2003). In Hela cells, IR-A showed greater and more sustained phosphorylation than IR-B following insulin stimulation and preferentially activated the MAP kinase pathway, whereas IR-B more strongly activated the Akt pathway. Additionally, membrane internalization of IR-A was observed to occur more rapidly than IR-B (Giudice, Leskow, Arndt-Jovin, Jovin, & Jares-Erijman, 2011).

The IR is 80% homologous to the IGF-IR and the two receptors readily form hybrids (Bailyes et al., 1997). The IGF-IR ligands (IGF-I and -II) also interact with the IR and IR/IGF-IR hybrids, adding further complexity to insulin signaling. IR-B has a high affinity only for insulin, whereas IR-A has a high affinity for insulin and IGF-II and a very low affinity for IGF-I (Frasca et al., 1999). The IR-A/IGF-IR and IR-B/IGF-IR hybrids also differ in their affinity to the different ligands, with IR-A/IGF-IR strongly activated by both IGF-II and IGF-I, and IR-B/IGF-IR only activated significantly by IGF-I (Benyoucef, Surinya, Hadaschik, & Siddle, 2007; Frasca et al., 1999; Yamaguchi, Flier, Benecke, Ransil, & Moller, 1993). Both the hybrid receptors bind insulin with very low affinity (Slaaby et al., 2006), although recently IR-A was found to bind and respond mitogenically to proinsulin (Malaguarnera et al., 2012).

Because high IR-A expression is associated with cancer cells, it follows that a high IR-A:IR-B ratio and thus more IR-A homodimers and IR-A/IGF-IR hybrids could be expressed in tumors. This receptor expression profile would not only drive cells to become "mitogenic" but would also confer responsiveness to multiple ligands, thus increasing the likelihood of neoplastic growth. In a panel of breast cancer cell lines, IR-A:IR-B ratios were found to lie between 64% and 100%, while in a panel of breast tumor tissues, the ratios were in the range of 40–80%, suggesting an increased expression of the IR-A in breast cancer (Sciacca et al., 1999). In a recent study, it was found that the relative expression of IR-A was higher in tumor tissue, but this was largely due to a reduction in IR-B expression rather than an increase in IR-A itself. A reduction in IR-B in tumor tissue could, however, have major effects on dimerization configurations, such as increasing the relative abundance of IR-A homodimers and IR-A/IGF-IR heterodimers. The IR-A/IR-B ratio was directly compared in two subtypes of ER-positive/PR-positive breast cancer, namely, luminal A and luminal B. Luminal B-subtype, which is associated with higher grade/larger tumors and more lymphatic invasion as well as tamoxifen resistance and shorter relapse-free survival, demonstrated a higher IR-A:IR-B differential as well as higher expression of a prominent cell proliferation gene signature known to be involved in tamoxifen resistance (NMK167, CCNB1, and MYBL2) (Huang et al., 2011). Interestingly, one study has suggested that the IR-A:IR-B ratio may also differ with respect to the ethnic group of type 2 diabetics, with African-American women expressing higher levels of IR-A than their Caucasian counterparts (Kalla Singh, Brito, Tan, De Leon, & De Leon, 2011). The formation of IR/IGF-IR hybrids also adds complexity to the design of treatment strategies which target IGF-IR signaling in breast cancer (Hendrickson & Haluska, 2009). Recently, it has been shown that antibody targeting of the IGF-I and IGF-II ligands may be more effective than targeting the IGF-IR. In mice, a human monoclonal antibody to IGF-I and IGF-II inhibited growth of xenograft tumors initiated from two different cell lines, both of which expressed high levels of IR and IGF-IR. Further, the antibody inhibited IGF-induced phosphorylation of IGF-IR, IR-A, IRS-1, Akt, and Erk (Gao et al., 2011), suggesting that inhibiting IR/IGF-IR ligands may be a promising strategy for the inhibition of insulin/IGF-related cancers.

2.2.5 Insulin resistance, hyperinsulinemia, and breast cancer

Insulin resistance is caused by defects in the IR signaling pathways that mediate glucose uptake and is a central feature of both the metabolic syndrome and type 2 diabetes. Such signaling defects may be due to mutations or by interference from several types of obesity-related adipocytokine-mediated inflammatory responses (reviewed in Muoio & Newgard, 2008). Ineffective glucose uptake results in persistent and increasingly severe hyperglycemia that, despite increased pancreatic insulin output, cannot be fully controlled. Thus, a state of chronic hyperinsulinemia and glucose intolerance may persist for prolonged periods prior to the development of hyperglycemia and frank type 2 diabetes. This could potentially impact cancer progression by several mechanisms involving the innate and highly sensitive IR/IGF-IR signaling system. First, insulin has a high affinity for IR-A and could thus promote cell proliferation through its cognate receptor. Second, hyperinsulinemia increases IGF-I bioavailability by (i) increasing hepatic growth hormone receptor expression, which leads to growth hormone-mediated increases in IGF-I production by the liver (Rhoads et al., 2004) and (ii) repressing hepatic production of IGF-binding proteins (IGFBP)-1 and -2 (Calle & Kaaks, 2004). This increase in IGF-I could lead to increased signaling via IR-A/IGF-IR hybrids and the IGF-IR. Third, hyperinsulinemia reduces hepatic secretion of sex hormone-binding globulin (SHBG) (Meirow et al., 1995; Pasquali et al., 1991), which leads to elevated circulation of free estrogen which can act as a mitogen for estrogen-dependent cancers of breast and endometrial origin (as discussed below) (Pike, Pearce, & Wu, 2004).

Over 30 years ago, breast epithelial cells growing in culture were found to express relatively high levels of the IR (Osborne, Monaco, Lippman, & Kahn, 1978). In breast tumor tissues, significantly higher levels of IR protein were found than in normal breast tissue (Frittitta et al., 1993; Papa et al., 1990), which also exhibited greater sensitivity toward insulin (Frittitta et al., 1993). Phosphorylated IR/IGF-IR has also been found to be a prognostic marker of poor outcome in breast cancer (Law et al., 2008). Interestingly, the study described previously by Huang et al. (2011) did not find increased expression of total IR mRNA in tumor tissues, suggesting that posttranslational modifications likely play a role in regulating IR protein expression. Expression of IR may also be regulated by the tumor suppressor gene *p53* which normally acts as a transcriptional repressor of the IR (Webster et al., 1996). In breast cancer, *p53* is commonly mutated, which could contribute to the elevated expression of the IR (Jones et al., 2004). In mouse models, transgenic overexpression of *Neu*, *Wnt1*, or *Ret* oncogenes were accompanied by spontaneous mammary tumor formation that were all found to harbor significant elevations of the IR (Frittitta et al., 1997). Mice overexpressing a dominant negative IGF-IR in skeletal muscle (the MKR$^{+/+}$ mouse model) develop insulin resistance and hyperinsulinemia while remaining lean

(Fernandez et al., 2001). When mouse mammary tumor cell lines, Met1 and MCNeuA, were orthotopically injected into $MKR^{+/+}$ and control mice, tumors developed more rapidly in $MKR^{+/+}$ mice, a phenomenon which could be abolished by use of the dual IR/IGF-IR inhibitor BMS-536924 (Novosyadlyy et al., 2010) or insulin-sensitizing therapy (Fierz, Novosyadlyy, Vijayakumar, Yakar, & LeRoith, 2010). Crossing transgenic female polyoma virus middle T antigen (PyVmT) mice with $MKR^{+/+}$ mice resulted in a bitransgenic model which exhibited increased mammary gland ductal hyperplasia at 6 weeks of age when compared to PyVmT alone (Novosyadlyy et al., 2009). Meanwhile, orthotopic injection of metastatic mammary tumor cell line Mvt1 into $MKR^{+/+}$ mice resulted in larger mammary tumors as well as significantly more lung metastases when compared to control animals (Ferguson et al., 2012). In the breast cancer cell line LCC6, shRNA knockdown of the IR decreased LCC6 xenograft tumor size and resulted in less dissemination of cells from the primary tumor. Further, intravenously injected LCC6 cells lacking functional IR failed to form metastases in the lung to the same levels as normal LCC6 cells, suggesting a critical role of the IR in breast tumor metastasis (Zhang et al., 2010).

2.3. IGF signaling and breast cancer

The growth factors IGF-I and IGF-II bind their cognate IGF-IR receptor with high affinity and thereby execute a highly conserved and crucial role in mediating the development and growth of mammals. As potent growth factors, the aberrant overexpression of both IGF-I and IGF-II has been linked to the development and progression of many types of cancer, including breast cancer (Sachdev & Yee, 2001). The IGFs may act in a paracrine or autocrine manner within tissues. Several clinical studies suggest a positive association between circulating IGF-I and breast cancer (Renehan et al., 2004; Rinaldi et al., 2006; Schernhammer, Holly, Pollak, & Hankinson, 2005), although one recent study did not report a positive correlation (Goodwin et al., 2002). In breast cancer, locally produced IGF-I is generally restricted to the surrounding normal breast tissue (Chong, Williams, Elkak, Sharma, & Mokbel, 2006; Marshman & Streuli, 2002; Yee et al., 1989). The *igf-II* gene is imprinted, but in several cancers, including breast cancer, biallelic expression of *igf-II* has been observed which may contribute to malignant progression (McCann et al., 1996). Although some studies have found no association between circulating IGF-II and breast cancer (Kaulsay et al., 1999; Yu et al., 2002), a study which focused specifically on early-stage breast cancer patients reported a significant elevation in free IGF-II compared to healthy controls (Espelund, Cold, Frystyk, Orskov, & Flyvbjerg, 2008). Local IGF-II may be a potent driver of breast cancer, with expression in both tumor tissue and stromal cells surrounding tumors (Giani et al., 2002; Giani, Cullen, Campani, & Rasmussen, 1996). The expression of local IGF-II has been linked to low histological tumor grade and early-stage tumors, suggesting that the IGF-II may be involved in the early stages of breast cancer development (Toropainen, Lipponen, & Syrjanen, 1995). Immunohistochemical studies on a large proportion of breast tumor specimens have revealed IGF-II expression in both stromal and tumor epithelial cells, a finding which was positively correlated with stromal cell proliferation and progesterone receptor expression, respectively. No association was observed between IGF-II levels and lymph node metastasis (Giani et al., 2002). However, a recent study carried out on a cohort of 1000 women in China reported that IGF-II expression was positively correlated with invasiveness, histological tumor grade, and ER expression (Qiu, Yang, Rao, Du, & Kalembo, 2012), showing that although locally produced IGF-II is likely to affect breast tumor progression, the stage of malignancy at which it has the most potent effect may differ depending on the subtype of breast cancer and other additional factors which need further clarification.

Upon receptor binding, IGF-I and IGF-II not only stimulate PI3K/Akt/mTOR-mediated mitogenic pathways in a similar way to the IR but, importantly, also upregulate pathways which promote loss of cell adhesion (Lynch, Vodyanik, Boettiger, & Guvakova, 2005) and increased cell motility (Kiely, O'Gorman, Luong, Ron, & O'Connor, 2006) which could lead to more invasive breast cancer phenotypes. The breast cancer cell line MDA-MB-231 also upregulated the expression of VEGF-C in response to IGF-I in a dose-dependent manner, a phenomenon which could be ablated by both PI3K and MAPK inhibitors, suggesting a further role of IGF-I in mediating tumor progression through angiogenesis (Zhu et al., 2011). During the progression of type 2 diabetes, the hyperinsulinemia-mediated increases in insulin, IGF-I, and IGF-II could therefore significantly contribute to worse outcome in breast cancers, particularly those undergoing a shifting IR-A:IR-B ratio, due to the increased relative abundance of exposed binding sites for these ligands. Altered IR-A:IR-B ratio in breast cancer may also increase sensitivity to the autocrine action of IGF-II in the various stages of tumorigenesis.

3. THE ROLE OF CHOLESTEROL IN CANCER GROWTH

Cholesterol is an essential structural component of mammalian cell membranes, ensuring their structural integrity and modulating their fluidity. It plays a functional role in cell osmolarity, pinocytosis, and activity and regulates membrane-associated proteins (Broitman, Cerda, & Wilkinson, 1993). Moreover, cholesterol is a precursor to several biochemical pathways, including the synthesis of steroid hormones and vitamin D. It has an integral role in cell growth and division, in stabilizing the DNA double helix, and in controlling the activity of membrane-bound enzymes, and as such cholesterol has been proposed to be involved in the etiology of cancer (Bielecka-Dabrowa, Hannam, Rysz, & Banach, 2011).

Lipid disorders or dyslipidemias frequently occur in those with obesity and type 2 diabetes. The most common type of dyslipidemia is hyperlipidemia, which includes hypercholesterolemia, hypertriglyceridemia, or combined hyperlipidemia. Increased levels of low-density lipoprotein (LDL) cholesterol in the circulation may be a consequence of obesity, diet, inherited diseases such as mutations in LDL receptor in familial hypercholesterolemia (FH), or the presence of other diseases such as diabetes, polycystic ovary syndrome, kidney disease, and hypothyroidism (Daniels & Greer, 2008). The prevalence of the heterozygous form of FH in the United States, Western Europe, and China is approximately 1 per 500 persons; the homozygous form is rare (approximately one per million). FH is characterized by tendinous xanthomas, premature coronary heart disease, and stroke. In contrast, higher levels of high-density lipoprotein (HDL) cholesterol are considered to have protective effects against cardiovascular disease (Shepherd et al., 1995). Two of the defining features of the metabolic syndrome, which is common in obese individuals and those with type 2 diabetes, are low HDL cholesterol (<40 mg/dL in men and <50 mg/dL in women) and hypertriglyceridemia (>250 mg/dL). The most effective class of drugs for lowering serum LDL cholesterol concentrations are the 3-hydroxy-3-methylglutaryl-coenzyme (HMG-CoA) reductase inhibitors, also known as statins. In previous years, several trials have demonstrated the efficacy and safety of statin therapy in children and adults (Rodenburg et al., 2007).

3.1. Epidemiological studies linking cholesterol and cancer

The relationship between cholesterol and the risk of cancer remains controversial; while some data point to a relationship between high cholesterol levels and cancer risk, it is difficult to find clear relationships in

epidemiological studies due to the strong association between high cholesterol and cardiovascular disease mortality and the association between low
cholesterol with chronic diseases. In 1985, the Seven Countries Study conducted in Finland, Greece, Italy, Japan, the Netherlands, the United States,
and Yugoslavia reported an increased risk of lung cancer death at cholesterol
levels under 170 mg/dl. However, the same study they showed that Northern Europe had higher rates of cancer and these populations have higher
cholesterol levels (Keys et al., 1985).

3.1.1 Breast cancer

Two cohort studies conducted on Norwegian women found that low serum
HDL is independently associated with increased postmenopausal breast cancer risk among women who are overweight or obese. The relationship
between HDL and the risk of postmenopausal breast cancer was strongest
among those who gained weight during follow-up, when analyses were
adjusted for BMI. Their findings suggest an interaction between metabolic
disturbances and postmenopausal breast carcinogenesis (Furberg, Veierod,
Wilsgaard, Bernstein, & Thune, 2004). The authors suggest that low serum
HDL could be an independent predictor of increased postmenopausal breast
cancer risk among overweight and obese women (Furberg et al., 2004). In a
follow-up study, these authors followed women aged around 30, demonstrating for the first time that a metabolic profile with low serum HDL is related to
increased levels of free, biologically active estradiol throughout the entire
menstrual cycle (Furberg et al., 2005). They found that women with high
BMI and high LDL/HDL serum ratio had higher free estradiol levels
(Furberg et al., 2005). Based on their overall results, they suggested using
low HDL serum levels in overweight and obese women as biomarker for
breast cancer risk. The United States-based Atherosclerosis Risk in Communities Study (ARIC) prospective cohort study carried out between 1987 and
2000 on women aged 45–64 observed at baseline a modest association of low
HDL cholesterol with increased incidence of breast cancer among
premenopausal women. The observation of a modest association of low
HDL cholesterol with increased incidence of breast cancer among women
who were pre- and perimenopausal at baseline, but not among postmenopausal women, can perhaps be explained in the context of the hormonal regulation of breast cancer (Kucharska-Newton et al., 2008). It could be
suggested that one of the strongest risk factors for breast cancer are high
endogenous estrogen levels (Hankinson & Hunter, 2002). High estrogen
levels, observed during premenopause, are inversely associated with low

HDL cholesterol (Furberg et al., 2005). These results suggest that low HDL cholesterol among premenopausal women serves as a prediction tool for increased breast cancer risk (Kucharska-Newton et al., 2008).

3.1.2 Prostate cancer

A large, prospective cohort study performed by Mondul failed to find an association between serum total cholesterol and risk for prostate cancer (PCa) when an adjustment was made for age alone (Mondul, Weinstein, Virtamo, & Albanes, 2011). However, when they used multivariable adjustment, it was suggested that men with high serum cholesterol were at higher risk of developing PCa, which is in agreement with other studies. They also suggested an inverse association between serum HDL levels and the risk of PCa development. Similar results were found when the ratio of total/HDL cholesterol was calculated (Mondul et al., 2011). It should be noted that all the subjects who participated in this study were heavy smokers for more than 30 years, a factor that can influence the baseline risk of cancer development. The results and conclusions were different from previous studies on the same cohort, and the authors suggest the adjustment for baseline serum α-tocopherol (α-TEA) as the main reason (Mondul et al., 2011). This work was also supported by another perspective work from men that confirmed in PCa patients versus healthy men that hypercholesterolemia is associated with a high risk of PCa (Magura et al., 2008). Another cohort study conducted by Kok (Kok et al., 2011) on men never treated with cholesterol-lowering drugs found a correlation between high serum LDL cholesterol and the risk of developing PCa. A similar correlation was also found with aggressive PCa, while a significant association was found between HDL cholesterol and nonaggressive PCa, suggesting that blood lipid levels may play a role in PCa development. However, the authors could not explain the role of each cholesterol fraction on PCa aggressiveness (Kok et al., 2011). Other studies demonstrated the correlation between hypercholesterolemia and the progression of PCa (Henriksson et al., 1989), and it was suggested that a western diet rich in cholesterol content promotes prostatic cancer development as suggested by epidemiological evidence (Di Vizio, Solomon, & Freeman, 2008).

3.2. Molecular mechanisms linking cholesterol to cancer growth

3.2.1 Cholesterol and breast cancer

As cholesterol has been reported to affect sex steroids regulation, the correlation between cholesterol and breast cancer was studied. When lipidic emulsion, which has the same lipid structure as LDL and may bind to LDL receptors, was injected into bloodstream, it was found to concentrate in breast cancer tumors but not in normal surrounding breast tissues (Graziani et al., 2002). One study which aimed to find an antitumorigenic therapy for breast cancer used a vitamin E analog named α-TEA. They found that this derivative acts as a good antitumor agent by causing apoptosis of breast cancer cells both *in vitro* and *in vivo* (mice or humans). Further, α-TEA inhibited lung cancer metastasis (in mice or humans). It had no toxicity on normal cells and tissues *in vivo*. In contrast to these findings, administration of vitamin E did not have any antitumor effect on breast cancer cells (Lawson et al., 2003).

Cholesterol has been demonstrated to play a central role in the expression of macrophage tumoricidal activity. Cholesterol-enriched macrophages lose their ability to become tumoricidal (Chapman & Hibbs, 1977). Further, reducing serum LDL-cholesterol levels may reduce endothelial activation and prevent interference with the immune system. Therefore, anti-inflammatory drugs may play an important role in chemoprevention of metastasis (Mehta, Hordines, Volpe, Doerr, & Cohen, 1997).

We have previously described that hypercholesterolemia, regardless of hyperglycemia or hyperinsulinemia, affects mammary tumor growth and metastasis (Alikhani et al., 2013). ApoE glycoprotein functions as a regulator of plasma lipid levels and has a role in the uptake of lipids into different tissues and in delivering cholesterol and triglycerides into cells. We injected breast cancer cells into ApoE$^{-/-}$ and WT female mice. When these mice were fed with a HF/HC diet, tumors in the ApoE$^{-/-}$ mice tended to be more aggressive, with larger volume and subsequent formation of more lung metastatic lesions. When breast cancer cells were injected into the tail vein of ApoE$^{-/-}$ and WT mice, we also found a larger number of metastases in the lungs of the ApoE$^{-/-}$ mice compared to WT (Alikhani et al., 2013). Stimulation of the same breast cancer cells with cholesterol *in vitro* led to a dose-dependent increase in cell proliferation as well as to stimulation of the PI3K pathway, demonstrated by robust Akt phosphorylation (Alikhani et al., 2013), which is in agreement with previous studies suggesting the effect of cholesterol on PI3K/Akt activation (Li, Park, Ye, Kim, & Kim, 2006). In summary, we and others propose that one potential mechanism whereby cholesterol can promote tumor growth and metastasis in breast cancer is through a mechanistic link between dyslipidemia and the PI3K/Akt pathway, and thus suggest that reducing total cholesterol levels may be an important therapeutic modality in the prevention and treatment of breast cancer (Alikhani et al., 2013).

3.2.2 Cholesterol and prostate cancer

Cells from the prostate, as well as cells from other tissues, synthesize endogenous cholesterol through the mevalonate pathway. However, most of the cholesterol located in the cell membrane originates from circulating cholesterol (Simons & Ikonen, 2000). Therefore, there is an equilibrium between the intrinsic synthesis of cholesterol by the cell and the regulatory functions of cholesterol in the blood circulation (Freeman & Solomon, 2004). This balance breaks down in the case of cancer as well as in the aging of the prostate. It was found that benign prostatic hyperplasia (BPH) tissue contains more cholesterol than normal prostatic tissue (Swyer, 1942). Later studies have found higher levels of cholesterol in the prostate and prostatic secretions in humans as well as in animals. These findings were correlated with age, disease, or malignant cells (Schaffner, 1981). On the other hand, population studies found that low cholesterol levels are associated with less aggressive PCa and a lower risk of PCa-related mortality (Batty, Kivimaki, Clarke, Davey Smith, & Shipley, 2011; Huxley, 2007; Mondul, Clipp, Helzlsouer, & Platz, 2010; Platz et al., 2009). It was suggested that cholesterol accumulation could be more common in malignant cases and was found in several cancer tumor types (Dessi, Batetta, Anchisi, et al., 1992; Dessi et al., 1994; Kolanjiappan, Ramachandran, & Manoharan, 2003; Rudling & Collins, 1996; Yoshioka et al., 2000). Several mechanisms are probably involved in the elevated levels of cholesterol content in tumors such as amplified absorption of circulating cholesterol (Graziani et al., 2002; Tatidis, Masquelier, & Vitols, 2002), downregulation of LDL resulting in loss of feedback regulation (Caruso, Notarnicola, Santillo, Cavallini, & Di Leo, 1999), and upregulation of HMG-CoA reductase (Caruso, Notarnicola, Cavallini, & Di Leo, 2002; Caruso et al., 1999). Increased transcription of fatty acid synthase and HMG-CoA reductase, stimulated by androgens, results in lipogenesis in human PCa cells (Heemers et al., 2001). As cholesterol synthesis and cholesterol uptake are linked to the cell cycle (Wadsack et al., 2003), it was suggested by Freeman and Solomon that the link between cholesterol, other lipogenic mechanisms, and androgen could be the pathways by which lipid production is involved in androgenic stimulation of PCa cell growth (Freeman & Solomon, 2004). Recently, it was demonstrated that circulating cholesterol is directly responsible for upregulating androgens (especially testosterone), causing increased angiogenesis in a castrated mouse model injected with the well-established PCa cell line, LNCaP (Mostaghel, Solomon, Pelton, Freeman, & Montgomery, 2012).

Several studies demonstrated that lowering circulating cholesterol in dogs and rodents using oral administration of hypocholesterolemic agents such as polyene macrolide candicidin resulted in prostate regression (Fisher et al., 1975; Gordon & Schaffner, 1968; Schaffner, 1981; Schaffner & Gordon, 1968). It was suggested that oral administration of candicidin lowered circulating cholesterol by inhibiting its absorption from the gut (Schaffner & Gordon, 1968). Several human studies reported an improvement of BPH with oral candicidin administration (Keshin, 1973; Orkin, 1974; Sporer, Cohen, Kamat, & Seebode, 1975) without changes in androgen levels (Orkin, 1974), suggesting that it is not the result of suppression of androgen production (Keshin, 1973).

3.2.3 Cholesterol in other tumor types

Studies on cervical and endometrial cancer cell lines demonstrated that an increased cholesterol concentration correlated with proliferation rate (Gal, MacDonald, Porter, & Simpson, 1981). An elevated uptake of LDL has been shown in lung cancer tissues and different leukemias. The LDL receptor levels were also shown to be increased on some epithelial carcinomas, hepatoma, malignant gliomas, endometrial cancers, and cervical cancer cell lines. Studies on breast cancer have shown an increased LDL concentration in tumor tissue which correlated with a dismal prognosis (Dessi, Batetta, Pulisci, et al., 1992; Gal et al., 1981; Menrad & Anderer, 1991; Rudling, Angelin, Peterson, & Collins, 1990; Stopeck, Nicholson, Mancini, & Hajjar, 1993; Vitols, Norgren, Juliusson, Tatidis, & Luthman, 1994).

Additionally, there are some *in vivo* studies which suggest an association between cholesterol and cancer metastasis. It has been shown that inducing colon cancer in rats by dimethylhydrazine correlated with reduced incidences of metastasis after deprivation of dietary cholesterol (Cruse, Lewin, & Clark, 1982). It was also demonstrated in breast cancer that hyperlipidemia is significantly associated with the distant metastasis (Liu et al., 2012). Interestingly, cohort studies found a correlation between elevated serum iron coupled with either high VLDL or low HDL to increase cancer risk. This was explained by iron-mediated oxidation of cholesterol that increases oxidative stress, and may lead to cancer development (Mainous, Wells, Koopman, Everett, & Gill, 2005).

3.3. Cholesterol and statins

Epidemiological studies have shown that statins may lower the risk for PCa development and progression (Bonovas, Filioussi, & Sitaras, 2008; Flick et al., 2007; Graaf, Beiderbeck, Egberts, Richel, & Guchelaar, 2004; Murtola, Tammela, Lahtela, & Auvinen, 2007; Platz, Clinton, & Giovannucci, 2008; Platz et al., 2006; Shannon et al., 2005).

When tested in rodents, statins failed to lower circulating cholesterol, but they reduced sterol synthesis in peripheral tissues (Germershausen et al., 1989; Koga et al., 1990; Sirtori, 1993). These results suggest a direct effect of the drug on peripheral tissues. It should be noted that the researchers used suprapharmacological doses in the range of 5–10 mg/kg/day (Monetti et al., 2007; Ozacmak, Sayan, Igdem, Cetin, & Ozacmak, 2007), whereas human doses range from 0.1 to 1.6 mg/kg/day (Solomon & Freeman, 2008). It was demonstrated *in vitro* that chronic administration of atorvastatin inhibited cancer cell proliferation and, even after 3 weeks of statin withdrawal, not all the changes associated with the treatment, such as a reduction in insulin signaling, were reversible (Miraglia, Hogberg, & Stenius, 2012). Several meta-analyses compared statin versus placebo treatment and claimed that statin failed to prevent cancer development in multiple organ sites (Baigent et al., 2005; Browning & Martin, 2007; Dale, Coleman, Henyan, Kluger, & White, 2006). On the other hand, other investigators claim these conclusions are incorrect, as the end points chosen were cancer incidence and disease-specific mortality, which are poor measurements of antitumor efficacy for some malignancies which develop slowly (Freeman, Solomon, & Moyad, 2006). Thus, while there is no consensus, there remains strong evidence of a statin effect.

4. OBESITY, ESTROGEN, AND BREAST CANCER

4.1. Obesity and circulating estrogens

The increased risk of postmenopausal breast cancer that is associated with increased BMI has been recognized for many years (Bergstrom, Pisani, Tenet, Wolk, & Adami, 2001). In women with breast cancer, the relationship between all-cause mortality and BMI after diagnosis appears to be U-shaped, while a more linear relationship between BMI and breast cancer mortality exists (Nichols et al., 2009). In a U.S. study of almost 4000 women, each 5 kg increase in weight after breast cancer diagnosis was associated with a 13% increase in breast cancer-specific mortality (Nichols et al., 2009). In younger women, obesity is associated with a greater risk of ER-negative tumors, and more advanced stage; however, in obese post-menopausal women, there is a greater risk of hormone-dependent ER-positive breast cancers (Rose & Vona-Davis, 2009). Among the many factors that may contribute to the increased breast cancer risk associated with excess weight is increased endogenous estrogen production by the adipose tissue. Estrogen is known to be important both for the normal mammary gland development and for the growth of breast cancers. A greater cumulative exposure to estrogen over the lifetime of a woman is known to increase her risk of postmenopausal breast cancer (Yager & Davidson, 2006). Antiestrogens, including aromatase inhibitors that reduce the synthesis of estrogen, and selective ER modulators have been used for many years in the treatment of breast cancer.

Obese women are known to have significantly higher circulating levels of estrogen than lean women (Key et al., 2003; Toniolo et al., 1995). Epidemiological studies have reported that higher circulating endogenous estrogen increases the RR of postmenopausal breast cancer approximately twofold (Key et al., 2003). The higher circulating levels of estrogen are due to increased aromatase activity in the adipose tissue of obese women, leading to the peripheral conversion of androstenedione and testosterone to estrone and estradiol, respectively (Kirschner, Schneider, Ertel, & Worton, 1982). Additionally, obese, insulin-resistant women have lower circulating levels of SHBG, due to the suppression of hepatic SHBG production (Le, Nestler, Strauss, & Wickham, 2012). SHBG binds circulating estrogens and androgens, and a reduction in SHBG results in more bioavailable estrogens and androgens in the circulation (Kopelman, Pilkington, White, & Jeffcoate, 1980). The increase in circulating estrogens may only be of clinical importance after the menopause, when ovarian estrogen production has declined. In obese postmenopausal women, increased aromatization of androgens and lower SHBG may result in more bioavailable estrogens in the circulation that could promote the growth and proliferation of breast cancers.

4.2. Obesity and breast aromatase activity

Circulating levels of endogenous estrogens, however, may not accurately reflect the local levels of estrogen in the breast (Pasqualini & Chetrite, 2005). Breast stromal tissue also expresses aromatase, and in postmenopausal women, estrogen levels are 10–50 times higher in the breast tissue than in blood (Pasqualini & Chetrite, 2005; Simpson, Ackerman, Smith, & Mendelson, 1981). In breast tissue from obese individuals, aromatase expression is increased approximately twofold compared to that of normal weight individuals. In tumor-bearing breast tissue, aromatase expression is further increased approximately four- to fivefold, compared to nontumor bearing breast tissue of the same breast. This increase in aromatase may explain the higher estrogen concentrations that have been found in breast tumors than nontumorous parts of the breast (Agarwal, Bulun, Leitch, Rohrich, & Simpson, 1996; Suzuki, Miki, Ohuchi, & Sasano, 2008; van Landeghem, Poortman, Nabuurs, & Thijssen, 1985).

Aromatase is encoded by the gene Cyp19A1, under the control of a number of promoters. In human breast cancer cells lines, its expression is largely controlled by two promoters, I.3 and II (Zhou, Clarke, Wang, & Chen, 1996). Recent studies have shown that proinflammatory cytokines from breast tissue are associated with increased aromatase expression in the mammary fat pad. In an animal model of postmenopausal (ovariecto-mized) high-fat diet–induced and genetically (leptin resistant, ob/ob) induced obesity, increased macrophage infiltration into the mammary fat pad with associated increased expression of inflammatory mediators (TNFα, IL-1β, COX-2) in mammary adipose tissue (Subbaramaiah et al., 2011). Additionally, the same group demonstrated that aromatase expression is increased in the breast tissue of obese women with breast cancer and is associated with increased levels of COX-2 and prostaglandin E2 (PGE2) in the breast tissue (Morris et al., 2011). Aromatase mRNA expression, derived from promoters 1.3 and II, correlated with COX-2 and PGE2 levels in this study (Morris et al., 2011). Therefore, the production of inflamma-tory cytokines in the breast tissue of obese women may explain the increased aromatase activity found in the breasts of obese women. The increase in aro-matase activity may increase local estrogen synthesis in the breast tissue of obese women and lead to a greater risk of postmenopausal hormone receptor-positive breast cancer (Morris et al., 2011).

Aromatase is regulated by a number of other factors that are altered in obe-sity and have been linked to breast cancer. The nutrient-sensing molecule, AMP-activated protein kinase (AMPK), is also a regulator of aromatase expres-sion. Activated AMPK is a negative regulator of the Akt/mTOR signaling pathway that is frequently increased in breast cancer due to oncogenes, the loss of tumor suppressor genes, or in the setting of hyperinsulinemia (Ferguson et al., 2012; Levine & Puzio-Kuter, 2010; Novosyadlyy et al., 2010). The serine-threonine kinase, liver kinase B1 (LKB1), is the kinase that phosphor-ylates AMPK in the setting of nutrient deprivation and is additionally a major tumor suppressor gene (Shackelford & Shaw, 2009). LKB1 and AMPK are negative regulators of aromatase expression in human breast tissue and may provide the link between obesity, inflammation, and aromatase expression in breast cancer (Brown et al., 2009; McInnes, Brown, Hunger, & Simpson,

2011). In the liver, AMPK inhibits gluconeogenesis by phosphorylating the c-AMP response element-binding protein (CREB) and the CREB-regulated transcription coactivator 2 (CRTC2) (He et al., 2009; Koo et al., 2005). In human adipose stromal cells, CRTC2 binds to the aromatase promoter PII leading to increased aromatase expression (Brown et al., 2009). AMPK phosphorylation of CRTC2 prevents its entry into the nucleus, decreasing aromatase expression. Many inflammatory and metabolic factors alter aromatase expression through their effect on LKB1/AMPK. PGE2 downregulates LKB1 and AMPK phosphorylation, resulting in increased nuclear localization of CRTC2 and increased aromatase expression (Brown et al., 2009). The adipokine leptin is increased in obese individuals due to leptin resistance and correlates with increased risk of breast cancer in epidemiological studies (Wu et al., 2009). Leptin increases aromatase expression by decreasing LKB1 protein expression and phosphorylation, resulting in increased nuclear localization of CRTC2 and subsequent binding to the PII promoter of aromatase (Brown et al., 2009). Adiponectin, in contrast to leptin, is decreased in the circulation of obese individuals and has been associated with a decreased risk of postmenopausal breast cancer in some epidemiological studies (Tworoger et al., 2007). *In vitro* studies have shown that adiponectin stimulates LKB1 and its activity, leading to decreased aromatase expression (Brown et al., 2009).

In recent years, the antidiabetic medication, metformin, has received attention after epidemiological studies reported decreased cancer incidence and mortality in patients with diabetes using metformin (Bodmer, Meier, Krahenbuhl, Jick, & Meier, 2010; Currie, Poole, & Gale, 2009; Evans, Donnelly, Emslie-Smith, Alessi, & Morris, 2005; Landman et al., 2010). There are many potential mechanisms through which metformin may reduce tumor growth, including its ability to improve insulin resistance, reduce insulin levels, and decrease blood glucose as discussed below in section 5 on diabetes medication and cancer. Metformin is an activator of AMPK and increases LKB1 protein and RNA levels by increasing LKB1 promoter activity in breast cancer adipose cells. Through this increase in LKB1/AMPK activity, metformin inhibits the nuclear translocation of CRTC2 and thereby decreases the expression of aromatase (Brown, Hunger, Docanto, & Simpson, 2010). Through these mechanisms, metformin may reduce local estrogen levels in the breast and may therefore protect against estrogen-stimulated breast cancer growth or may be beneficial as an adjuvant therapy for the treatment of breast cancer.

4.3. Estrogen receptor and breast cancer in obesity and type 2 diabetes

4.3.1 Estrogen receptor signaling

The effects of estrogen in the breast are mediated through ERα, ERβ, and the G protein-coupled estrogen receptor (GPER) (Bartella, De Marco, Malaguarnera, Belfiore, & Maggiolini, 2012). ERα and ERβ are transcribed from two genes, ESR1 and ESR2. They have 96% homology in their DNA-binding domains, but only 58% homology in their ligand-binding domains (Yager & Davidson, 2006). Multiple ERβ isoforms exist and their functions have recently been reviewed elsewhere (Leung, Lee, Lam, Tarapore, & Ho, 2012). Classically, estrogen signaling occurs through the binding of estrogen to the ERα, leading to dimerization of ERα, translocation to the nucleus, and the regulation of gene transcription. The ER regulation of gene transcription is a complex process. After ligand binding to the ERα or ERβ and nuclear translocation, a complex is formed, comprising the ER with corepressors, coactivators, histone acetyltransferases, and histone deacetylases. Additionally, ERβ may recruit ERα to the complex, and certain genes may only be transcribed in the presence of ERα and ERβ in the complex. The ER complex binds to ER response elements in the promoter regions of various ER-regulated genes, and depending upon the corepressors and coactivators present in the ER complex, gene transcription may be activated or repressed (Ariazi et al., 2007; Malik et al., 2010; Pearce & Jordan, 2004). The ER may also interact with other transcription factors, including Runx1, FOXA1, members of the activation protein 1 (AP1), and specificity protein 1 (Sp1) families, to facilitate binding to the serum response elements leading to transcription (Bartella et al., 2012; Musgrove & Sutherland, 2009). However, ER is not only a transcription factor. Studies have shown that in human breast cancer cell lines, activation of the ER also leads to the phosphorylation of proteins within minutes of stimulation, demonstrating that this signaling was not related to changes in gene transcription and translation which would take hours. These effects were demonstrated to be due to activation of the ER at the plasma membrane. The membrane-bound ER interacts with other growth factor receptors, including the IGF-IR (Kelly & Levin, 2001). Additionally, the GPER is involved in many of the rapid effects of estrogens, including transactivation of EGF receptors, the activation of MAPK and PI3K transduction pathways, adenylyl cyclase stimulation, and mobilization of intracellular calcium (Bartella et al., 2012). The ER has also been found in the mitochondria, where it is thought to play a role in resisting apoptosis

(Yang et al., 2004). ERβ is predominantly localized in the mitochondria and regulates mitochondrial gene expression and ATP production (Richardson, Hamilton, Davis, Brito, & De Leon, 2011). The ER status of a tumor is designated as ER negative if there is <10% nuclear staining for ERα on immunohistochemistry. However, "ER-negative" breast cancer cells may still express ERα at low levels or in extranuclear sites of the cell such as the cytoplasm or membrane, additionally, ERβ expression is higher in some "ER-negative" breast cancer cell lines than in ER-positive cell lines (Richardson et al., 2011). Therefore, even in breast cancers traditionally considered as ER negative and unresponsive to hormone therapy, the ERs may be playing a role in cell signaling, growth, and survival.

4.3.2 ER and IGF-1R cross talk in breast cancer

IGF-I and IGF-IR signaling may play an important role in breast cancer growth in the setting of obesity and type 2 diabetes, as described in Section 2. IGF-IR and ER signaling are known to interact in normal mammary gland development and breast cancer (Cui et al., 2003; Lee et al., 1999; Molloy, May, & Westley, 2000). In human breast cancer specimens, there is a correlation between IGF-IR/IRS-1 and ERα expression (Lee et al., 1999). Components of IGF-IR signaling are estrogen regulated, while IGF-I signaling can phosphorylate ERα as well as receptor coactivators and other regulatory proteins, leading to potentiation of ERα signaling (Bartella et al., 2012; Cui et al., 2003). Cross talk between the IGF-IR and ERα signaling pathways has been hypothesized as a mechanism of resistance to hormone receptor-targeted therapy (Fagan & Yee, 2008). *In vitro* studies using ER-positive MCF7 and T47D human breast cancer cell lines stably expressing aromatase demonstrated that treating the cells with both the aromatase inhibitor letrozole and the IGF-IR inhibitor NVP-AEW541 led to a synergistic increase in apoptosis, compared to treatment with either agent alone (Lisztwan, Pornon, Chen, Chen, & Evans, 2008). In MCF7 cells, IGF-IR signaling has been shown to mediate resistance to antiestrogen and antiprogestin therapy by activation of the MEK1/MAPK and PI3K signaling pathways (Periyasamy-Thandavan et al., 2012; Zhang et al., 2011). Gene expression profiling of MCF-7 cells treated with IGF-I, estrogen, or their inhibitors reported that estrogen and IGF-I signaling result in the repression of many common target genes, and for many of the genes, the estrogen- and IGF-I-mediated repression occurred independent of IGF-IR and ERα signaling (Casa et al., 2012). Therefore, because of this cross talk and independent regulation of common genes, it has been hypothesized that inhibiting IGF-IR signaling in addition to ER signaling would prevent or overcome breast cancer resistance to hormone therapy. However, breast cancer clinical trials studying the effects of targeting IGF-IR signaling in addition to the ER have thus far been disappointing. One such phase III clinical trial compared 5 years treatment of tamoxifen alone versus 5 years of tamoxifen treatment with 2 years treatment with the somatostatin analog, octreotide. Despite lower circulating IGF-I levels in the octreotide-treated group, no differences in event-free survival, recurrence-free survival, or overall survival were found (Pritchard et al., 2011). These results may seem surprising as *in vitro* and *in vivo* studies have shown that targeting the IGF-IR with monoclonal antibodies alone or in combination with other therapy reduced tumor growth (Goetsch et al., 2005; Sachdev et al., 2003). However, many of these *in vitro* studies were performed in hormone-sensitive cells and orthografts. More recent *in vitro* studies examining tamoxifen-resistant MCF-7 cells and an *in vivo* study of MCF-7 xenografts demonstrated that adding an IGF-IR inhibitor to tamoxifen treatment did not lead to any additional inhibition of tumor growth (Fagan, Uselman, Sachdev, & Yee, 2012). Tamoxifen-treated xenografts were found to have reduced IGF-IR expression, potentially explaining the lack of response to the addition of IGF-IR monoclonal antibody therapy (Fagan et al., 2012). Similarly, recurrent tumors from patients with tamoxifen-resistant breast cancer also were found to have decreased IGF-IR expression (Drury et al., 2011). As ERα is known to increase IGF-IR expression, the decrease in IGF-1R expression and lack of response to IGF-IR-targeted therapy in breast cancers treated with tamoxifen or resistant to tamoxifen may not be unexpected. In contrast, however, using a tyrosine kinase inhibitor (TKI) that blocks both IR and IGF-IR signaling in tamoxifen-resistant MCF7 cells inhibited their growth. The TKI had acted synergistically with tamoxifen and letrozole to inhibit tumor growth in MCF7 aromatase expressing xenografts (Fagan et al., 2012). These findings suggest that the IR may be playing an important role in the growth of hormone refractory breast cancers.

4.3.3 ER and IR signaling in hormone refractory breast cancers

In human breast cancer cell lines, IR signaling provides an escape mechanism allowing cells to resist the effects of IGF-IR monoclonal antibodies, as discussed in section 2.2.4 on IR and IR hybrids in breast cancer (Ulanet, Ludwig, Kahn, & Hanahan, 2010). An increased IR to IGF-IR ratio in human breast cancer cell lines has been associated with resistance to IGF-IR-targeted therapy (Ulanet et al., 2010). IR signaling may also affect the response to hormone receptor-targeted therapy. Two recent studies have reported an increase in the IR-A:IR-B ratio in hormone refractory ER-positive or luminal B-type breast cancers that are known to be less responsive to hormonal therapies (Harrington et al., 2012; Huang et al., 2011). In human ER-negative breast cancer cell lines, IGF-II, which acts through the IGF-IR and IR-A, led to phosphorylation of ERα and ERβ, in the absence of estrogen (Richardson et al., 2011). By separately knocking down the IGF-IR and IR in the ER-negative cell lines (CRL-2335 and Hs578t), Richardson and colleagues demonstrated that in Hs578t cells knocking down the IGF-IR decreased phosphorylation of both ERα and ERβ, but IGF-II treatment restored phosphorylation of both ERs, by acting through IR-A. In contrast, knocking down the IGF-IR in CRL-2335 had no effect on ERα or ERβ1 phosphorylation, but decreased phosphorylation of the ERβ5 variant. Knocking down the IR in the CRL-2335 cells decreased phosphorylation of ERα, ERβ1, and ERβ5; however, phosphorylation of the ERs was restored upon treatment with IGF-II. These studies demonstrated that both the IR and IGF-IR are important in mediating the effects of IGF-II on ERα and ERβ phosphorylation in ER-negative breast cancer cells (Richardson et al., 2011). IGF-II stimulation in these cells led to translocation of the ERs to the mitochondria. Mitochondrial localization of the ER is thought to be important in resisting apoptosis (Yang et al., 2004). Insulin acts through both isoforms of the IR; therefore, it is possible that insulin may also increase ER phosphorylation in breast cancer cells that express high levels of IR-A. However, to date, insulin has not been shown to stimulate ERα or ERβ phosphorylation in the absence of estrogen. Other differences in cross talk between the ER, IR, and IGF-IR signaling pathways may exist. While ER signaling increases IGF-IR expression (Fagan & Yee, 2008), studies have shown that, in nonmammary cells (human promonocytic cells), estrogen acting through ERβ inhibits IR gene expression (Garcia-Arencibia, Molero, Davila, Carranza, & Calle, 2005). Therefore, different ratios of ERα, ERβ, and the ERβ variants in breast cancer cells may affect their response to IR signaling. How obesity and diabetes affect the cross talk between the ERs and the signaling pathways of the IR isoforms remains to be determined.

5. CURRENT MEDICATIONS FOR TYPE 2 DIABETES: RELATIONSHIP TO BREAST CANCER

Medications for type 2 diabetes focus on the control of hyperglycemia mediated by insulin deprivation. Treatments for type 2 diabetes include those that use insulin or insulin analogs to replace physiological insulin and others which sensitize tissues to insulin action. As many type 2 diabetes medications are used as long-term solutions for glycemic control, but may have altered binding kinetics for the IR or increased affinity for the IGF-IR, it is important to investigate how antidiabetic drugs that affect IR action could also affect the outcome of breast cancer.

5.1. Recombinant insulin and insulin analogs

Several studies have investigated the risk of recombinant human insulin on cancer incidence as compared to insulin analogs. Three short-acting analogs (lispro, aspart, and glulisine) and two long-acting analogs (glargine and detemir) have been approved for human use. The breast cancer cell line MCF-7 showed higher proliferation rates in response to glargine than to human insulin (Mayer, Shukla, & Enzmann, 2008) and also demonstrated increased mitogenesis in response to glargine, detemir, and lispro as compared to insulin (Weinstein, Simon, Yehezkel, Laron, & Werner, 2009). In agreement with these studies, serum from diabetic patients receiving insulin glargine (accompanied by lispro, aspart, and glulisine) caused a significant increase in MCF-7 cell proliferation in culture compared to serum from diabetic patients receiving human insulin alone. Serum containing detemir (again accompanied by lispro, aspart, and glulisine) resulted in similar proliferation rates of MCF7 cells as those treated with serum containing insulin alone (Mayer & Chantelau, 2010). Clinical studies on the risk of insulin glargine versus human insulin have produced some conflicting data. Two studies showed that no difference in cancer risk existed in users of insulin versus insulin glargine (Colhoun & Group, 2009; Currie, 2009). Another study found that insulin glargine compared to human insulin use was associated with an increased risk of breast cancer specifically, but stated that results were not statistically significant and that several confounding factors had not been accounted for (Jonasson et al., 2009). A follow-up of this study then reported no increased risk for breast cancer for insulin glargine versus insulin (Ljung et al., 2012). Conversely, one study has reported a dose-dependent increase in overall cancer risk from insulin glargine compared to insulin (Hemkens, Grouven, et al., 2009), although this report has been the subject of some controversy (Hemkens, Bender, Grouven, & Sawicki, 2009). More recently, a study examined the effect of insulin glargine compared to insulin over a 3.5-year period and found no increased association between insulin glargine and breast cancer (Lind, Fahlen, Eliasson, & Oden,

2012). A study that followed breast cancer incidence in insulin glargine users observed no significant risk of tumors within the first 5 years of treatment. However, after between 5 and 8 years of insulin glargine use, the risk of breast cancer incidence became significantly greater than with insulin alone, particularly in women who had used other types of insulin prior to starting insulin glargine (Suissa et al., 2011). However, results from the recent ORIGIN trial found no difference in any cancer incidence in glargine users compared to regular insulin users over a period of 6 years (Gerstein et al., 2012), suggesting that the risk of breast cancer incidence and mortality from the use of insulin analogs, such as glargine, may be the same as that for human insulin. However, further studies on the effect of treatment length on tumor occurrence may be necessary to assess the effects of long-term use on breast cancer development.

5.2. Insulin secretagogues

Insulin secretagogues, such as the sulfonylureas and the glitinides, increase systemic insulin levels by stimulating pancreatic β-cells to release insulin into the circulation. Secretagogues target ATP-dependent potassium channels in pancreatic β-cells by attaching to the sulfonylurea receptor subunit of the channel. This results in closure of the channel followed by membrane depolarization, which triggers the opening of voltage-gated Ca^{2+} channels and an influx of Ca^{2+} into the cell. Increased intracellular Ca^{2+} then mediates the exocytosis of insulin-containing vesicles and the release of insulin (Ashcroft & Rorsman, 1989). As well as controlling endocytosis, ATP-dependent potassium channels are intricately involved in mediating cell proliferation and mitochondrial function and, as such, have been studied as possible antitumor agents *in vitro* with promising results, particularly, on the inhibition of the growth of bladder, liver, and gastric cancer cell lines (Malaguarnera et al., 2012; Qian et al., 2008; Wondergem, Cregan, Strickler, Miller, & Suttles, 1998), and more recently, for the suppression of lung and colon tumors in mice (Lee et al., 2002). Conversely, an epidemiological study has reported a significantly increased risk of cancer-related mortality in type 2 diabetic patients receiving sulfonylureas compared to patients receiving metformin (Bowker, Majumdar, Veugelers, & Johnson, 2006). Other studies report different effects on malignancies according to the type of sulfonylureas being used such as a study which found glibenclamide use to be associated with increased cancer risk (Monami et al., 2007), while gliclazide conferred a protective effect (Monami,

Lamanna, Balzi, Marchionni, & Mannucci, 2009). Thus, further clinical trials are required to establish how sulfonylurea treatments in type 2 diabetes affect tumor incidence or progression, particularly for breast cancer, where data are very limited.

5.3. Insulin sensitizers (biguanides and thiazolidinediones)

The biguanide metformin has proved a highly effective medication for type 2 diabetes due to its capacity to target multiple aspects of the disease. Meformin acts as an insulin sensitizer, thus improving glucose uptake into cells (Bikman et al., 2010; Edgerton, Johnson, & Cherrington, 2009), but also suppresses hepatic gluconeogenesis, thereby lowering glucose output from the liver (Caton et al., 2010; Hundal et al., 2000; Kim et al., 2008). Regarding metformin and cancer development, metformin attenuates cell growth by interacting with the mitochondrial respiratory chain complex I and thereby causing an imbalance in ATP production and consumption which leads to an altered AMP:ATP ratio in the cell (Owen, Doran, & Halestrap, 2000). Increased AMP levels then activate AMP kinase (AMPK) which dampens signaling by the mTOR pathway (Dowling, Zakikhani, Fantus, Pollak, & Sonenberg, 2007). For breast cancer, specifically, *in vitro* studies have shown that metformin effectively inhibits proliferation and colony-forming ability and induces cell cycle arrest in ER-positive, Her2-positive, and triple-negative breast tumor cell lines (Alimova et al., 2009; Liu et al., 2009). Further, siRNA knockdown of AMPK in MCF7 cells rescued cells from metformin-induced growth inhibition (Zakikhani, Dowling, Fantus, Sonenberg, & Pollak, 2006). Metformin has also been reported to inhibit cell proliferation more potently than rapamycin, most likely due to its AMPK-mediated negative phosphorylation of IRS1 at Ser^{789} which attenuates AKT Ser^{473} phosphorylation, reducing downstream mitogenic signals via mTOR (Zakikhani, Blouin, Piura, & Pollak, 2010). Epidemiological studies on the effects of metformin in tumor development in type 2 diabetes are numerous and have been subject to a recent meta-analysis which reports a 30% decrease in cancer incidence in patients with type 2 diabetes using metformin compared with other diabetic therapies (DeCensi et al., 2010). Recently, mortality from overall cancer was also found to be reduced in type 2 diabetics receiving metformin treatment (Bo et al., 2012). For breast cancer, specifically, two studies have recently reported a reduction in breast cancer incidence for type 2 diabetic women using metformin compared to those not using metformin (Bodmer et al.,

2010). One study, however, has shown no effect of metformin on breast cancer incidence (Currie, 2009) and another has highlighted that type 2 diabetic patients receiving metformin alone were more likely to exhibit a shift to a PR-positive subtype of breast cancer, a phenomenon which was not observed in women receiving sulfonylureas or sulfonylureas in addition to insulin (Berstein, Boyarkina, Tsyrlina, Turkevich, & Semiglazov, 2011). However, another study on postmenopausal participants of the Women's Health Initiative Trial which followed 68,000 women for almost 12 years has just reported that use of metformin was associated with breast tumors which were more likely to express Her2 and also less likely to be both ER and PR positive. Overall, lower incidence of invasive breast cancer was found in diabetic users of metformin compared to women without type 2 diabetes. Type 2 diabetic women who received other antidiabetic therapies had a small increased risk of breast cancer when compared to women without type 2 diabetes (Chlebowski et al., 2012).

Thiazolidinediones (TZDs) are another type of insulin-sensitizing drug which act by binding peroxisome proliferator-activator nuclear receptor (PPAR)-γ, a transcription factor which is abundant in adipose cells. Activation of (PPAR)-γ allows its interaction with peroxisome proliferator response elements that are present on the promoters of (PPAR)-γ target genes, thus stimulating their transcription (Straus & Glass, 2007). Genes controlled by (PPAR)-γ are physiologically important for adipogenesis, adipose differentiation, and lipogenesis (Cariou, Charbonnel, & Staels, 2012). Activation of (PPAR)-γ by TZDs in insulin-resistant mouse models was found to decrease systemic hyperglycemia and hyperinsulinemia while improving insulin sensitivity in the liver, skeletal muscle, and adipose tissue (Fujita et al., 1983; Fujiwara, Yoshioka, Yoshioka, Ushiyama, & Horikoshi, 1988). Similarly, in humans, TZDs have been reported to improve whole-body insulin sensitivity (Miyazaki et al., 2002; Tiikkainen et al., 2004), decrease liver fat (Juurinen, Kotronen, Graner, & Yki-Jarvinen, 2008; Tiikkainen et al., 2004), lower fasting-free fatty acid concentrations (Juurinen et al., 2008; Miyazaki et al., 2002), and decrease hepatic glucose production (Phielix, Szendroedi, & Roden, 2011). A limited number of preclinical studies have assessed the proliferative effect of TZDs on breast cancer cell proliferation. Troglitazone inhibited the proliferation of breast cancer cell line MCF7 as well as the growth of breast cancer cell lines derived from human tissue. Additionally, growth of MCF7 tumors was delayed by troglitazone in immunodeficient mice (Elstner et al., 1998). Conflicting studies, however, have reported that mammary tumors grew more rapidly in mice receiving

TZD treatment (Saez et al., 2004). Clinical trials specifically investigating the relationship between breast cancer incidence and TZD usage in type 2 diabetics are also sparse. The Prospective Pioglitazone Clinical Trial in Macrovascular Events (PROACTIVE) trial reported that pioglitazone resulted in reduced breast cancer incidence, but this reduction failed to reach significance (Dormandy et al., 2005). A more recent trial has implicated that TZDs in tandem with metformin have improved the outcome of Her2-positive breast cancer specifically, although the effects of TZDs alone on this type of breast cancer as well as other subtypes are still to be determined (He et al., 2012). The PROACTIVE trial and subsequently a study conducted in the Kaiser Permanente Northern California reported increased rates of bladder cancer in those taking pioglitazone (Dormandy et al., 2005; Lewis et al., 2011). This increased risk appears to increase with duration of treatment; however, whether it is an effect that is common to all TZDs remains unclear (Colmers, Bowker, Majumdar, & Johnson, 2012; Mamtani et al., 2012).

6. CONCLUSIONS AND FUTURE DIRECTIONS

Insulin, IGF-I, cholesterol, their receptors, signaling pathways, and interactions with other hormones such as estrogens and androgens appear to play important roles in the development and growth of many cancers. These pathways likely explain part of the increased risk of cancer seen in individuals with diabetes, obesity, and the metabolic syndrome; however, other factors including adipokines, cytokines, and inflammatory cells are also known to interact with these pathways. Understanding how these factors increase cancer risk is essential to understand why these individuals are at greater risk of mortality, resistance to treatment, and cancer recurrence. Additionally, a greater understanding is necessary for the development of targeted therapies in individuals who develop cancer in association with diabetes and obesity.

REFERENCES

Accili, D., Drago, J., Lee, E. J., Johnson, M. D., Cool, M. H., Salvatore, P., et al. (1996). Early neonatal death in mice homozygous for a null allele of the insulin receptor gene. *Nature Genetics*, *12*, 106–109.

Agarwal, V. R., Bulun, S. E., Leitch, M., Rohrich, R., & Simpson, E. R. (1996). Use of alternative promoters to express the aromatase cytochrome P450 (CYP19) gene in breast adipose tissues of cancer-free and breast cancer patients. *The Journal of Clinical Endocrinology and Metabolism*, *81*, 3843–3849.

Alessi, D. R., James, S. R., Downes, C. P., Holmes, A. B., Gaffney, P. R., Reese, C. B., et al. (1997). Characterization of a 3-phosphoinositide-dependent protein kinase which phosphorylates and activates protein kinase Balpha. *Current Biology, 7*, 261–269.

Alikhani, N., Ferguson, R. D., Novosyadlyy, R., Gallagher, E. J., Scheinman, E. J., Yakar, S., et al. (2013). Mammary tumor growth and pulmonary metastasis are enhanced in a hyperlipidemic mouse model. *Oncogene, 32*, 961–967.

Alimova, I. N., Liu, B. L., Fan, Z. Y., Edgerton, S. M., Dillon, T., Lind, S. E., et al. (2009). Metformin inhibits breast cancer cell growth, colony formation and induces cell cycle arrest in vitro. *Cell Cycle, 8*, 909–915.

Ariazi, E. A., Leitao, A., Oprea, T. I., Chen, B., Louis, T., Bertucci, A. M., et al. (2007). Exemestane's 17-hydroxylated metabolite exerts biological effects as an androgen. *Molecular Cancer Therapeutics, 6*, 2817–2827.

Ashcroft, F. M., & Rorsman, P. (1989). Electrophysiology of the pancreatic beta-cell. *Progress in Biophysics and Molecular Biology, 54*, 87–143.

Baigent, C., Keech, A., Kearney, P. M., Blackwell, L., Buck, G., Pollicino, C., et al. (2005). Efficacy and safety of cholesterol-lowering treatment: Prospective meta-analysis of data from 90,056 participants in 14 randomised trials of statins. *The Lancet, 366*, 1267–1278.

Bailyes, E. M., Nave, B. T., Soos, M. A., Orr, S. R., Hayward, A. C., & Siddle, K. (1997). Insulin receptor/IGF-I receptor hybrids are widely distributed in mammalian tissues: Quantification of individual receptor species by selective immunoprecipitation and immunoblotting. *The Biochemical Journal, 327*(Pt 1), 209–215.

Bartella, V., De Marco, P., Malaguarnera, R., Belfiore, A., & Maggiolini, M. (2012). New advances on the functional cross-talk between insulin-like growth factor-I and estrogen signaling in cancer. *Cellular Signalling, 24*, 1515–1521.

Batty, G. D., Kivimaki, M., Clarke, R., Davey Smith, G., & Shipley, M. J. (2011). Modifiable risk factors for prostate cancer mortality in London: Forty years of follow-up in the Whitehall study. *Cancer Causes & Control, 22*, 311–318.

Benecke, H., Flier, J. S., & Moller, D. E. (1992). Alternatively spliced variants of the insulin receptor protein. Expression in normal and diabetic human tissues. *The Journal of Clinical Investigation, 89*, 2066–2070.

Benyoucef, S., Surinya, K. H., Hadaschik, D., & Siddle, K. (2007). Characterization of insulin/IGF hybrid receptors: Contributions of the insulin receptor L2 and Fn1 domains and the alternatively spliced exon 11 sequence to ligand binding and receptor activation. *The Biochemical Journal, 403*, 603–613.

Berggreen, C., Gormand, A., Omar, B., Degerman, E., & Goransson, O. (2009). Protein kinase B activity is required for the effects of insulin on lipid metabolism in adipocytes. *American Journal of Physiology. Endocrinology and Metabolism, 296*, E635–E646.

Bergstrom, A., Pisani, P., Tenet, V., Wolk, A., & Adami, H. O. (2001). Overweight as an avoidable cause of cancer in Europe. *International Journal of Cancer, 91*, 421–430.

Berstein, L. M., Boyarkina, M. P., Tsyrlina, E. V., Turkevich, E. A., & Semiglazov, V. F. (2011). More favorable progesterone receptor phenotype of breast cancer in diabetics treated with metformin. *Medical Oncology, 28*, 1260–1263.

Bielecka-Dabrowa, A., Hannam, S., Rysz, J., & Banach, M. (2011). Malignancy-associated dyslipidemia. *The Open Cardiovascular Medicine Journal, 5*, 35–40.

Bikman, B. T., Zheng, D., Kane, D. A., Anderson, E. J., Woodlief, T. L., Price, J. W., et al. (2010). Metformin improves insulin signaling in obese rats via reduced IKKbeta action in a fiber-type specific manner. *Journal of Obesity, 2010*, 1–8.

Bo, S., Ciccone, G., Rosato, R., Villois, P., Appendino, G., Ghigo, E., et al. (2012). Cancer mortality reduction and metformin: A retrospective cohort study in type 2 diabetic patients. *Diabetes, Obesity & Metabolism, 14*, 23–29.

Bodmer, M., Meier, C., Krahenbuhl, S., Jick, S. S., & Meier, C. R. (2010). Long-term metformin use is associated with decreased risk of breast cancer. *Diabetes Care, 33*, 1304–1308.

Bonovas, S., Filioussi, K., & Sitaras, N. M. (2008). Statin use and the risk of prostate cancer: A metaanalysis of 6 randomized clinical trials and 13 observational studies. *International Journal of Cancer, 123*, 899–904.

Bosetti, C., Rosato, V., Polesel, J., Levi, F., Talamini, R., Montella, M., et al. (2012). Diabetes mellitus and cancer risk in a network of case–control studies. *Nutrition and Cancer, 64*, 643–651.

Bowker, S. L., Majumdar, S. R., Veugelers, P., & Johnson, J. A. (2006). Increased cancer-related mortality for patients with type 2 diabetes who use sulfonylureas or insulin. *Diabetes Care, 29*, 254–258.

Bowker, S. L., Richardson, K., Marra, C. A., & Johnson, J. A. (2011). Risk of breast cancer after onset of type 2 diabetes: Evidence of detection bias in postmenopausal women. *Diabetes Care, 34*, 2542–2544.

Broitman, S. A., Cerda, S., & Wilkinson, J. T. (1993). Cholesterol metabolism and colon cancer. *Progress in Food & Nutrition Science, 17*, 1–40.

Brown, K. A., Hunger, N. I., Docanto, M., & Simpson, E. R. (2010). Metformin inhibits aromatase expression in human breast adipose stromal cells via stimulation of AMP-activated protein kinase. *Breast Cancer Research and Treatment, 123*, 591–596.

Brown, K. A., McInnes, K. J., Hunger, N. I., Oakhill, J. S., Steinberg, G. R., & Simpson, E. R. (2009). Subcellular localization of cyclic AMP-responsive element binding protein-regulated transcription coactivator 2 provides a link between obesity and breast cancer in postmenopausal women. *Cancer Research, 69*, 5392–5399.

Browning, D. R., & Martin, R. M. (2007). Statins and risk of cancer: A systematic review and metaanalysis. *International Journal of Cancer, 120*, 833–843.

Byrnes, K., White, S., Chu, Q., Meschonat, C., Yu, H., Johnson, L. W., et al. (2006). High eIF4E, VEGF, and microvessel density in stage I to III breast cancer. *Annals of Surgery, 243*, 684–690 (discussion 691–692).

Calle, E. E., & Kaaks, R. (2004). Overweight, obesity and cancer: Epidemiological evidence and proposed mechanisms. *Nature Reviews. Cancer, 4*, 579–591.

Cariou, B., Charbonnel, B., & Staels, B. (2012). Thiazolidinediones and PPAR gamma agonists: Time for a reassessment. *Trends in Endocrinology and Metabolism, 23*, 205–215.

Carstensen, B., Witte, D. R., & Friis, S. (2012). Cancer occurrence in Danish diabetic patients: Duration and insulin effects. *Diabetologia, 55*, 948–958.

Caruso, M. G., Notarnicola, M., Cavallini, A., & Di Leo, A. (2002). 3-Hydroxy-3-methylglutaryl coenzyme A reductase activity and low-density lipoprotein receptor expression in diffuse-type and intestinal-type human gastric cancer. *Journal of Gastroenterology, 37*, 504–508.

Caruso, M. G., Notarnicola, M., Santillo, M., Cavallini, A., & Di Leo, A. (1999). Enhanced 3-hydroxy-3-methyl-glutaryl coenzyme A reductase activity in human colorectal cancer not expressing low density lipoprotein receptor. *Anticancer Research, 19*, 451–454.

Casa, A. J., Potter, A. S., Malik, S., Lazard, Z., Kuiatse, I., Kim, H. T., et al. (2012). Estrogen and insulin-like growth factor-I (IGF-I) independently down-regulate critical repressors of breast cancer growth. *Breast Cancer Research and Treatment, 132*, 61–73.

Caton, P. W., Nayuni, N. K., Kieswich, J., Khan, N. Q., Yaqoob, M. M., & Corder, R. (2010). Metformin suppresses hepatic gluconeogenesis through induction of SIRT1 and GCN5. *The Journal of Endocrinology, 205*, 97–106.

Chapman, H. A., Jr., & Hibbs, J. B., Jr. (1977). Modulation of macrophage tumoricidal capability by components of normal serum: A central role for lipid. *Science, 197*, 282–285.

Chen, W. W., Shao, Y. Y., Shau, W. Y., Lin, Z. Z., Lu, Y. S., Chen, H. M., et al. (2012). The impact of diabetes mellitus on prognosis of early breast cancer in Asia. *The Oncologist, 17*, 485–491.

Chlebowski, R. T., McTiernan, A., Wactawski-Wende, J., Manson, J. E., Aragaki, A. K., Rohan, T., et al. (2012). Diabetes, metformin, and breast cancer in postmenopausal women. *Journal of Clinical Oncology, 30*, 2844–2852.

Chong, Y. M., Williams, S. L., Elkak, A., Sharma, A. K., & Mokbel, K. (2006). Insulin-like growth factor 1 (IGF-1) and its receptor mRNA levels in breast cancer and adjacent nonneoplastic tissue. *Anticancer Research, 26,* 167–173.

Cleveland, R. J., North, K. E., Stevens, J., Teitelbaum, S. L., Neugut, A. I., & Gammon, M. D. (2012). The association of diabetes with breast cancer incidence and mortality in the Long Island Breast Cancer Study Project. *Cancer Causes & Control, 23,* 1193–1203.

Colhoun, H. M., & Group, S. E. (2009). Use of insulin glargine and cancer incidence in Scotland: A study from the Scottish Diabetes Research Network Epidemiology Group. *Diabetologia, 52,* 1755–1765.

Colmers, I. N., Bowker, S. L., Majumdar, S. R., & Johnson, J. A. (2012). Use of thiazolidinediones and the risk of bladder cancer among people with type 2 diabetes: A meta-analysis. *CMAJ, 184,* E675–E683.

Cruse, J. P., Lewin, M. R., & Clark, C. G. (1982). Dietary cholesterol deprivation improves survival and reduces incidence of metastatic colon cancer in dimethylhydrazine-pretreated rats. *Gut, 23,* 594–599.

Cui, X., Zhang, P., Deng, W., Oesterreich, S., Lu, Y., Mills, G. B., et al. (2003). Insulin-like growth factor-I inhibits progesterone receptor expression in breast cancer cells via the phosphatidylinositol 3-kinase/Akt/mammalian target of rapamycin pathway: Progesterone receptor as a potential indicator of growth factor activity in breast cancer. *Molecular Endocrinology, 17,* 575–588.

Currie, C. J. (2009). The longest ever randomised controlled trial of insulin glargine: Study design and HbA(1c) findings. *Diabetologia, 52,* 2234–2235 (author reply 2236–2239).

Currie, C. J., Poole, C. D., & Gale, E. A. M. (2009). The influence of glucose-lowering therapies on cancer risk in type 2 diabetes. *Diabetologia, 52,* 1766–1777.

Dale, K. M., Coleman, C. I., Henyan, N. N., Kluger, J., & White, C. M. (2006). Statins and cancer risk: A meta-analysis. *JAMA: The Journal of the American Medical Association, 295,* 74–80.

Daniels, S. R., & Greer, F. R. (2008). Lipid screening and cardiovascular health in childhood. *Pediatrics, 122,* 198–208.

DeCensi, A., Puntoni, M., Goodwin, P., Cazzaniga, M., Gennari, A., Bonanni, B., et al. (2010). Metformin and cancer risk in diabetic patients: A systematic review and meta-analysis. *Cancer Prevention Research (Philadelphia, PA), 3,* 1451–1461.

Dessi, S., Batetta, B., Anchisi, C., Pani, P., Costelli, P., Tessitore, L., et al. (1992). Cholesterol metabolism during the growth of a rat ascites hepatoma (Yoshida AH-130). *British Journal of Cancer, 66,* 787–793.

Dessi, S., Batetta, B., Pulisci, D., Spano, O., Anchisi, C., Tessitore, L., et al. (1994). Cholesterol content in tumor tissues is inversely associated with high-density lipoprotein cholesterol in serum in patients with gastrointestinal cancer. *Cancer, 73,* 253–258.

Dessi, S., Batetta, B., Pulisci, D., Spano, O., Cherchi, R., Lanfranco, G., et al. (1992). Altered pattern of lipid metabolism in patients with lung cancer. *Oncology, 49,* 436–441.

Di Cristofano, A., & Pandolfi, P. P. (2000). The multiple roles of PTEN in tumor suppression. *Cell, 100,* 387–390.

Di Vizio, D., Solomon, K. R., & Freeman, M. R. (2008). Cholesterol and cholesterol-rich membranes in prostate cancer: An update. *Tumori, 94,* 633–639.

Dormandy, J. A., Charbonnel, B., Eckland, D. J., Erdmann, E., Massi-Benedetti, M., Moules, I. K., et al. (2005). Secondary prevention of macrovascular events in patients with type 2 diabetes in the PROactive Study (PROspective pioglitAzone Clinical Trial In macroVascular Events): A randomised controlled trial. *Lancet, 366,* 1279–1289.

Dowling, R. J. O., Zakikhani, M., Fantus, I. G., Pollak, M., & Sonenberg, N. (2007). Metformin inhibits mammalian target of rapamycin-dependent translation initiation in breast cancer cells. *Cancer Research, 67,* 10804–10812.

Drury, S. C., Detre, S., Leary, A., Salter, J., Reis-Filho, J., Barbashina, V., et al. (2011). Changes in breast cancer biomarkers in the IGF1R/PI3K pathway in recurrent breast cancer after tamoxifen treatment. *Endocrine-Related Cancer, 18*, 565–577.

Duggan, C., Irwin, M. L., Xiao, L., Henderson, K. D., Smith, A. W., Baumgartner, R. N., et al. (2011). Associations of insulin resistance and adiponectin with mortality in women with breast cancer. *Journal of Clinical Oncology, 29*, 32–39.

Edgerton, D. S., Johnson, K. M. S., & Cherrington, A. D. (2009). Current strategies for the inhibition of hepatic glucose production in type 2 diabetes. *Frontiers in Bioscience, 14*, 1169–1181.

Elstner, E., Muller, C., Koshizuka, K., Williamson, E. A., Park, D., Asou, H., et al. (1998). Ligands for peroxisome proliferator-activated receptorgamma and retinoic acid receptor inhibit growth and induce apoptosis of human breast cancer cells in vitro and in BNX mice. *Proceedings of the National Academy of Sciences of the United States of America, 95*, 8806–8811.

Espelund, U., Cold, S., Frystyk, J., Orskov, H., & Flyvbjerg, A. (2008). Elevated free IGF2 levels in localized, early-stage breast cancer in women. *European Journal of Endocrinology, 159*, 595–601.

Evans, J. M., Donnelly, L. A., Emslie-Smith, A. M., Alessi, D. R., & Morris, A. D. (2005). Metformin and reduced risk of cancer in diabetic patients. *BMJ, 330*, 1304–1305.

Fagan, D. H., Uselman, R. R., Sachdev, D., & Yee, D. (2012). Acquired resistance to tamoxifen is associated with loss of the type I insulin-like growth factor receptor: Implications for breast cancer treatment. *Cancer Research, 72*, 3372–3380.

Fagan, D. H., & Yee, D. (2008). Crosstalk between IGF1R and estrogen receptor signaling in breast cancer. *Journal of Mammary Gland Biology and Neoplasia, 13*, 423–429.

Ferguson, R. D., Novosyadlyy, R., Fierz, Y., Alikhani, N., Sun, H., Yakar, S., et al. (2012). Hyperinsulinemia enhances c-Myc-mediated mammary tumor development and advances metastatic progression to the lung in a mouse model of type 2 diabetes. *Breast Cancer Research, 14*, R8.

Fernandez, A. M., Kim, J. K., Yakar, S., Dupont, J., Hernandez-Sanchez, C., Castle, A. L., et al. (2001). Functional inactivation of the IGF-I and insulin receptors in skeletal muscle causes type 2 diabetes. *Genes & Development, 15*, 1926–1934.

Fierz, Y., Novosyadlyy, R., Vijayakumar, A., Yakar, S., & LeRoith, D. (2010). Insulin-sensitizing therapy attenuates type 2 diabetes-mediated mammary tumor progression. *Diabetes, 59*, 686–693.

Fisher, P. B., Goldstein, N. I., Bonner, D. P., Mechlinski, W., Bryson, V., & Schaffner, C. P. (1975). Toxicity of amphotericin B and its methyl ester toward normal and tumor cell lines. *Cancer Research, 35*, 1996–1999.

Flick, E. D., Habel, L. A., Chan, K. A., Van Den Eeden, S. K., Quinn, V. P., Haque, R., et al. (2007). Statin use and risk of prostate cancer in the California Men's Health Study cohort. *Cancer Epidemiology, Biomarkers & Prevention: A Publication of the American Association for Cancer Research, Cosponsored by the American Society of Preventive Oncology, 16*, 2218–2225.

Formica, V., Tesauro, M., Cardillo, C., & Roselli, M. (2012). Insulinemia and the risk of breast cancer and its relapse. *Diabetes, Obesity & Metabolism*.

Frasca, F., Pandini, G., Scalia, P., Sciacca, L., Mineo, R., Costantino, A., et al. (1999). Insulin receptor isoform A, a newly recognized, high-affinity insulin-like growth factor II receptor in fetal and cancer cells. *Molecular and Cellular Biology, 19*, 3278–3288.

Freeman, M. R., & Solomon, K. R. (2004). Cholesterol and prostate cancer. *Journal of Cellular Biochemistry, 91*, 54–69.

Freeman, M. R., Solomon, K. R., & Moyad, M. (2006). Statins and the risk of cancer. *JAMA: The Journal of the American Medical Association, 295*, 2720–2721 (author reply 2721–2722).

Frittitta, L., Cerrato, A., Sacco, M. G., Weidner, N., Goldfine, I. D., & Vigneri, R. (1997). The insulin receptor content is increased in breast cancers initiated by three different oncogenes in transgenic mice. *Breast Cancer Research and Treatment, 45,* 141–147.

Frittitta, L., Vigneri, R., Papa, V., Goldfine, I. D., Grasso, G., & Trischitta, V. (1993). Structural and functional studies of insulin receptors in human breast cancer. *Breast Cancer Research and Treatment, 25,* 73–82.

Fujita, T., Sugiyama, Y., Taketomi, S., Sohda, T., Kawamatsu, Y., Iwatsuka, H., et al. (1983). Reduction of insulin resistance in obese and/or diabetic animals by 5-[4-(1-methylcyclohexylmethoxy)benzyl]-thiazolidine-2,4-dione (ADD-3878, U-63,287, ciglitazone), a new antidiabetic agent. *Diabetes, 32,* 804–810.

Fujiwara, T., Yoshioka, S., Yoshioka, T., Ushiyama, I., & Horikoshi, H. (1988). Characterization of new oral antidiabetic agent CS-045. Studies in KK and ob/ob mice and Zucker fatty rats. *Diabetes, 37,* 1549–1558.

Furberg, A. S., Jasienska, G., Bjurstam, N., Torjesen, P. A., Emaus, A., Lipson, S. F., et al. (2005). Metabolic and hormonal profiles: HDL cholesterol as a plausible biomarker of breast cancer risk. The Norwegian EBBA Study. *Cancer Epidemiology, Biomarkers & Prevention, 14,* 33–40.

Furberg, A. S., Veierod, M. B., Wilsgaard, T., Bernstein, L., & Thune, I. (2004). Serum high-density lipoprotein cholesterol, metabolic profile, and breast cancer risk. *Journal of the National Cancer Institute, 96,* 1152–1160.

Gal, D., MacDonald, P. C., Porter, J. C., & Simpson, E. R. (1981). Cholesterol metabolism in cancer cells in monolayer culture. III. Low-density lipoprotein metabolism. *International Journal of Cancer, 28,* 315–319.

Gao, J., Chesebrough, J. W., Cartlidge, S. A., Ricketts, S. A., Incognito, L., Veldman-Jones, M., et al. (2011). Dual IGF-I/II-neutralizing antibody MEDI-573 potently inhibits IGF signaling and tumor growth. *Cancer Research, 71,* 1029–1040.

Garcia-Arencibia, M., Molero, S., Davila, N., Carranza, M. C., & Calle, C. (2005). 17beta-Estradiol transcriptionally represses human insulin receptor gene expression causing cellular insulin resistance. *Leukemia Research, 29,* 79–87.

Germershausen, J. I., Hunt, V. M., Bostedor, R. G., Bailey, P. J., Karkas, J. D., & Alberts, A. W. (1989). Tissue selectivity of the cholesterol-lowering agents lovastatin, simvastatin and pravastatin in rats in vivo. *Biochemical and Biophysical Research Communications, 158,* 667–675.

Gerstein, H. C., Bosch, J., Dagenais, G. R., Diaz, R., Jung, H., Maggioni, A. P., et al. (2012). Basal insulin and cardiovascular and other outcomes in dysglycemia. *The New England Journal of Medicine, 367,* 319–328.

Giani, C., Campani, D., Rasmussen, A., Fierabracci, P., Miccoli, P., Bevilacqua, G., et al. (2002). Insulin-like growth factor II (IGF-II) immunohistochemistry in breast cancer: Relationship with the most important morphological and biochemical prognostic parameters. *The International Journal of Biological Markers, 17,* 90–95.

Giani, C., Cullen, K. J., Campani, D., & Rasmussen, A. (1996). IGF-II mRNA and protein are expressed in the stroma of invasive breast cancers: An in situ hybridization and immunohistochemistry study. *Breast Cancer Research and Treatment, 41,* 43–50.

Gingras, A. C., Raught, B., & Sonenberg, N. (2001). Regulation of translation initiation by FRAP/mTOR. *Genes & Development, 15,* 807–826.

Giudice, J., Leskow, F. C., Arndt-Jovin, D. J., Jovin, T. M., & Jares-Erijman, E. A. (2011). Differential endocytosis and signaling dynamics of insulin receptor variants IR-A and IR-B. *Journal of Cell Science, 124,* 801–811.

Glidden, E. J., Gray, L. G., Vemuru, S., Li, D., Harris, T. E., & Mayo, M. W. (2012). Multiple site acetylation of Rictor stimulates mammalian target of rapamycin complex 2 (mTORC2)-dependent phosphorylation of Akt protein. *The Journal of Biological Chemistry, 287,* 581–588.

Goetsch, L., Gonzalez, A., Leger, O., Beck, A., Pauwels, P. J., Haeuw, J. F., et al. (2005). A recombinant humanized anti-insulin-like growth factor receptor type I antibody (h7C10) enhances the antitumor activity of vinorelbine and anti-epidermal growth factor receptor therapy against human cancer xenografts. *International Journal of Cancer, 113*, 316–328.

Gonzalez, E., & McGraw, T. E. (2009). The Akt kinases: Isoform specificity in metabolism and cancer. *Cell Cycle, 8*, 2502–2508.

Goodwin, P. J., Ennis, M., Pritchard, K. I., Trudeau, M. E., Koo, J., Madarnas, Y., et al. (2002). Fasting insulin and outcome in early-stage breast cancer: Results of a prospective cohort study. *Journal of Clinical Oncology, 20*, 42–51.

Goodwin, P. J., Ennis, M., Pritchard, K. I., Trudeau, M. E., Koo, J., Taylor, S. K., et al. (2012). Insulin- and obesity-related variables in early-stage breast cancer: Correlations and time course of prognostic associations. *Journal of Clinical Oncology, 30*, 164–171.

Gordon, H. W., & Schaffner, C. P. (1968). The effect of polyene macrolides on the prostate gland and canine prostatic hyperplasia. *Proceedings of the National Academy of Sciences of the United States of America, 60*, 1201–1208.

Graaf, M. R., Beiderbeck, A. B., Egberts, A. C., Richel, D. J., & Guchelaar, H. J. (2004). The risk of cancer in users of statins. *Journal of Clinical Oncology: Official Journal of the American Society of Clinical Oncology, 22*, 2388–2394.

Graziani, S. R., Igreja, F. A., Hegg, R., Meneghetti, C., Brandizzi, L. I., Barboza, R., et al. (2002). Uptake of a cholesterol-rich emulsion by breast cancer. *Gynecologic Oncology, 85*, 493–497.

Gunter, M. J., Hoover, D. R., Yu, H., Wassertheil-Smoller, S., Rohan, T. E., Manson, J. E., et al. (2009). Insulin, insulin-like growth factor-I, and risk of breast cancer in postmenopausal women. *Journal of the National Cancer Institute, 101*, 48–60.

Hankinson, S. E., & Hunter, D. J. (2002). Breast cancer. In H. O. Adami, D. Hunter, & D. Trichopoulos (Eds.), *Textbook of cancer epidemiology* (pp. 301–339). New York, NY: Oxford University Press.

Harrington, S. C., Weroha, S. J., Reynolds, C., Suman, V. J., Lingle, W. L., & Haluska, P. (2012). Quantifying insulin receptor isoform expression in FFPE breast tumors. *Growth Hormone & IGF Research, 22*, 108–115.

Haruta, T., Uno, T., Kawahara, J., Takano, A., Egawa, K., Sharma, P. M., et al. (2000). A rapamycin-sensitive pathway down-regulates insulin signaling via phosphorylation and proteasomal degradation of insulin receptor substrate-1. *Molecular Endocrinology, 14*, 783–794.

Hay, N., & Sonenberg, N. (2004). Upstream and downstream of mTOR. *Genes & Development, 18*, 1926–1945.

He, X., Esteva, F. J., Ensor, J., Hortobagyi, G. N., Lee, M. H., & Yeung, S. C. (2012). Metformin and thiazolidinediones are associated with improved breast cancer-specific survival of diabetic women with HER2+ breast cancer. *Annals of Oncology, 23*, 1771–1780.

He, L., Sabet, A., Djedjos, S., Miller, R., Sun, X., Hussain, M. A., et al. (2009). Metformin and insulin suppress hepatic gluconeogenesis through phosphorylation of CREB binding protein. *Cell, 137*, 635–646.

Heemers, H., Maes, B., Foufelle, F., Heyns, W., Verhoeven, G., & Swinnen, J. V. (2001). Androgens stimulate lipogenic gene expression in prostate cancer cells by activation of the sterol regulatory element-binding protein cleavage activating protein/sterol regulatory element-binding protein pathway. *Molecular Endocrinology, 15*, 1817–1828.

Hemkens, L. G., Bender, R., Grouven, U., & Sawicki, P. T. (2009). Insulin glargine and cancer. *Lancet, 374*, 1743–1744 (author reply 1/44).

Hemkens, L. G., Grouven, U., Bender, R., Gunster, C., Gutschmidt, S., Selke, G. W., et al. (2009). Risk of malignancies in patients with diabetes treated with human insulin or insulin analogues: A cohort study. *Diabetologia, 52*, 1732–1744.

Hendrickson, A. W., & Haluska, P. (2009). Resistance pathways relevant to insulin-like growth factor-1 receptor-targeted therapy. *Current Opinion in Investigational Drugs, 10*, 1032–1040.

Henriksson, P., Eriksson, M., Ericsson, S., Rudling, M., Stege, R., Berglund, L., et al. (1989). Hypocholesterolaemia and increased elimination of low-density lipoproteins in metastatic cancer of the prostate. *Lancet, 2*, 1178–1180.

Hou, Z., He, L., & Qi, R. Z. (2007). Regulation of s6 kinase 1 activation by phosphorylation at ser-411. *The Journal of Biological Chemistry, 282*, 6922–6928.

Huang, J., Morehouse, C., Streicher, K., Higgs, B. W., Gao, J., Czapiga, M., et al. (2011). Altered expression of insulin receptor isoforms in breast cancer. *PLoS One, 6*, e26177.

Hudson, C. C., Liu, M., Chiang, G. G., Otterness, D. M., Loomis, D. C., Kaper, F., et al. (2002). Regulation of hypoxia-inducible factor 1alpha expression and function by the mammalian target of rapamycin. *Molecular and Cellular Biology, 22*, 7004–7014.

Hundal, R. S., Krssak, M., Dufour, S., Laurent, D., Lebon, V., Chandramouli, V., et al. (2000). Mechanism by which metformin reduces glucose production in type 2 diabetes. *Diabetes, 49*, 2063–2069.

Huxley, R. (2007). The impact of modifiable risk factors on mortality from prostate cancer in populations of the Asia-Pacific region. *Asian Pacific Journal of Cancer Prevention, 8*, 199–205.

Irwin, M. L., Duggan, C., Wang, C. Y., Smith, A. W., McTiernan, A., Baumgartner, R. N., et al. (2011). Fasting C-peptide levels and death resulting from all causes and breast cancer: The health, eating, activity, and lifestyle study. *Journal of Clinical Oncology, 29*, 47–53.

Jonasson, J. M., Ljung, R., Talback, M., Haglund, B., Gudbjornsdottir, S., & Steineck, G. (2009). Insulin glargine use and short-term incidence of malignancies-a population-based follow-up study in Sweden. *Diabetologia, 52*, 1745–1754.

Jones, B. A., Kasl, S. V., Howe, C. L., Lachman, M., Dubrow, R., Curnen, M. M., et al. (2004). African-American/White differences in breast carcinoma: p53 alterations and other tumor characteristics. *Cancer, 101*, 1293–1301.

Juurinen, L., Kotronen, A., Graner, M., & Yki-Jarvinen, H. (2008). Rosiglitazone reduces liver fat and insulin requirements and improves hepatic insulin sensitivity and glycemic control in patients with type 2 diabetes requiring high insulin doses. *The Journal of Clinical Endocrinology and Metabolism, 93*, 118–124.

Kalla Singh, S., Brito, C., Tan, Q. W., De Leon, M., & De Leon, D. (2011). Differential expression and signaling activation of insulin receptor isoforms A and B: A link between breast cancer and diabetes. *Growth Factors, 29*, 278–289.

Kaplan, S. A. (1984). The insulin receptor. *The Journal of Pediatrics, 104*, 327–336.

Kaplan, M. A., Pekkolay, Z., Kucukoner, M., Inal, A., Urakci, Z., Ertugrul, H., et al. (2012). Type 2 diabetes mellitus and prognosis in early stage breast cancer women. *Medical Oncology, 29*, 1576–1580.

Kaulsay, K. K., Ng, E. H., Ji, C. Y., Ho, G. H., Aw, T. C., & Lee, K. O. (1999). Serum IGF-binding protein-6 and prostate specific antigen in breast cancer. *European Journal of Endocrinology, 140*, 164–168.

Kelly, M. J., & Levin, E. R. (2001). Rapid actions of plasma membrane estrogen receptors. *Trends in Endocrinology and Metabolism, 12*, 152–156.

Keshin, J. G. (1973). Effect of candicidin on the human benign hypertrophied prostate gland. *International Surgery, 58*, 116–122.

Key, T. J., Appleby, P. N., Reeves, G. K., Roddam, A., Dorgan, J. F., Longcope, C., et al. (2003). Body mass index, serum sex hormones, and breast cancer risk in postmenopausal women. *Journal of the National Cancer Institute, 95*, 1218–1226.

Keys, A., Aravanis, C., Blackburn, H., Buzina, R., Dontas, A. S., Fidanza, F., et al. (1985). Serum cholesterol and cancer mortality in the Seven Countries Study. *American Journal of Epidemiology, 121,* 870–883.

Kiely, P. A., O'Gorman, D., Luong, K., Ron, D., & O'Connor, R. (2006). Insulin-like growth factor I controls a mutually exclusive association of RACK1 with protein phosphatase 2A and beta1 integrin to promote cell migration. *Molecular and Cellular Biology, 26,* 4041–4051.

Kim, Y. D., Park, K. G., Lee, Y. S., Park, Y. Y., Kim, D. K., Nedumaran, B., et al. (2008). Metformin inhibits hepatic gluconeogenesis through AMP-activated protein kinase-dependent regulation of the orphan nuclear receptor SHP. *Diabetes, 57,* 306–314.

Kirschner, M. A., Schneider, G., Ertel, N. H., & Worton, E. (1982). Obesity, androgens, estrogens, and cancer risk. *Cancer Research, 42,* 3281s–3285s.

Kitamura, T., Kitamura, Y., Kuroda, S., Hino, Y., Ando, M., Kotani, K., et al. (1999). Insulin-induced phosphorylation and activation of cyclic nucleotide phosphodiesterase 3B by the serine-threonine kinase Akt. *Molecular and Cellular Biology, 19,* 6286–6296.

Koga, T., Shimada, Y., Kuroda, M., Tsujita, Y., Hasegawa, K., & Yamazaki, M. (1990). Tissue-selective inhibition of cholesterol synthesis in vivo by pravastatin sodium, a 3-hydroxy-3-methylglutaryl coenzyme A reductase inhibitor. *Biochimica et Biophysica Acta, 1045,* 115–120.

Kok, D. E., van Roermund, J. G., Aben, K. K., den Heijer, M., Swinkels, D. W., Kampman, E., et al. (2011). Blood lipid levels and prostate cancer risk; a cohort study. *Prostate Cancer and Prostatic Diseases, 14,* 340–345.

Kolanjiappan, K., Ramachandran, C. R., & Manoharan, S. (2003). Biochemical changes in tumor tissues of oral cancer patients. *Clinical Biochemistry, 36,* 61–65.

Koo, S. H., Flechner, L., Qi, L., Zhang, X., Screaton, R. A., Jeffries, S., et al. (2005). The CREB coactivator TORC2 is a key regulator of fasting glucose metabolism. *Nature, 437,* 1109–1111.

Kopelman, P. G., Pilkington, T. R., White, N., & Jeffcoate, S. L. (1980). Abnormal sex steroid secretion and binding in massively obese women. *Clinical Endocrinology, 12,* 363–369.

Kucharska-Newton, A. M., Rosamond, W. D., Mink, P. J., Alberg, A. J., Shahar, E., & Folsom, A. R. (2008). HDL-cholesterol and incidence of breast cancer in the ARIC cohort study. *Annals of Epidemiology, 18,* 671–677.

Landman, G. W., Kleefstra, N., van Hateren, K. J., Groenier, K. H., Gans, R. O., & Bilo, H. J. (2010). Metformin associated with lower cancer mortality in type 2 diabetes: ZODIAC-16. *Diabetes Care, 33,* 322–326.

Larsson, S. C., Mantzoros, C. S., & Wolk, A. (2007). Diabetes mellitus and risk of breast cancer: A meta-analysis. *International Journal of Cancer, 121,* 856–862.

Law, J. H., Habibi, G., Hu, K., Masoudi, H., Wang, M. Y., Stratford, A. L., et al. (2008). Phosphorylated insulin-like growth factor-I/insulin receptor is present in all breast cancer subtypes and is related to poor survival. *Cancer Research, 68,* 10238–10246.

Lawson, K. A., Anderson, K., Menchaca, M., Atkinson, J., Sun, L., Knight, V., et al. (2003). Novel vitamin E analogue decreases syngeneic mouse mammary tumor burden and reduces lung metastasis. *Molecular Cancer Therapeutics, 2,* 437–444.

Le, T. N., Nestler, J. E., Strauss, J. F., 3rd., & Wickham, E. P., 3rd. (2012). Sex hormone-binding globulin and type 2 diabetes mellitus. *Trends in Endocrinology and Metabolism, 23,* 32–40.

Lee, C. W., Hong, D. H., Han, S. B., Jung, S. H., Kim, H. C., Fine, R. L., et al. (2002). A novel stereo-selective sulfonylurea, 1-[1-(4-aminobenzoyl)-2,3-dihydro-1H indol-6-sulfonyl]-4-phenyl imidazolidin-2-on e, has antitumor efficacy in in vitro and in vivo tumor models. *Biochemical Pharmacology, 64,* 473–480.

Lee, A. V., Jackson, J. G., Gooch, J. L., Hilsenbeck, S. G., Coronado-Heinsohn, E., Osborne, C. K., et al. (1999). Enhancement of insulin-like growth factor signaling in human breast cancer: Estrogen regulation of insulin receptor substrate-1 expression in vitro and in vivo. *Molecular Endocrinology, 13*, 787–796.

Leung, Y. K., Lee, M. T., Lam, H. M., Tarapore, P., & Ho, S. M. (2012). Estrogen receptor-beta and breast cancer: Translating biology into clinical practice. *Steroids, 77*, 727–737.

Levine, A. J., & Puzio-Kuter, A. M. (2010). The control of the metabolic switch in cancers by oncogenes and tumor suppressor genes. *Science, 330*, 1340–1344.

Lewis, J. D., Ferrara, A., Peng, T., Hedderson, M., Bilker, W. B., Quesenberry, C. P., Jr., et al. (2011). Risk of bladder cancer among diabetic patients treated with pioglitazone: Interim report of a longitudinal cohort study. *Diabetes Care, 34*, 916–922.

Li, B. D., Liu, L., Dawson, M., & De Benedetti, A. (1997). Overexpression of eukaryotic initiation factor 4E (eIF4E) in breast carcinoma. *Cancer, 79*, 2385–2390.

Li, B. D., McDonald, J. C., Nassar, R., & De Benedetti, A. (1998). Clinical outcome in stage I to III breast carcinoma and eIF4E overexpression. *Annals of Surgery, 227*, 756–761 (discussion 761–763).

Li, X., Monks, B., Ge, Q., & Birnbaum, M. J. (2007). Akt/PKB regulates hepatic metabolism by directly inhibiting PGC-1alpha transcription coactivator. *Nature, 447*, 1012–1016.

Li, Y. C., Park, M. J., Ye, S. K., Kim, C. W., & Kim, Y. N. (2006). Elevated levels of cholesterol-rich lipid rafts in cancer cells are correlated with apoptosis sensitivity induced by cholesterol-depleting agents. *The American Journal of Pathology, 168*, 1107–1118 (quiz 1404–1405).

Lind, M., Fahlen, M., Eliasson, B., & Oden, A. (2012). The relationship between the exposure time of insulin glargine and risk of breast and prostate cancer: An observational study of the time-dependent effects of antidiabetic treatments in patients with diabetes. *Primary Care Diabetes, 6*, 53–59.

Lisztwan, J., Pornon, A., Chen, B., Chen, S., & Evans, D. B. (2008). The aromatase inhibitor letrozole and inhibitors of insulin-like growth factor I receptor synergistically induce apoptosis in in vitro models of estrogen-dependent breast cancer. *Breast Cancer Research, 10*, R56.

Liu, B. L., Fan, Z. Y., Edgerton, S. M., Deng, X. S., Alimova, I. N., Lind, S. E., et al. (2009). Metformin induces unique biological and molecular responses in triple negative breast cancer cells. *Cell Cycle, 8*, 2031–2040.

Liu, Y. L., Qian, H. X., Qin, L., Zhou, X. J., Zhang, B., & Chen, X. (2012). Association of serum lipid profile with distant metastasis in breast cancer patients. *Zhonghua Zhong Liu Za Zhi, 34*, 129–131.

Ljung, R., Talback, M., Haglund, B., Jonasson, J. M., Gudbjornsdottir, S., & Steineck, G. (2012). Insulin glargine use and short-term incidence of breast cancer—A four-year population-based observation. *Acta Oncologica, 51*, 400–402.

Lynch, L., Vodyanik, P. I., Boettiger, D., & Guvakova, M. A. (2005). Insulin-like growth factor I controls adhesion strength mediated by alpha5beta1 integrins in motile carcinoma cells. *Molecular Biology of the Cell, 16*, 51–63.

Maehama, T., & Dixon, J. E. (1998). The tumor suppressor, PTEN/MMAC1, dephosphorylates the lipid second messenger, phosphatidylinositol 3,4,5-trisphosphate. *The Journal of Biological Chemistry, 273*, 13375–13378.

Magura, L., Blanchard, R., Hope, B., Beal, J. R., Schwartz, G. G., & Sahmoun, A. E. (2008). Hypercholesterolemia and prostate cancer: A hospital-based case–control study. *Cancer Causes & Control, 19*, 1259–1266.

Mainous, A. G., 3rd., Wells, B. J., Koopman, R. J., Everett, C. J., & Gill, J. M. (2005). Iron, lipids, and risk of cancer in the Framingham Offspring cohort. *American Journal of Epidemiology, 161*, 1115–1122.

Malaguarnera, R., Sacco, A., Voci, C., Pandini, G., Vigneri, R., & Belfiore, A. (2012). Pro-insulin binds with high affinity the insulin receptor isoform A and predominantly activates the mitogenic pathway. *Endocrinology, 153,* 2152–2163.

Malik, S., Jiang, S., Garee, J. P., Verdin, E., Lee, A. V., O'Malley, B. W., et al. (2010). Histone deacetylase 7 and FoxA1 in estrogen-mediated repression of RPRM. *Molecular and Cellular Biology, 30,* 399–412.

Mamillapalli, R., Gavrilova, N., Mihaylova, V. T., Tsvetkov, L. M., Wu, H., Zhang, H., et al. (2001). PTEN regulates the ubiquitin-dependent degradation of the CDK inhibitor p27(KIP1) through the ubiquitin E3 ligase SCF(SKP2). *Current Biology, 11,* 263–267.

Mamtani, R., Haynes, K., Bilker, W. B., Vaughn, D. J., Strom, B. L., Glanz, K., et al. (2012). Association between longer therapy with thiazolidinediones and risk of bladder cancer: A cohort study. *Journal of the National Cancer Institute, 104,* 1411–1421.

Marshman, E., & Streuli, C. H. (2002). Insulin-like growth factors and insulin-like growth factor binding proteins in mammary gland function. *Breast Cancer Research, 4,* 231–239.

Mayer, D., & Chantelau, E. (2010). Treatment with insulin glargine (Lantus) increases the proliferative potency of the serum of patients with type-1 diabetes: A pilot study on MCF-7 breast cancer cells. *Archives of Physiology and Biochemistry, 116,* 73–78.

Mayer, D., Shukla, A., & Enzmann, H. (2008). Proliferative effects of insulin analogues on mammary epithelial cells. *Archives of Physiology and Biochemistry, 114,* 38–44.

McCann, A. H., Miller, N., O'Meara, A., Pedersen, I., Keogh, K., Gorey, T., et al. (1996). Biallelic expression of the IGF2 gene in human breast disease. *Human Molecular Genetics, 5,* 1123–1127.

McInnes, K. J., Brown, K. A., Hunger, N. I., & Simpson, E. R. (2011). Regulation of LKB1 expression by sex hormones in adipocytes. *International Journal of Obesity, 36,* 982–985.

Mehta, N., Hordines, J., Volpe, C., Doerr, R., & Cohen, S. A. (1997). Cellular effects of hypercholesterolemia in modulation of cancer growth and metastasis: A review of the evidence. *Surgical Oncology, 6,* 179–185.

Meirow, D., Yossepowitch, O., Rosler, A., Brzezinski, A., Schenker, J. G., Laufer, N., et al. (1995). Insulin resistant and non-resistant polycystic ovary syndrome represent two clinical and endocrinological subgroups. *Human Reproduction, 10,* 1951–1956.

Menrad, A., & Anderer, F. A. (1991). Expression of LDL receptor on tumor cells induced by growth factors. *Anticancer Research, 11,* 385–390.

Miller, T. W., Perez-Torres, M., Narasanna, A., Guix, M., Stal, O., Perez-Tenorio, G., et al. (2009). Loss of Phosphatase and Tensin homologue deleted on chromosome 10 engages ErbB3 and insulin-like growth factor-I receptor signaling to promote antiestrogen resistance in breast cancer. *Cancer Research, 69,* 4192–4201.

Miraglia, E., Hogberg, J., & Stenius, U. (2012). Statins exhibit anticancer effects through modifications of the pAkt signaling pathway. *International Journal of Oncology, 40,* 867–875.

Miyazaki, Y., Mahankali, A., Matsuda, M., Mahankali, S., Hardies, J., Cusi, K., et al. (2002). Effect of pioglitazone on abdominal fat distribution and insulin sensitivity in type 2 diabetic patients. *The Journal of Clinical Endocrinology and Metabolism, 87,* 2784–2791.

Moller, D. E., Yokota, A., Caro, J. F., & Flier, J. S. (1989). Tissue-specific expression of two alternatively spliced insulin receptor mRNAs in man. *Molecular Endocrinology, 3,* 1263–1269.

Molloy, C. A., May, F. E., & Westley, B. R. (2000). Insulin receptor substrate-1 expression is regulated by estrogen in the MCF-7 human breast cancer cell line. *The Journal of Biological Chemistry, 275,* 12565–12571.

Monami, M., Balzi, D., Lamanna, C., Barchielli, A., Masotti, G., Buiatti, E., et al. (2007). Are sulphonylureas all the same? A cohort study on cardiovascular and cancer-related mortality. *Diabetes/Metabolism Research and Reviews, 23,* 479–484.

Monami, M., Lamanna, C., Balzi, D., Marchionni, N., & Mannucci, E. (2009). Sulphonylureas and cancer: A case–control study. *Acta Diabetologica, 46*, 279–284.

Mondul, A. M., Clipp, S. L., Helzlsouer, K. J., & Platz, E. A. (2010). Association between plasma total cholesterol concentration and incident prostate cancer in the CLUE II cohort. *Cancer Causes & Control, 21*, 61–68.

Mondul, A. M., Weinstein, S. J., Virtamo, J., & Albanes, D. (2011). Serum total and HDL cholesterol and risk of prostate cancer. *Cancer Causes & Control, 22*, 1545–1552.

Monetti, M., Canavesi, M., Camera, M., Parente, R., Paoletti, R., Tremoli, E., et al. (2007). Rosuvastatin displays anti-atherothrombotic and anti-inflammatory properties in apoE-deficient mice. *Pharmacological Research: The Official Journal of the Italian Pharmacological Society, 55*, 441–449.

Morris, P. G., Hudis, C. A., Giri, D., Morrow, M., Falcone, D. J., Zhou, X. K., et al. (2011). Inflammation and increased aromatase expression occur in the breast tissue of obese women with breast cancer. *Cancer Prevention Research (Philadelphia, PA), 4*, 1021–1029.

Mostaghel, E. A., Solomon, K. R., Pelton, K., Freeman, M. R., & Montgomery, R. B. (2012). Impact of circulating cholesterol levels on growth and intratumoral androgen concentration of prostate tumors. *PLoS One, 7*, e30062.

Mosthaf, L., Grako, K., Dull, T. J., Coussens, L., Ullrich, A., & McClain, D. A. (1990). Functionally distinct insulin receptors generated by tissue-specific alternative splicing. *The EMBO Journal, 9*, 2409–2413.

Muoio, D. M., & Newgard, C. B. (2008). Mechanisms of disease: Molecular and metabolic mechanisms of insulin resistance and beta-cell failure in type 2 diabetes. *Nature Reviews. Molecular Cell Biology, 9*, 193–205.

Murtola, T. J., Tammela, T. L., Lahtela, J., & Auvinen, A. (2007). Cholesterol-lowering drugs and prostate cancer risk: A population-based case–control study. *Cancer Epidemiology, Biomarkers & Prevention: A Publication of the American Association for Cancer Research, Cosponsored by the American Society of Preventive Oncology, 16*, 2226–2232.

Musgrove, E. A., & Sutherland, R. L. (2009). Biological determinants of endocrine resistance in breast cancer. *Nature Reviews. Cancer, 9*, 631–643.

Nichols, H. B., Trentham-Dietz, A., Egan, K. M., Titus-Ernstoff, L., Holmes, M. D., Bersch, A. J., et al. (2009). Body mass index before and after breast cancer diagnosis: Associations with all-cause, breast cancer, and cardiovascular disease mortality. *Cancer Epidemiology, Biomarkers & Prevention, 18*, 1403–1409.

Novosyadlyy, R., Lann, D. E., Vijayakumar, A., Rowzee, A., Lazzarino, D. A., Fierz, Y., et al. (2010). Insulin-mediated acceleration of breast cancer development and progression in a nonobese model of type 2 diabetes. *Cancer Research, 70*, 741–751.

Novosyadlyy, R., Vijayakumar, A., Lann, D., Fierz, Y., Kurshan, N., & LeRoith, D. (2009). Physical and functional interaction between polyoma virus middle T antigen and insulin and IGF-I receptors is required for oncogene activation and tumour initiation. *Oncogene, 28*, 3477–3486.

Orkin, L. A. (1974). Efficacy of candicidin in benign prostatic hypertrophy. *Urology, 4*, 80–84.

Ormandy, C. J., Musgrove, E. A., Hui, R., Daly, R. J., & Sutherland, R. L. (2003). Cyclin D1, EMS1 and 11q13 amplification in breast cancer. *Breast Cancer Research and Treatment, 78*, 323–335.

Osborne, C. K., Monaco, M. E., Lippman, M. E., & Kahn, C. R. (1978). Correlation among insulin binding, degradation, and biological activity in human breast cancer cells in long-term tissue culture. *Cancer Research, 38*, 94–102.

Owen, M. R., Doran, E., & Halestrap, A. P. (2000). Evidence that metformin exerts its anti-diabetic effects through inhibition of complex 1 of the mitochondrial respiratory chain. *The Biochemical Journal, 348*(Pt 3), 607–614.

Ozacmak, V. H., Sayan, H., Igdem, A. A., Cetin, A., & Ozacmak, I. D. (2007). Attenuation of contractile dysfunction by atorvastatin after intestinal ischemia reperfusion injury in rats. *European Journal of Pharmacology, 562*, 138–147.

Papa, V., Pezzino, V., Costantino, A., Belfiore, A., Giuffrida, D., Frittitta, L., et al. (1990). Elevated insulin receptor content in human breast cancer. *The Journal of Clinical Investigation, 86*, 1503–1510.

Pasquali, R., Casimirri, F., Cantobelli, S., Melchionda, N., Morselli Labate, A. M., Fabbri, R., et al. (1991). Effect of obesity and body fat distribution on sex hormones and insulin in men. *Metabolism, 40*, 101–104.

Pasqualini, J. R., & Chetrite, G. S. (2005). Recent insight on the control of enzymes involved in estrogen formation and transformation in human breast cancer. *The Journal of Steroid Biochemistry and Molecular Biology, 93*, 221–236.

Peairs, K. S., Barone, B. B., Snyder, C. F., Yeh, H. C., Stein, K. B., Derr, R. L., et al. (2011). Diabetes mellitus and breast cancer outcomes: A systematic review and meta-analysis. *Journal of Clinical Oncology, 29*, 40–46.

Pearce, S. T., & Jordan, V. C. (2004). The biological role of estrogen receptors alpha and beta in cancer. *Critical Reviews in Oncology/Hematology, 50*, 3–22.

Periyasamy-Thandavan, S., Takhar, S., Singer, A., Dohn, M. R., Jackson, W. H., Welborn, A. E., et al. (2012). Insulin-like growth factor 1 attenuates antiestrogen- and antiprogestin-induced apoptosis in ER+ breast cancer cells by MEK1 regulation of the BH3-only pro-apoptotic protein Bim. *Breast Cancer Research, 14*, R52.

Phielix, E., Szendroedi, J., & Roden, M. (2011). The role of metformin and thiazolidinediones in the regulation of hepatic glucose metabolism and its clinical impact. *Trends in Pharmacological Sciences, 32*, 607–616.

Pike, M. C., Pearce, C. L., & Wu, A. H. (2004). Prevention of cancers of the breast, endometrium and ovary. *Oncogene, 23*, 6379–6391.

Pisani, P. (2008). Hyper-insulinaemia and cancer, meta-analyses of epidemiological studies. *Archives of Physiology and Biochemistry, 114*, 63–70.

Platz, E. A., Clinton, S. K., & Giovannucci, E. (2008). Association between plasma cholesterol and prostate cancer in the PSA era. *International Journal of Cancer, 123*, 1693–1698.

Platz, E. A., Leitzmann, M. F., Visvanathan, K., Rimm, E. B., Stampfer, M. J., Willett, W. C., et al. (2006). Statin drugs and risk of advanced prostate cancer. *Journal of the National Cancer Institute, 98*, 1819–1825.

Platz, E. A., Till, C., Goodman, P. J., Parnes, H. L., Figg, W. D., Albanes, D., et al. (2009). Men with low serum cholesterol have a lower risk of high-grade prostate cancer in the placebo arm of the prostate cancer prevention trial. *Cancer Epidemiology, Biomarkers & Prevention: A Publication of the American Association for Cancer Research, Cosponsored by the American Society of Preventive Oncology, 18*, 2807–2813.

Pritchard, K. I., Shepherd, L. E., Chapman, J. A., Norris, B. D., Cantin, J., Goss, P. E., et al. (2011). Randomized trial of tamoxifen versus combined tamoxifen and octreotide LAR Therapy in the adjuvant treatment of early-stage breast cancer in postmenopausal women: NCIC CTG MA.14. *Journal of Clinical Oncology, 29*, 3869–3876.

Qian, X., Li, J., Ding, J., Wang, Z., Duan, L., & Hu, G. (2008). Glibenclamide exerts an antitumor activity through reactive oxygen species-c-jun NH2-terminal kinase pathway in human gastric cancer cell line MGC-803. *Biochemical Pharmacology, 76*, 1705–1715.

Qiu, J., Yang, R., Rao, Y., Du, Y., & Kalembo, F. W. (2012). Risk factors for breast cancer and expression of insulin-like growth factor-2 (IGF-2) in women with breast cancer in Wuhan City, China. *PLoS One, 7*, e36497.

Renehan, A. G., Zwahlen, M., Minder, C., O'Dwyer, S. T., Shalet, S. M., & Egger, M. (2004). Insulin-like growth factor (IGF)-I, IGF binding protein-3, and cancer risk: Systematic review and meta-regression analysis. *Lancet, 363*, 1346–1353.

Rhoads, R. P., Kim, J. W., Leury, B. J., Baumgard, L. H., Segoale, N., Frank, S. J., et al. (2004). Insulin increases the abundance of the growth hormone receptor in liver and adipose tissue of periparturient dairy cows. *The Journal of Nutrition, 134*, 1020–1027.

Richardson, A. E., Hamilton, N., Davis, W., Brito, C., & De Leon, D. (2011). Insulin-like growth factor-2 (IGF-2) activates estrogen receptor-alpha and -beta via the IGF-1 and the insulin receptors in breast cancer cells. *Growth Factors, 29*, 82–93.

Rinaldi, S., Peeters, P. H., Berrino, F., Dossus, L., Biessy, C., Olsen, A., et al. (2006). IGF-I, IGFBP-3 and breast cancer risk in women: The European Prospective Investigation into Cancer and Nutrition (EPIC). *Endocrine-Related Cancer, 13*, 593–605.

Rodenburg, J., Vissers, M. N., Wiegman, A., van Trotsenburg, A. S., van der Graaf, A., de Groot, E., et al. (2007). Statin treatment in children with familial hypercholesterolemia: The younger, the better. *Circulation, 116*, 664–668.

Rose, D. P., & Vona-Davis, L. (2009). Influence of obesity on breast cancer receptor status and prognosis. *Expert Review of Anticancer Therapy, 9*, 1091–1101.

Rudling, M. J., Angelin, B., Peterson, C. O., & Collins, V. P. (1990). Low density lipoprotein receptor activity in human intracranial tumors and its relation to the cholesterol requirement. *Cancer Research, 50*, 483–487.

Rudling, M., & Collins, V. P. (1996). Low density lipoprotein receptor and 3-hydroxy-3-methylglutaryl coenzyme A reductase mRNA levels are coordinately reduced in human renal cell carcinoma. *Biochimica et Biophysica Acta, 1299*, 75–79.

Sachdev, D., Li, S. L., Hartell, J. S., Fujita-Yamaguchi, Y., Miller, J. S., & Yee, D. (2003). A chimeric humanized single-chain antibody against the type I insulin-like growth factor (IGF) receptor renders breast cancer cells refractory to the mitogenic effects of IGF-I. *Cancer Research, 63*, 627–635.

Sachdev, D., & Yee, D. (2001). The IGF system and breast cancer. *Endocrine-Related Cancer, 8*, 197–209.

Saez, E., Rosenfeld, J., Livolsi, A., Olson, P., Lombardo, E., Nelson, M., et al. (2004). PPAR gamma signaling exacerbates mammary gland tumor development. *Genes & Development, 18*, 528–540.

Salas, T. R., Reddy, S. A., Clifford, J. L., Davis, R. J., Kikuchi, A., Lippman, S. M., et al. (2003). Alleviating the suppression of glycogen synthase kinase-3beta by Akt leads to the phosphorylation of cAMP-response element-binding protein and its transactivation in intact cell nuclei. *The Journal of Biological Chemistry, 278*, 41338–41346.

Saltiel, A. R., & Pessin, J. E. (2002). Insulin signaling pathways in time and space. *Trends in Cell Biology, 12*, 65–71.

Sarbassov, D. D., Ali, S. M., Kim, D. H., Guertin, D. A., Latek, R. R., Erdjument-Bromage, H., et al. (2004). Rictor, a novel binding partner of mTOR, defines a rapamycin-insensitive and raptor-independent pathway that regulates the cytoskeleton. *Current Biology, 14*, 1296–1302.

Sarbassov, D. D., Ali, S. M., & Sabatini, D. M. (2005). Growing roles for the mTOR pathway. *Current Opinion in Cell Biology, 17*, 596–603.

Schaffner, C. P. (1981). Prostatic cholesterol metabolism: Regulation and alteration. *Progress in Clinical and Biological Research, 75A*, 279–324.

Schaffner, C. P., & Gordon, H. W. (1968). The hypocholesterolemic activity of orally administered polyene macrolides. *Proceedings of the National Academy of Sciences of the United States of America, 61*, 36–41.

Schernhammer, E. S., Holly, J. M., Pollak, M. N., & Hankinson, S. E. (2005). Circulating levels of insulin-like growth factors, their binding proteins, and breast cancer risk. *Cancer Epidemiology, Biomarkers & Prevention, 14*, 699–704.

Sciacca, L., Costantino, A., Pandini, G., Mineo, R., Frasca, F., Scalia, P., et al. (1999). Insulin receptor activation by IGF-II in breast cancers: Evidence for a new autocrine/paracrine mechanism. *Oncogene, 18*, 2471–2479.

Seino, S., & Bell, G. I. (1989). Alternative splicing of human insulin receptor messenger RNA. *Biochemical and Biophysical Research Communications, 159,* 312–316.

Shackelford, D. B., & Shaw, R. J. (2009). The LKB1-AMPK pathway: Metabolism and growth control in tumour suppression. *Nature Reviews. Cancer, 9,* 563–575.

Shannon, J., Tewoderos, S., Garzotto, M., Beer, T. M., Derenick, R., Palma, A., et al. (2005). Statins and prostate cancer risk: A case–control study. *American Journal of Epidemiology, 162,* 318–325.

Shen, W. H., Yang, X., Boyle, D. W., Lee, W. H., & Liechty, E. A. (2001). Effects of intravenous insulin-like growth factor-I and insulin administration on insulin-like growth factor-binding proteins in the ovine fetus. *The Journal of Endocrinology, 171,* 143–151.

Shepherd, J., Cobbe, S. M., Ford, I., Isles, C. G., Lorimer, A. R., MacFarlane, P. W., et al. (1995). Prevention of coronary heart disease with pravastatin in men with hypercholesterolemia. West of Scotland Coronary Prevention Study Group. *The New England Journal of Medicine, 333,* 1301–1307.

Simons, K., & Ikonen, E. (2000). How cells handle cholesterol. *Science, 290,* 1721–1726.

Simpson, E. R., Ackerman, G. E., Smith, M. E., & Mendelson, C. R. (1981). Estrogen formation in stromal cells of adipose tissue of women: Induction by glucocorticosteroids. *Proceedings of the National Academy of Sciences of the United States of America, 78,* 5690–5694.

Sirtori, C. R. (1993). Tissue selectivity of hydroxymethylglutaryl coenzyme A (HMG CoA) reductase inhibitors. *Pharmacology & Therapeutics, 60,* 431–459.

Slaaby, R., Schaffer, L., Lautrup-Larsen, I., Andersen, A. S., Shaw, A. C., Mathiasen, I. S., et al. (2006). Hybrid receptors formed by insulin receptor (IR) and insulin-like growth factor I receptor (IGF-IR) have low insulin and high IGF-1 affinity irrespective of the IR splice variant. *The Journal of Biological Chemistry, 281,* 25869–25874.

Solomon, K. R., & Freeman, M. R. (2008). Do the cholesterol-lowering properties of statins affect cancer risk? *Trends in Endocrinology and Metabolism, 19,* 113–121.

Spaventi, R., Antica, M., & Pavelic, K. (1990). Insulin and insulin-like growth factor I (IGF I) in early mouse embryogenesis. *Development, 108,* 491–495.

Sporer, A., Cohen, S., Kamat, M. H., & Seebode, J. J. (1975). Candicidin: Physiologic effect on prostate. *Urology, 6,* 298–304.

Sridharan, S., & Basu, A. (2011). S6 kinase 2 promotes breast cancer cell survival via Akt. *Cancer Research, 71,* 2590–2599.

Stopeck, A. T., Nicholson, A. C., Mancini, F. P., & Hajjar, D. P. (1993). Cytokine regulation of low density lipoprotein receptor gene transcription in HepG2 cells. *The Journal of Biological Chemistry, 268,* 17489–17494.

Straus, D. S., & Glass, C. K. (2007). Anti-inflammatory actions of PPAR ligands: New insights on cellular and molecular mechanisms. *Trends in Immunology, 28,* 551–558.

Subbaramaiah, K., Howe, L. R., Bhardwaj, P., Du, B., Gravaghi, C., Yantiss, R. K., et al. (2011). Obesity is associated with inflammation and elevated aromatase expression in the mouse mammary gland. *Cancer Prevention Research (Philadelphia, PA), 4,* 329–346.

Suissa, S., Azoulay, L., Dell'Aniello, S., Evans, M., Vora, J., & Pollak, M. (2011). Long-term effects of insulin glargine on the risk of breast cancer. *Diabetologia, 54,* 2254–2262.

Suzuki, T., Miki, Y., Ohuchi, N., & Sasano, H. (2008). Intratumoral estrogen production in breast carcinoma: Significance of aromatase. *Breast Cancer, 15,* 270–277.

Swyer, G. I. M. (1942). The cholesterol content of normal and enlarged prostates. *Cancer Research, 2,* 372–375.

Tatidis, L., Masquelier, M., & Vitols, S. (2002). Elevated uptake of low density lipoprotein by drug resistant human leukemic cell lines. *Biochemical Pharmacology, 63,* 2169–2180.

Tee, A. R., Manning, B. D., Roux, P. P., Cantley, L. C., & Blenis, J. (2003). Tuberous sclerosis complex gene products, Tuberin and Hamartin, control mTOR signaling by acting as a GTPase-activating protein complex toward Rheb. *Current Biology, 13,* 1259–1268.

Tiikkainen, M., Hakkinen, A. M., Korsheninnikova, E., Nyman, T., Makimattila, S., & Yki-Jarvinen, H. (2004). Effects of rosiglitazone and metformin on liver fat content, hepatic insulin resistance, insulin clearance, and gene expression in adipose tissue in patients with type 2 diabetes. *Diabetes, 53,* 2169–2176.

Toniolo, P. G., Levitz, M., Zeleniuch-Jacquotte, A., Banerjee, S., Koenig, K. L., Shore, R. E., et al. (1995). A prospective study of endogenous estrogens and breast cancer in postmenopausal women. *Journal of the National Cancer Institute, 87,* 190–197.

Toropainen, E. M., Lipponen, P. K., & Syrjanen, K. J. (1995). Expression of insulin-like growth factor II in female breast cancer as related to established prognostic factors and long-term prognosis. *Anticancer Research, 15,* 2669–2674.

Toschi, A., Lee, E., Gadir, N., Ohh, M., & Foster, D. A. (2008). Differential dependence of hypoxia-inducible factors 1 alpha and 2 alpha on mTORC1 and mTORC2. *The Journal of Biological Chemistry, 283,* 34495–34499.

Tworoger, S. S., Eliassen, A. H., Kelesidis, T., Colditz, G. A., Willett, W. C., Mantzoros, C. S., et al. (2007). Plasma adiponectin concentrations and risk of incident breast cancer. *The Journal of Clinical Endocrinology and Metabolism, 92,* 1510–1516.

Uhles, S., Moede, T., Leibiger, B., Berggren, P. O., & Leibiger, I. B. (2003). Isoform-specific insulin receptor signaling involves different plasma membrane domains. *The Journal of Cell Biology, 163,* 1327–1337.

Ulanet, D. B., Ludwig, D. L., Kahn, C. R., & Hanahan, D. (2010). Insulin receptor functionally enhances multistage tumor progression and conveys intrinsic resistance to IGF-1R targeted therapy. *Proceedings of the National Academy of Sciences of the United States of America, 107,* 10791–10798.

van Landeghem, A. A., Poortman, J., Nabuurs, M., & Thijssen, J. H. (1985). Endogenous concentration and subcellular distribution of estrogens in normal and malignant human breast tissue. *Cancer Research, 45,* 2900–2906.

Vitols, S., Norgren, S., Juliusson, G., Tatidis, L., & Luthman, H. (1994). Multilevel regulation of low-density lipoprotein receptor and 3-hydroxy-3-methylglutaryl coenzyme A reductase gene expression in normal and leukemic cells. *Blood, 84,* 2689–2698.

Wadsack, C., Hrzenjak, A., Hammer, A., Hirschmugl, B., Levak-Frank, S., Desoye, G., et al. (2003). Trophoblast-like human choriocarcinoma cells serve as a suitable in vitro model for selective cholesteryl ester uptake from high density lipoproteins. *European Journal of Biochemistry/FEBS, 270,* 451–462.

Webster, N. J., Resnik, J. L., Reichart, D. B., Strauss, B., Haas, M., & Seely, B. L. (1996). Repression of the insulin receptor promoter by the tumor suppressor gene product p53: A possible mechanism for receptor overexpression in breast cancer. *Cancer Research, 56,* 2781–2788.

Weinstein, D., Simon, M., Yehezkel, E., Laron, Z., & Werner, H. (2009). Insulin analogues display IGF-I-like mitogenic and anti-apoptotic activities in cultured cancer cells. *Diabetes/Metabolism Research and Reviews, 25,* 41–49.

Weng, L., Brown, J., & Eng, C. (2001). PTEN induces apoptosis and cell cycle arrest through phosphoinositol-3-kinase/Akt-dependent and -independent pathways. *Human Molecular Genetics, 10,* 237–242.

Weng, L. P., Smith, W. M., Brown, J. L., & Eng, C. (2001). PTEN inhibits insulin-stimulated MEK/MAPK activation and cell growth by blocking IRS-1 phosphorylation and IRS-1/Grb-2/Sos complex formation in a breast cancer model. *Human Molecular Genetics, 10,* 605–616.

Wolf, I., Sadetzki, S., Catane, R., Karasik, A., & Kaufman, B. (2005). Diabetes mellitus and breast cancer. *The Lancet Oncology, 6,* 103–111.

Wondergem, R., Cregan, M., Strickler, L., Miller, R., & Suttles, J. (1998). Membrane potassium channels and human bladder tumor cells: II. Growth properties. *The Journal of Membrane Biology, 161,* 257–262.

Wu, M. H., Chou, Y. C., Chou, W. Y., Hsu, G. C., Chu, C. H., Yu, C. P., et al. (2009). Circulating levels of leptin, adiposity and breast cancer risk. *British Journal of Cancer, 100*, 578–582.

Xu, J., Chen, Y., & Olopade, O. I. (2010). MYC and breast cancer. *Genes & Cancer, 1*, 629–640.

Xue, F., & Michels, K. B. (2007). Diabetes, metabolic syndrome, and breast cancer: A review of the current evidence. *The American Journal of Clinical Nutrition, 86*, s823–s835.

Yager, J. D., & Davidson, N. E. (2006). Estrogen carcinogenesis in breast cancer. *The New England Journal of Medicine, 354*, 270–282.

Yamaguchi, Y., Flier, J. S., Benecke, H., Ransil, B. J., & Moller, D. E. (1993). Ligand-binding properties of the two isoforms of the human insulin receptor. *Endocrinology, 132*, 1132–1138.

Yamnik, R. L., Digilova, A., Davis, D. C., Brodt, Z. N., Murphy, C. J., & Holz, M. K. (2009). S6 kinase 1 regulates estrogen receptor alpha in control of breast cancer cell proliferation. *The Journal of Biological Chemistry, 284*, 6361–6369.

Yang, S. H., Liu, R., Perez, E. J., Wen, Y., Stevens, S. M., Jr., Valencia, T., et al. (2004). Mitochondrial localization of estrogen receptor beta. *Proceedings of the National Academy of Sciences of the United States of America, 101*, 4130–4135.

Yee, D., Paik, S., Lebovic, G. S., Marcus, R. R., Favoni, R. E., Cullen, K. J., et al. (1989). Analysis of insulin-like growth factor I gene expression in malignancy: Evidence for a paracrine role in human breast cancer. *Molecular Endocrinology, 3*, 509–517.

Yoshioka, Y., Sasaki, J., Yamamoto, M., Saitoh, K., Nakaya, S., & Kubokawa, M. (2000). Quantitation by (1)H-NMR of dolichol, cholesterol and choline-containing lipids in extracts of normal and phathological thyroid tissue. *NMR in Biomedicine, 13*, 377–383.

Yu, H., Jin, F., Shu, X. O., Li, B. D., Dai, Q., Cheng, J. R., et al. (2002). Insulin-like growth factors and breast cancer risk in Chinese women. *Cancer Epidemiology, Biomarkers & Prevention, 11*, 705–712.

Zakikhani, M., Blouin, M. J., Piura, E., & Pollak, M. N. (2010). Metformin and rapamycin have distinct effects on the AKT pathway and proliferation in breast cancer cells. *Breast Cancer Research and Treatment, 123*, 271–279.

Zakikhani, M., Dowling, R., Fantus, I. G., Sonenberg, N., & Pollak, M. (2006). Metformin is an AMP kinase-dependent growth inhibitor for breast cancer cells. *Cancer Research, 66*, 10269–10273.

Zhang, H., Fagan, D. H., Zeng, X., Freeman, K. T., Sachdev, D., & Yee, D. (2010). Inhibition of cancer cell proliferation and metastasis by insulin receptor downregulation. *Oncogene, 29*, 2517–2527.

Zhang, Y., Moerkens, M., Ramaiahgari, S., de Bont, H., Price, L., Meerman, J., et al. (2011). Elevated insulin-like growth factor 1 receptor signaling induces antiestrogen resistance through the MAPK/ERK and PI3K/Akt signaling routes. *Breast Cancer Research, 13*, R52.

Zhou, D., Clarke, P., Wang, J., & Chen, S. (1996). Identification of a promoter that controls aromatase expression in human breast cancer and adipose stromal cells. *The Journal of Biological Chemistry, 271*, 15194–15202.

Zhou, S., Wang, G. P., Liu, C., & Zhou, M. (2006). Eukaryotic initiation factor 4E (eIF4E) and angiogenesis: Prognostic markers for breast cancer. *BMC Cancer, 6*, 231.

Zhu, C., Qi, X., Chen, Y., Sun, B., Dai, Y., & Gu, Y. (2011). PI3K/Akt and MAPK/ERK1/2 signaling pathways are involved in IGF-1-induced VEGF-C upregulation in breast cancer. *Journal of Cancer Research and Clinical Oncology, 137*, 1587–1594.

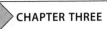

CHAPTER THREE

Sex Hormone Receptors in Breast Cancer

Nina D'Abreo[*,†,1], Alexander A. Hindenburg[*,†]

[*]Oncology/Hematology Division, Winthrop University Hospital, Mineola, New York, USA
[†]SUNY Stony Brook School of Medicine, Stony Brook, New York, USA
[1]Corresponding author: e-mail address: ndabreo@winthrop.org

Contents

Abstract

The dependency of certain breast cancers on estrogen is undeniably one of the most important observations in oncology. Since this early observation, there has been a tremendous effort to define the precise roles of the estrogen receptor (ER) in the pathogenesis of breast cancer. Estrogen signaling pathways can also be exploited as effective

Vitamins and Hormones, Volume 93
ISSN 0083-6729
http://dx.doi.org/10.1016/B978-0-12-416673-8.00001-0

99

targets for cancer treatment. Both ligand-dependent and ligand-independent receptor activation pathways have been successfully blocked by hormonal therapies including selective ER modulators such as tamoxifen, by blocking and accelerating the degradation of ER (fulvestrant), and by depleting tissue levels of estrogen (aromatase inhibitors). Because of the immense prognostic and predictive value of the ER and PR receptor, accurately defining hormone dependency is also of paramount importance. Despite this avalanche of discovery and development resulting in improved outcome for the patient, resistance to these therapies, both intrinsic and acquired, is well known. Uncovering the various mechanisms of resistance has deepened scientific understanding of posttranslational modifications of these receptors, as well as their cross talk with other receptor families such as the HER-2/neu receptor. The recent discovery that orphan estrogen-related receptors may also play an important role in breast cancer is just starting to be appreciated. A clear understanding of the historical perspective and the intricacies of ER structure and function is required to improve current therapeutic strategies for breast cancer.

1. INTRODUCTION

In 2001, the discovery of the drug Gleevac targeting $t(9;22)$, the causative abnormality of chronic myelogenous leukemia was heralded with a *TIME* magazine cover proclaiming a revolution in the war against cancer (Lemonick & Park, 2001). However, the idea of tumor-targeted therapy, with its promise of minimizing collateral damage to nonmalignant tissues, has been used for over a century, albeit in a more common and ultimately harder to treat malignancy, breast cancer. This distinction belongs to the antiestrogen drug Tamoxifen, which, since 1977, has been used as targeted therapy both in the treatment and in the prevention of breast cancer (EBCTCG, 1998; Fisher et al., 1998; Gradishar, 2004; Jordan, 2003). The steroid hormone estrogens, in particular, 17-β-estradiol (E2), the most potent human estrogen, and its less active metabolites estrone and estriol have a key role in the normal physiological development of mammary tissue as well as in the development of breast cancer (Heldring et al., 2007). Estrogen has morphogenetic properties and cumulative exposure to estrogens not only increases breast cancer risk but also stimulates proliferation of breast cancer cells (Colditz, 1998; Kelsey, Gammon, & John, 1993). These effects are mediated by signaling through the estrogen receptors ERα and ERβ, which represent antagonistic forces in terms of their tumorigenic properties (Pettersson, Delaunay, & Gustafsson, 2000) and their splice variants (Heldring et al., 2007; Levin, 2009; McDonnell & Norris, 2002). While only 15–25% of mammary epithelial cells express ERα, the vast majority of cells associated with atypical ductal hyperplasia, lobular carcinoma *in situ*, and 70–80% of both ductal and invasive breast cancers are ERα expressing and their growth is regulated by estrogen (Clarke, Howell, Potten, & Anderson, 1997; Russo, Ao, Grill, & Russo, 1999). Overexpression of ERα even in benign mammary tissue has been shown to increase the risk of breast cancer, and this expression increases with age (Khan, Rogers, Khurana, Meguid, & Numann, 1998; Shoker et al., 1999). However, receptor signaling is infinitely more complex and involves both transcriptional regulation (genomic action) and direct activation of signaling cascades (nongenomic action), cross coupling with growth factor pathways as well as posttranslational modifications (PTMs) (Le Romancer et al., 2011; White & Parker, 1998). While ERα overexpression is a good prognostic factor and predicts response to endocrine therapies, this complexity of signaling translates into varying cellular responses to estrogens and also clinical resistance to antiestrogen therapy. Endocrine resistance, either *de novo* or acquired, is seen in 40–50% of women receiving endocrine therapies (Ali & Coombes, 2002). The aim of this chapter is to review the historical aspects and describe current knowledge of sex-hormone signaling pathways in breast cancer as well as summarize evolving understanding of the mechanisms of resistance and future therapeutic strategies. This chapter makes a modest attempt to review the progress that has been made to date and to hopefully inspire further research for the future.

2. HISTORICAL PERSPECTIVE

2.1. The relationship between sex steroids and breast cancer

In 1882, Thomas William Nunn first reported a case of a woman who had spontaneous breast cancer regression 6 months after menopause, thus suggesting a link between ovarian function and breast cancer (Love & Philips, 2002). In 1889, Albert Schinzinger proposed surgical oophorectomy both as treatment and as prophylaxis against local recurrence of breast cancer, but this was not adopted in practice (Schinzinger, 1889). In 1896, George Thomas Beatson reported on two patients who experienced a remission from inoperable breast cancer after bilateral oophorectomy. Castration of cattle was popularly used to extend the duration of lactation, and Beatson felt that fatty degeneration of the malignant breast would result after oophorectomy, analogous to the observation in spayed cows. However, he also administered thyroid extract before and after oophorectomy, believing that this might also influence the growth of cancer cells (Beatson, 1896a, 1896b). The latter contention was disputed by another surgeon, Stanley Boyd, who had observed Beatson's work and also that of A. Pearce Gould, who had reported on a case of spontaneous remission of metastatic breast cancer in a woman undergoing menopause. Boyd reported the outcomes with 54 patients undergoing oophorectomy for breast cancer including one of his own cases, the first adjuvant oophorectomy, in 1897. He was the first to hypothesize that the effect of this treatment was related to some ovarian secretion. He also astutely observed that only a third of the patients benefited from oophorectomy and that, in the majority of cases, cancer recurred or progressed in 6–12 months (Boyd, 1897, 1899, 1900). A long hiatus ensued, however, as oophorectomy was associated with a high mortality rate (Love & Philips, 2002) especially after the introduction of radiation castration in 1905. In the 1950s, Charles Huggins reintroduced oophorectomy in combination with adrenalectomy as therapy for patients with locally advanced or metastatic cancer (Huggins & Dao, 1953).

2.2. Sex steroids and their targets

Simultaneously, since the early half of the twentieth century, there was a growing interest in nonsurgical methods of hormonal suppression. In 1923, using ovariectomized mice, Allen and Doisy showed that vaginal cornification developed in the presence of a principle found in ovarian follicular fluid, that they called estrogen, later identified as 17-β estradiol (E2). The Allen–Doisy vaginal cornification assay was a major advance that set the stage for development of synthetic estrogens and the study of their effects on target tissues (Allen & Doisy, 1983; Jordan, 2009). Sir Alexander Haddow introduced the first chemical therapy for advanced breast cancer in 1944, when he used nonsteroidal triphenylethylene-based estrogens as high-dose estrogen therapy to treat postmenopausal breast cancer, a seeming paradox to effect of ovarian ablation in achieving tumor regression (Haddow, Watkinson, Paterson, & Koller, 1944; Jordan, 2008). The first nonsteroidal antiestrogen was serendipitously discovered by Lerner, who tested a potential estrogen-like triphenylethylene compound, later named MER 25, which surprisingly proved to be antiestrogenic, but not potent enough for clinical use. He also was instrumental in the discovery of another antiestrogen, clomiphene, which found use eventually as an ovulation inducer (Jordan, 2003, 2009; Lerner, Holthaus, & Thompson, 1958).

In the 1960s, there was increasing demand for antifertility and contraceptive drugs and another nonsteroidal triphenylethylene, I.C.I. 46,474, the *trans*-isomer of 1(*p*-β-dimethylaminoeth-oxyphenyl)-1,2-diphenylbut-1-ene, was developed originally for this purpose (Jordan, 2009). In female rats, its antiestrogenic activity was demonstrated by its inhibitory effect on vaginal cornification and in the presence of exogenous estrogens. It was felt that its efficacy in preventing implantation of the fertilized ova on day 4 of pregnancy was either due to inhibition of estrogen production or by inhibition of estrogen uptake by some specific receptors in the target tissue. In the same species, however, this compound was also found to have a peculiar property, a weaker estrogenic effect shown by actually inducing vaginal cornification and having an uterotrophic effect at higher doses. This atypical behavior was important for the later recognition of selective ER modulation (Harper & Walpole, 1967; Jordan, 2009). This compound fell out of favor as a postcoital contraceptive, but was eventually reintroduced in the 1970s as an anticancer drug for advanced breast cancer. During a time when treatment for breast cancer involved the use of cytotoxic chemotherapy combinations often with devastating side effects, this compound produced remissions with relatively few adverse effects (Cole, Jones, & Todd, 1971). This drug, later known as tamoxifen, approved in 1977 by the Food and Drug Administration, was not only the first targeted therapy for metastatic breast cancer but also the first chemopreventive to be approved for the reduction of breast cancer incidence in both pre- and postmenopausal women at high risk (Fisher et al., 1998; Jordan, 2003, 2009).

The use of tamoxifen as adjuvant therapy for early-stage breast cancer evolved in the 1970s. Early trials limited the use of the drug to 1 year to avoid premature drug resistance based on the observed duration of efficacy of tamoxifen in controlling metastatic disease (Cole et al., 1971). Using the dimethyl-benzanthracene-treated rat mammary carcinoma model, the standard of 5 years was established (Jordan, Dix, & Allen, 1979). Since then, numerous clinical trials have confirmed that 5 years of tamoxifen treatment reduces annual recurrence rates by nearly half and mortality from breast cancer by a third compared to control groups, with no difference in the recurrence or mortality due to tamoxifen in the ERα-negative patients (EBCTCG, 2005). With this tremendous advance, also came the realization that tamoxifen had estrogenic activity in certain target tissues which were both beneficial and potentially dangerous. In particular, this drug not only lowered cholesterol and improved bone density but also showed an increase in the risk of developing thromboembolism and endometrial cancer (EBCTCG, 1998; Gottardis, Robinson, Satyaswaroop, & Jordan, 1988; Jordan, Phelps, & Lindgren, 1987). At the time of its discovery as an effective targeted agent for late breast cancer, however, the actual mechanism of estrogen action on target tissues remained a mystery and early trials did not select participants based on ER expression. This reinvention of sorts was made possible by the discovery of the target, the ER.

2.3. The estrogen receptor

In the late 1950s, Elwood Jensen and Jacobsen at the Ben–May Laboratories at the University of Chicago, synthesized 6,7-(^{3}H)-estradiol, a highly specific estrogen, which they injected into immature female rats. They demonstrated that the labeled compound was retained unchanged in estrogen target tissues in uterus, vagina, and anterior pituitary, but not in nontarget tissues such as muscle, heart, and lung by a heretofore unknown entity. This component, a protein that was extractable from the rat uterus, and bound cytosolic (^{3}H)-estradiol which then promoted uterine cell growth without undergoing chemical alteration, was identified as the ER in 1960 (Jensen & Jacobsen, 1960; Jordan, 2009; Osborne, 1996; Toft & Gorski, 1966). Subsequently, it was also shown that the trophic effects of estrogen on the uterus could be inhibited by blocking estradiol uptake by an antiestrogen, providing further evidence that the binding entity was a true receptor, recognized today as ERα (Jensen, 1996).

The creation of knockout mice models almost three decades later was instrumental in the discovery of ERβ, which was cloned from a rat prostate DNA library in 1995 (Kuiper, Enmark, Pelto-Huikko, Nilsson, & Gustafsson, 1996; Lubahn et al., 1993). In normal mammary tissue, ERβ is widely expressed in various tissues including the luminal and myoepithelial cellular compartments, but only infrequent ERα staining is reported in the luminal epithelium (Clarke et al., 1997; Speirs, Skliris, Burdall, & Carder, 2002). Experiments with ER null mice also demonstrated that the ER receptors were not essential to life, but ERα knockout mouse models do not show development of mammary gland, while ERβ knockout models show very little effect on mammary gland differentiation and no effect on its function (Couse & Korach, 1999; Forster et al., 2002). Extensive studies in using knockout and transgenic mice have demonstrated that ERα is required for proliferation, whereas ERβ in contrast plays an antiproliferative role (Hewitt, Harrell, & Korach, 2005).

3. RECEPTOR STRUCTURE AND FUNCTION

3.1. ER structure

ERα and ERβ are members of the steroid hormone superfamily of nuclear receptors (NRs), which share a common architecture and contain evolutionarily conserved structurally and functionally distinct but interacting domains (Evans, 1998; Heldring et al., 2007). Structurally, the receptor core consists of a central DNA-binding domain (DBD) flanked by transactivation function domains AF-1 and AF-2. More specifically, the five main domains are the N-terminal or A/B domain; the C domain which is the DBD; the D domain, a hinge region containing a nuclear localization signal; E domain which harbors the ligand-binding domain (LBD), and the ligand-dependent transactivation function (AF-2) (see Fig. 3.1; Le Romancer et al., 2011; Nilsson et al., 2001). The C-terminal F domain is a variable domain whose function is still to be clarified (Beato, 1989; Le Romancer et al., 2011). The DBD is composed of two zinc fingers and is the central and most conserved domain, while the N-terminal A/B domain, which bears the constitutively active ligand-independent activation function (AF-1), is not conserved and is the most variable in length and sequence (Heldring et al., 2007; Nilsson et al., 2001). Binding of estrogen or another ligand to ER triggers a conformational change in the receptor, which via a series of complex interactions results in a cell-specific transcriptional response in estrogen response elements (EREs). This process involves receptor dimerization, recruitment, and interaction with coactivators and other transcription factors (genomic action) as well as activation of signaling cascades (nongenomic action) (Beato, 1989; Beekman, Allan, Tsai, Tsai, & O'Malley, 1993; Nilsson et al., 2001; see Figs. 3.2 and 3.3).

NH$_2$	AF-1	DBD	HINGE	LBD/AF-2	COOH
	AB	C	D	E	F

Figure 3.1 ER structure: Five main domains are the N-terminal or A/B domain harboring the activation function (AF-1) region; the C domain, which is the DNA-binding domain (DBD); the D domain, a hinge region containing a nuclear localization signal; E domain, which harbors the ligand-binding domain (LBD); and the ligand-dependent trans-activation function (AF-2). The C-terminal F domain is a variable domain whose function is still to be clarified. (See Color Insert.)

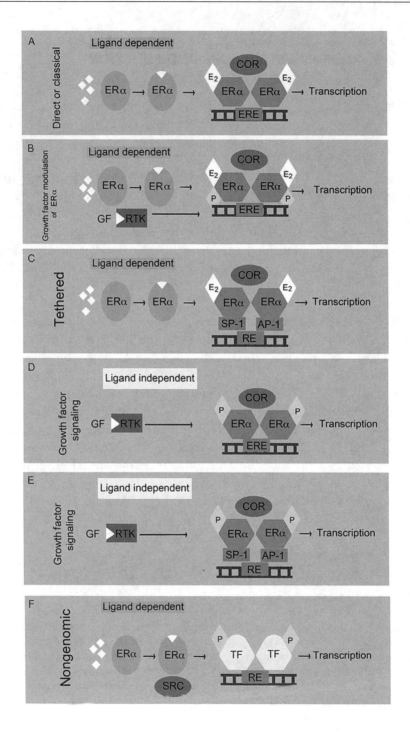

3.2. ERα and ERβ: Similarities and differences

The 66 kDa ERα and 60 kDa ERβ are gene products of two separate chromosomes (Enmark et al., 1997; Tsai & O'Malley, 1994). Both ERs display less than 15% homology in their N-terminal sequences, but their DBDs are virtually identical. The LBDs of ERα and ERβ, which harbor AF-2, share about 56% homology and are very similar in their tertiary structure (Heldring et al., 2007; Katzenellenbogen & Katzenellenbogen, 2000; Nilsson et al., 2001). They have similar affinities for E2 (see Fig. 3.4A) and other major compounds and similar potencies in their interaction with DNA response elements, but exhibit different physiological functions (Hyder, Chiappetta, & Stancel, 1999; Kuiper et al., 1998; Menasce, White, Harrison, & Boyd, 1995; Mosselman, Polman, & Dijkema, 1996). However, dissimilarities in AF-2 homology may also account for the notable

---

Figure 3.2 ER signaling pathways. (A) The classical genomic mechanism of estrogen hormone action involves the binding of E2 to the estrogen receptor (ER) releasing it from its dormant inactive but protected complex with heat-shock proteins (HSP). This induces a conformational change allowing the estrogen receptor to bind to estrogen response elements (ERE) and to induce transcription. This is further modulated by a number of coregulatory cofactors (COR). Maximal transcription activity requires the concerted efforts of AF-1 and AF-2. (B) Variation on the classical genomic pathway. ER and CORs are targets for multiple posttranslational modifications (PRM). Various growth factors (GR) can modify the action of ER by affecting phosphorylation (P) shown, and methylation, acetylation, SUMOylation, and ubiquitination (not shown but can substitute M, A, S, or U for P). (C) The alternative genomic mechanism, also ligand and ER dependent, involves the tethering of ER to regulatory DNA sequences such as activating protein (AP1) or specific protein (SP1) which induces a transcription factor cross talk and induction of nonestrogen response elements (RE) transcription. (D) ER action can be induced and regulated by estrogen-independent and ligand-independent pathways involving growth factors that activate various receptor tyrosine kinases (RTKs). Similar to what is described in (B), some of the actions may involve P, M, A, S, and U of the ER inducing the estrogen receptor to bind to ERE and to induce transcription. (E) In addition to what is described in (D), ER can be tethered to other transcription factors inducing transcription which in contrast to (D) is not mediated by ERE. (F) Nongenomic pathways. There is a small pool of ER which is associated with the membrane which can be rapidly recruited to alter the expression of genes normally regulated by GF. This pathway is independent of gene transcription. The ligand binds to ER which forms dimers and activates signal cascades involving steroid receptor coactivator (SRC) and phosphatidylinositol 3-kinase (PI3K). This activates pathways both dependent and independent of transcription. The transcription pathways that are involved here are also not mediated by ERE. The fact that most of the nongenomic effects are rapid points to the importance of posttranslational modifications involved in these pathways. (See Color Insert.)

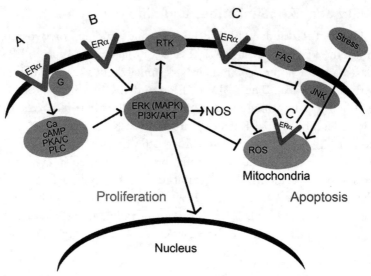

Figure 3.3 Nongenomic pathways. ER signaling by nongenomic pathways is mediated by membrane bound, cytoplasmic and mitochondrial pools of ER. E2 signaling leads to rapid regulation of cellular functions. The genomic and nongenomic pathways are not independent and ultimately converge to modulate nuclear transcription-dependent processes (activation depicted by arrows, downregulation by blocked lines). (A) Signaling by E2 leads to modulation of G protein-linked membrane receptors, which can lead to a variety of cellular actions such as mobilization of intracellular calcium, protein kinase C (PKC), C-AMP generation via protein kinase A (PKA) activation, as well as activation of phospholipase C (PLC). (B) E2 exposure leads to rapid activation of two main signaling cascades, the RAS/MEK/ERK (MAPK) pathway and the PI3K/Akt/mTOR pathway. MAPKs can also lead to ligand-independent phosphorylation of receptor tyrosine kinases (RTK). E2 activation of the p38 MAPK cascade. Activation of Akt mediates several downstream cellular effects including rapid activation of nitric oxide synthase (NOS), leading to increased NO synthesis which has a vascular protective function. (C) Apoptotic pathways are depicted. Estrogen binding to E2 can downregulate the activity of FAS and JNK cascades (extrinsic pathway). E2 as well as stress in the microenvironment can activate the mitochondrial pathway (intrinsic pathway) and lead to formation of reactive oxygen species (ROS), ultimately activating proapoptotic pathways. ER receptors in the mitochondrial membrane may also play a role in inhibition of ROS. The PI3k/Akt signaling pathway has a negative effect on generation of proapoptotic proteins in the mitochondria, an effect that can be blocked by E2. (See Color Insert.)

differences in the ability of the ERs to bind with other naturally occurring ligands such as the phytoestrogens genistein, quercetin, or coumestrol. Genistein, for example, has about a 30-fold higher affinity for ERβ, despite having a very similar molecular structure to E2 (Magee & Rowland, 2004;

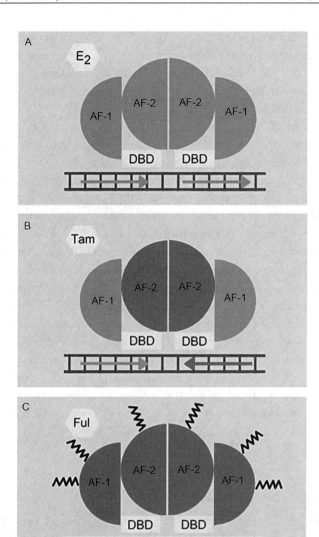

Figure 3.4 Differential action of ligands at the AF-1 and AF-2 domains of the ER. (A) Estrogen (E2) is an agonist at the AF-1 and AF-2 sites, leading to interaction with EREs and modulation of gene transcription (green arrows). The activity of the AF-1 region is reduced in ERβ, which has lower transcriptional activity compared to ERα. (B) Tamoxifen (Tam) has dual agonist/antagonist properties, being agonists at the AF-1 domain and antagonists at the AF-2 site. In breast cancer cells, where AF-2 activity is dominant, tamoxifen and other SERMs (selective estrogen receptor modulator) act as antagonists, but in the uterus where AF-1 activity is dominant, tamoxifen acts as an agonist. (C) Fulvestrant (Ful), a SERD (selective estrogen receptor downregulator), is a complete antagonist at both AF-1 and AF-2, thus completely blocking transcription (red arrows)

Miodini, Fioravanti, Di Fronzo, & Cappelletti, 1999). This difference may be due to subtle variations in conformational changes within the tertiary structure of the ERs induced by specific ligand binding (Gee, Carlson, Martini, Katzenellenbogen, & Katzenellenbogen, 1999; Tremblay, Tremblay, Labrie, & Giguere, 1999).

A significant difference between the ERs is in the activity of the AF-1 region encoded by the N-terminal domain, which is markedly reduced in ERβ. Thus, despite equal affinity for E2, ERβ has markedly lower transcriptional activity in part due to this difference (Zwart et al., 2010). E2 and other antiestrogens thus differentially regulate ER receptor–regulatory elements (Levy et al., 2008; Tee et al., 2004). E2 binding results in the formation of homodimers, which interact with EREs and modulate rates of gene transcription. However, functional heterodimers of the ER receptor can bind to steroid receptor coactivator (SRC-1) and may lead to differences in ER-dependent gene expression and subsequent transcription of gene (Cowley, Hoare, Mosselman, & Parker, 1997). Transient cotransfection experiments have shown that ERβ can act as dominant regulator of ERα function in response to E2 and to tamoxifen and coexpression of both ERs can modulate ERα AF-1 activity and result in receptor activity distinct from that of ER homodimers (Pettersson et al., 2000). ERα and ERβ have antagonistic actions at proproliferative target genes, suggesting that the morphogenetic response to estrogen in the mammary tissues, which leads to carcinogenesis, is due to a balance between ERα and ERβ signaling (Liu et al., 2002).

3.3. ER isoforms and splice variants

ER variants resulting from alternative splicing of exons or alternative promoters have been reported in addition to the classical ERα and ERβ transcripts. These either transcriptionally active in the absence of E2 and have dominant positive actions or are transcriptionally inactive but have dominant-negative actions on classic ER. However, in some cases, their biological functions remain to be clarified (Kos, Reid, Denger, & Gannon, 2001; McGuire, Chamness, & Fuqua, 1991). Shorter isoforms that lack the first-coding exon (exon1A) of the *ERα* gene and thus lack the AF-1

---

of ER-regulated genes. In addition, it lowers the amount of ER available for ligand binding by mediating rapid degradation of the ER by uncoupling it from heat-shock protein complex (zigzag lines). (See Color Insert.)

domain such as hERα 46 and hERα 36 have been identified in various cell lines including MCF-7 and HEK 293 breast cancer cells (Flouriot et al., 2000; Wang et al., 2005). hERα 46 can heterodimerize with full-length ERα or directly compete for the ERα DNA-binding site and thus repress its AF-1 activity. By virtue of its inhibitory action on full-length ER in terms of E2 binding and transcription, this variant may also mediate endocrine resistance (Flouriot et al., 2000). hERα 36 also has the potential to localize to the plasma membrane and initiate nongenomic pathways of ER function such as E2-dependent activation of the mitogen-activated protein kinase (MAPK) pathway (Wang et al., 2005; Zhang et al., 2011). These and other variants such as ERα polymorphisms may have important implications however in our understanding of mechanisms of breast tumor behavior and endocrine resistance (Klinge et al., 2010; Li, Lambert, & Xu, 2003; McGuire et al., 1991; Zhang et al., 2011).

ERβ1, the full-length ligand-binding isoform has antiproliferative and proapoptotic properties. Splice variants of ERβ have been described in breast cancer cells that may also mediate resistance. ERβcx, a receptor with a variation in exon 8, has no transcriptive activity, as it cannot bind E2. However, it preferentially heterodimerizes with ERα and inhibits DNA binding, thus exerting a negative effect on ligand-dependent ERα-mediated transcription (Ogawa et al., 1998).

4. ER AGONISTS AND ANTAGONISTS

ER activity at the LBD has been pharmacologically exploited, leading to the development of two distinct classes of synthetic ER ligands with tissue-selective agonist/antagonist activity that are extensively used for prevention and treatment of breast cancer (Gradishar, 2004; Le Romancer et al., 2011; see Fig. 3.4A).

SERMs (selective estrogen receptor modulators) such as tamoxifen and raloxifene inhibit AF-2-dependent activation of the ER and thus function as antagonists in breast cancer cells where AF-2 activity is the dominant mechanism of ER function (see Fig. 3.4B). In the uterus, where AF-1 function is dominant, tamoxifen acts as an agonist (Jordan & O'Malley, 2007; Smith & O'Malley, 2004). Structural studies of the ER using crystallography have largely focused on the LBD. These have demonstrated that ligand binding alters the position of amino acids in helix 12, which is a key element on the interaction surface of AF-2. Differences in helix 12 positioning induced by different synthetic ligands are responsible for the receptor conformation changes that result either an agonist or an antagonist function. Agonists such as E2 and diethylstilbestrol, upon binding to the LBD of ERα, result in exposure of a hydrophobic groove formed by α-helices 3, 4, 5, and 12, which is an agonistic positioning forming a surface for association of transcriptional coactivators such as GRIP1 (Ali, Buluwela, & Coombes, 2011). Antagonists such as tamoxifen and raloxifene displace helix 12 from its agonist position and position it over the coactivator-binding groove which blocks coactivator recruitment (Nilsson et al., 2001). *In vitro*, binding of an agonist thus induces conformational changes in the ER that promote and stabilize ER–coactivator interactions, which in turn limits dissociation of the ER-bound ligand (Gee et al., 1999; Nilsson et al., 2001; Tremblay et al., 1999). Another class of drugs is the selective estrogen receptor downregulators (SERDs) exemplified by the drug fulvestrant that have a 100-fold greater affinity for ERα compared to tamoxifen. Fulvestrant blocks both AF-1 and AF-2 functions and thus completely blocks transcription of ER-regulated genes. SERDs thus inhibit receptor dimerization and are antagonists in all tissues (Le Romancer et al., 2011; Wakeling, Dukes, & Bowler, 1991). Binding of fulvestrant to the LBD results in occupation of the coactivator pocket by a bulky side chain that prevents helix 12 from assuming an agonistic position (Ali et al., 2011). In a dose-dependent fashion, fulvestrant also mediates rapid degradation of ER from the target tissue, by uncoupling it from the heat-shock protein complex, thus reducing the amount of ER available for ligand binding (Le Romancer et al., 2011; see Fig. 3.4C).

5. MOLECULAR MECHANISMS OF ESTROGEN SIGNALING

ER signaling is a complex biological pathway driven by estrogen that is exploited by breast cancer cells and enables cell proliferation, survival, apoptosis, invasion, and angiogenesis (Osborne & Schiff, 2011). Mechanistically, there are distinct molecular pathways that regulate ER function and are either driven by E2 or independent of ligand action, namely, genomic and nongenomic pathways.

5.1. Ligand-dependent genomic pathways

The classical or direct genomic pathway involves the binding of a ligand such as E2 to the receptors in the nucleus resulting in dissociation from the heat-shock protein receptor complex and phosphorylation (see Fig. 3.2A). This leads to receptor dimerization resulting in cell-specific transcriptional response depending on the properties of the unique EREs located in the promoters of target genes (Heldring et al., 2007; Le Romancer et al., 2011; Nilsson et al., 2001). In addition, ligand binding induces a conformational change within the LBD that allows recruitment of coregulatory complexes and histone-modifying enzymes, such as histone acetyl and methyl transferases, deacetylases, and demethylases that modulate transcription (Bannister & Kouzarides, 1996; Robyr, Wolffe, & Wahli, 2000). Growth factor receptor pathways active within a target cell can also determine the outcome of ligand-mediated transcription of the ER in the presence of physiological doses of E2 (see Fig. 3.2B). PTM of the ER occurs mainly via phosphorylation, while other mechanisms such as acetylation, ubiquination SUMOylation, and lysine methylation are also involved (Le Romancer et al., 2011; Nilsson et al., 2001).

A nonclassical mechanism of genomic action is the ligand-dependent pathway involving the tethering of ER via protein–protein interactions with transcription factors, such as Fos/Jun and AP-1 (activator protein-1) or SP-1 (specificity protein-1), and nuclear factor-κB (NF-κB) which function as coregulators and thus affect transcription of genes that do not harbor EREs by indirect DNA binding (Kushner et al., 2000; Quaedackers, van den Brink, van der Saag, & Tertoolen, 2007; Saville et al., 2000). This mechanism, known as transcriptional cross talk, can be used to regulate hundreds of estrogen-responsive genes that do not contain EREs (Gottlicher, Heck, & Herrlich, 1998; see Fig. 3.2C).

5.2. Ligand-independent genomic pathways

In the absence of E2, ERs can also be activated by alternate signaling pathways regulated by membrane receptor tyrosine kinases such as the epidermal growth factor receptor (EGFR), HER2, and insulin-like growth factor receptor (IGF1-R) (McKenna, Lanz, & O'Malley, 1999; Schiff et al., 2004) (see Fig. 3.2D and E). In turn, cross talk between these receptors also influences the ultimate transcriptional function of the ER. Increased expression of ligands such as transforming growth factor-α (TGF-α) and IGF-1 induced by E2 can in turn activate the growth factor receptor pathway (Schiff et al., 2004; Vyhlidal, Samudio, Kladde, & Safe, 2000).

5.3. Nongenomic pathways

ERs can also be regulated by E2 via nontranscriptional actions (see Figs. 3.3 and 3.2F). These actions are too rapid, usually occurring within seconds to minutes, to be accounted for by RNA activation and protein synthesis (Bjornstrom & Sjoberg, 2005). ER pools have been found localized to the cytoplasm, plasma membrane, and mitochondria of breast cancer cells (Levin & Pietras, 2008; Pedram, Razandi, Wallace, & Levin, 2006). Plasma membrane ERs have been found to be involved in regulation of cell membrane ion channels via activation of G protein-coupled receptors leading to mobilization of intracellular calcium, C-AMP production via the adenylate cyclase/protein kinase A pathway, activation of protein kinase C, and regulation of the phospholipase C/diacylglycerol/inositol 1,4,5-trisphosphate cascade. These effects lead to rapid transduction of signals that affect cellular function, proliferation, migration, and differentiation (Aronica, Kraus, & Katzenellenbogen, 1994; Simoncini & Genazzani, 2003; Fig. 3.3 ER pathways A).

Dimerization of nonnuclear ERα upon ligand binding activates multiple signal transduction cascades through direct interactions with various proteins such as Src kinase, ras, G proteins, Shc (SH2-containing protein), and the p85 α-regulatory subunit of PI3-kinase, thus activating two major pathways: the Src/ras/MAPK and the PI3/AKT/mTOR pathways (Kumar et al., 2007; Migliaccio et al., 1996, 1998; Simoncini et al., 2000; Song et al., 2002; Song, Zhang, & Santen, 2005; Fig. 3.3 ER pathways B). Activation of MAPK leads to either downstream cytoplasmic or transcriptional events that potentiate AF-1 activation. In turn, MAPKs can directly catalyze the phosphorylation of ER at serine 118 as well as indirectly phosphorylate serine 167 via its downstream target RSK (p90 ribosomal-S6-kinase) and increase their transcriptional efficacy (Lorenzo, 2003). Activation of the PI3K/AKT pathway leads to downstream activation of nitric oxide synthase (NOS). NOS enhances release of the vasodilator nitric oxide (NO) that is vascular protective. AKT can directly phosphorylate ER also and enhance the ligand-dependent transcriptional activity of EREs (Simoncini, Rabkin, & Liao, 2003). ERβ has also been discovered near the plasma membrane and also participates in nongenomic regulation via the Src protein (Migliaccio et al., 2000; Pappas, Gametchu, & Watson, 1995).

ERs located at the plasma membrane also associate with scaffold protein caveolin-1. In endothelial cells, among others, ERs have also been found in caveolae, which are caveolin-1-enriched membrane invaginations that serve as a surface for molecules involved in signal transduction (Chambliss et al., 2000; Lu et al., 2004; Razandi, Oh, Pedram, Schnitzer, & Levin, 2002).

The interaction of E2-activated membrane ERα is also enhanced by MNAR, another scaffold protein, which then leads to activation of the

MAPK pathway via increased Src-kinase activity (Wong, McNally, Nickbarg, Komm, & Cheskis, 2002).

Membrane-associated ERα activated by E2 can also activate various receptor tyrosine kinases directly such as the IGF-1 receptor and the Her-2/neu receptor, leading to activation of the MAPK pathway (Chung, Sheu, Yang, Lin, & Yen, 2002; Kahlert et al., 2000). Signaling from the tumor microenvironment can be modulated by the stress kinase pathway or via integrins which trigger downstream activation of p38 MAPK, c-Jun N-terminal kinase (JNK), and FAK (focal adhesion kinase) which can further modulate transcription by phosphorylation of ER and its coregulators (Lee & Bai, 2002; Osborne & Schiff, 2011; Fig. 3.3C).

The genomic and nongenomic pathways are not mutually exclusive but have myriad points of convergence and interaction with each other, resulting in a complementary effect on the regulation of transcription (Bjornstrom & Sjoberg, 2005; Le Romancer et al., 2011; Ordonez-Moran & Munoz, 2009).

5.4. Proapoptotic nongenomic pathways

E2 in low doses is a potent stimulator of cell proliferation and inhibitor of apoptosis. However, high-dose estrogen was used in the 1940s as an effective treatment for postmenopausal patients with metastatic breast cancer (Haddow et al., 1944; Jordan, 2008). The mechanism of estrogen-induced tumor regression *in vivo* has been shown by *in vitro* studies to be paradoxically due to estrogen-induced apoptosis (Lewis, Osipo, Meeke, & Jordan, 2005). These signaling pathways can be extrinsic, involving the Fas/Fas ligand or intrinsic (mitochondrial) (see Fig. 3.3C; Lewis-Wambi & Jordan, 2009; Peter & Krammer, 2003). The extrinsic pathway is mediated via the cell-surface Fas receptor which is activated by proapoptotic ligands including CD95l/Fasl ultimately resulting in the release of initiator caspases 8 and 10 into the cytoplasm where they activate caspases 3, 6, and 7 and converge on the intrinsic pathway.

The mitochondrial pathway is activated by various types of cell stress, including that induced by DNA damage from radiation and chemotherapy. These stressors stimulate the formation of mitochondrial reactive oxygen species (Benhar, Engelberg, & Levitzki, 2002) and ultimately activate the members of the proapoptotic Bcl-2 family proteins while inhibiting anti-apoptotic members of the same family. Suppression of Bcl-2 expression in MCF-7:2A cells that have a basal elevated Bcl-2 expression was found to increase E2-mediated apoptosis fivefold (Lewis-Wambi & Jordan, 2009).

6. IMPLICATIONS IN BREAST CANCER

6.1. ER antagonist activity

The varied and complex pathways of ER regulation have important clinical implications in the prognosis and treatment of breast cancer. The steroid receptor coactivator SRC (p160) family of coactivators plays an extremely important role in ER function (Heldring et al., 2007). The tethering of ERα to AP-1 induced by E2 requires the AF-2 domain, which binds p160 coactivators and stabilizes the protein–protein interaction (Teyssier, Belguise, Galtier, & Chalbos, 2001; Webb et al., 1999). ER activation has been found to be markedly disturbed in the absence of SRCs (McKenna et al., 1999).

ER B tethering to AP-1, however, does not have any transcriptional effect on reporter genes (Paech et al., 1997). This difference has been proposed as a mechanism behind differential response of the SERMs in specific tissues. Tamoxifen and raloxifene, which are antagonists at EREs, behave like agonists through indirect DNA-binding pathways. This effect of SERMs on an AP-1 reporter gene can be blocked by ERβ, but not ERα in the presence of E2 (Paech et al., 1997; Webb, Lopez, Uht, & Kushner, 1995). Similarly, SERMs can differentially activate ERα–SP-1 and ERβ–SP-1 complexes (Saville et al., 2000). Tamoxifen, raloxifene, and fulvestrant can also block the expression of EREs by inhibiting coactivator recruitment by ERα and promoting recruitment of corepressors such as nuclear receptor corepressor (NCoR) and silencing mediator of retinoic acid and thyroid hormone receptor (Shang & Brown, 2002; Webb, Nguyen, & Kushner, 2003).

6.2. Endocrine resistance

In addition to being exploited for clinical benefit, certain modifications of ER activation pathways can also mediate resistance to antagonist activity. The mechanisms are varied and can be *de novo* (intrinsic) or acquired during anti-E2 therapy after a period of response (Osborne & Schiff, 2011).

Phosphorylation of ERα may change the three-dimensional structure of the protein receptor. In breast cancer cells, phosphomodification of particular sites such as S118 and S305 within the AF-1 domain of ER can affect the binding of SRC-1 in the presence of tamoxifen, resulting in resistance to its action (de Leeuw, Neefjes, & Michalides, 2011; Zwart et al., 2007). Downregulation of the corepressor NCoR by long-term tamoxifen exposure in MCF-7 breast cancer cells transplanted in nude mice has been found to be associated with development of resistance to tamoxifen (Lavinsky et al., 1998). Increased AP-1 and NF-κB activity has also been described in breast cancer cells that develop resistance to tamoxifen (Johnston et al., 1999; Zhou et al., 2007). Downstream activation of the PI3K/AKT and the MAPK pathway by growth factor receptor activation can downregulate ER expression and may thus mediate endocrine resistance (Massarweh et al., 2008; Osborne et al., 2003).

Overexpression of the ER coactivator amplified in breast cancer 1 (AIB1 or SRC 3) is found in 5–10% of breast tumors. AIB1 can act as an oncogene, resulting in the development of ER-positive breast tumors in transgenic mice who overexpress this coactivator (Ali et al., 2011; Torres-Arzayus et al., 2004). High-level expression of AIB1 is associated with tamoxifen resistance (Osborne et al., 2003). Coexpression of AIB1 and Her2 or AIB1 and EGFR has been found to be associated with a very poor response to tamoxifen, especially seen in ER-positive/PR-negative tumors (Jordan & O'Malley, 2007; Kirkegaard et al., 2007; Osborne et al., 2003). E2 represses the *IL-6* gene through interaction of ERs with NF-κB and CCAAT/enhancer-binding protein B (Ray, Prefontaine, & Ray, 1994; Stein & Yang, 1995). Regulation of other transcription factors such as GATA-1 and STAT5 is also mediated by transcriptional cross talk in the presence of E2 (Bjornstrom, Kilic, Norman, Parker, & Sjoberg, 2001; Blobel, Sieff, & Orkin, 1995).

Fulvestrant, a SERD, a complete ER antagonist, can function as a potent agonist to both ERα and ERβ tethered to Ap-1, Sp-1, and Stat-5, but cannot exert nongenomic actions through classic ER receptors. Thus, this drug completely blocks the nongenomic actions of E2 but cannot block other signaling pathways (Bjornstrom & Sjoberg, 2005; Bjornstrom et al., 2001).

While E2 can indirectly impact mitochondrial function via NRs, high-affinity ER receptors have also been localized to the mitochondria of MCF-7 breast cancer cells and endothelial cells. Contrary to E2 effects described above, these mitochondrial ERs may in fact protect tumor cells from radiation-induced apoptosis by blocking ROS formation (Pedram et al., 2006).

6.3. Application of ER signaling mechanisms to current treatment strategies

Antihormonal therapy is currently widely used for treatment of ER-expressing breast cancer. Knowledge of some of the mechanisms of endocrine resistance has been successfully translated into effective alternative therapeutic strategies. In addition to SERM- and SERD-mediated ER antagonism to block E2-stimulated tumor cell growth, aromatase inhibitors (AIs) are also standard of care to block E2 synthesis in postmenopausal women. In the adjuvant treatment of breast cancer, AIs not only have a small but significant increase in efficacy in this population of patients but also avoid the tissue-specific adverse effects of tamoxifen, namely, endometrial cancer and thrombosis (Cuzick et al., 2010; Thurlimann et al., 2005). There is a significant rate of relapse seen after completion of 5 years of tamoxifen therapy (EBCTCG, 2005; Saphner, Tormey, & Gray, 1996), but recently, the international ATLAS (Adjuvant Tamoxifen, Longer Against Shorter) study demonstrated that extending tamoxifen from the standard of 5 years to 10 years lowered the risk for breast cancer recurrence and disease-specific death, a benefit that became most apparent in the next decade (Davies et al., 2013). This suggests that tamoxifen acts predominantly through a cytostatic effect on residual breast cancer and that prolonged and sustained exposure is necessary for maximal effect. This has to be tempered against tamoxifen's known partial agonist properties and its potential to increase sensitivity of breast cancer cells to its own estrogenic actions and to E2 after long-term use (Berstein et al., 2004). In addition, emergence of a hormone-independent tumor phenotype due to adaptive MAPK-mediated signaling in long-term estrogen-deprived tumor cells may also explain this clinical finding (Jeng, Yue, Eischeid, Wang, & Santen, 2000; Massarweh et al., 2008; Schiff et al., 2004). Sequential use of a non-cross-resistant therapy, an AI after tamoxifen, has been shown to be an effective strategy to combat this phenomenon of tamoxifen resistance (Long et al., 2004). Women who have completed 2–5 years of tamoxifen treatment are currently eligible to receive an additional 5 years of an AI (Goss, 2007; Mamounas, 2001). Recent evidence is also emerging that the AI letrozole improved outcomes when given to disease-free women for periods up to 5 years after completion of tamoxifen (Goss, 2007).

In athymic nude mice implanted with estrogen-dependent MCF-7 breast cancer cells which have developed resistance to tamoxifen, use of fulvestrant suppressed the growth of tumors twice as long as did the treatment with tamoxifen or estrogen withdrawal. Fulvestrant was also found to be more effective than tamoxifen in reducing the expression of E2-regulated genes (Osborne et al., 1995). E2-induced apoptosis can cause regression of tamoxifen-resistant breast cancer cells by inducing Fas expression and suppressing the antiapoptotic/prosurvival factors NF-κB and Her2/neu. Fulvestrant can inhibit this proapoptotic effect by blocking ERα signaling by E2 and thus paradoxically enhance tumor growth (Lewis-Wambi & Jordan, 2009; Osipo, Gajdos, Liu, Chen, & Jordan, 2003). In addition, there is evidence that a ligand-activated G protein GPR 30 may be involved in this effect via transactivation of EGFR rather than classic ERα (Mauriac, Pippen, Quaresma Albano, Gertler, & Osborne, 2003). Fulvestrant is currently approved for use in postmenopausal women who have experienced disease progression on other antiestrogen therapy. It was found to have no added clinical benefit over an AI alone in the second-line setting (Prossnitz, Arterburn, & Sklar, 2007). Recently, however, the combination of fulvestrant and an AI, anastrazole, has been shown to improve both progression-free and overall survival in postmenopausal women with previously untreated ER-positive metastatic breast cancer compared to anastrazole alone (Mehta et al., 2012).

The PI3K/Akt/mTOR pathway is a vital regulatory pathway which modulates ligand-driven signaling via the ER and the HER family of receptors (Campbell et al., 2001; Kurokawa & Arteaga, 2003; Stoica et al., 2003). MCF-7 breast cancer cells with aberrantly upregulated Akt signaling are resistant to endocrine therapy and to chemotherapy, but the sensitivity to tamoxifen can be restored by treatment with an mTOR inhibitor (deGraffenried et al., 2004). Preclinical studies have also demonstrated that in endocrine-resistant cells, cotreatment with the mTOR inhibitor everolimus and letrozole or fulvestrant restores the response of these cells to levels observed in responsive cells treated with letrozole or fulvestrant alone (Beeram et al., 2007). S6 kinase 1, a substrate of mTOR complex 1 (mTOR1), can mediate ligand-dependent ER activation by phosphorylation of the AF-1 domain (Yamnik et al., 2009). Clinical trials have since translated this science into practice and confirmed that the combination of mTOR inhibitors and AIs improves progression-free survival in postmenopausal women with endocrine-resistant breast cancer (Baselga et al., 2009, 2012).

The progesterone receptor (PR) consists of two isoforms PR-A and PR-B which are expressed from a single gene (Kraus, Montano, & Katzenellenbogen, 1993). PR also contains a DBD, an LBD, and AFs similar to ER. PR is an ER-regulated gene in the presence of E2, and the ratio of

PR-A to PR-B is critical for normal mammary gland development (Conneely, Jericevic, & Lydon, 2003). Overexpression of PR-A is associated with tamoxifen resistance and up to 50% of tamoxifen-treated tumors lose PR expression when resistance develops (Gross, Clark, Chamness, & McGuire, 1984; Hopp et al., 2004). Clinical studies have demonstrated that tamoxifen-treated patients with early-stage ER-positive/PR-positive tumors (Bardou, Arpino, Elledge, Osborne, & Clark, 2003) as well as metastatic cancer (Ravdin et al., 1992) have a significant improvement in overall survival compared to those with ER-positive/PR-negative tumors. The relative resistance of ER-positive/PR-negative tumors to SERMs has been considered to be a surrogate for nonfunctional PR (Cui, Schiff, Arpino, Osborne, & Lee, 2005; Horwitz & McGuire, 1975). However, selective resistance mechanisms in ER-positive/PR-negative tumors to SERMs have been recently described which implicate growth factor-mediated down-regulation of PR. ER-positive/PR-negative tumors which show a relatively high level of growth factor signaling may thus be best treated with an AI or a SERD (Cui et al., 2005).

7. FUTURE DIRECTIONS

The understanding of the complexities of the ER signaling system continues to evolve and generate new therapeutic possibilities. A few areas that are being actively explored are noted below.

7.1. Origin of ER-positive breast cancer as related to stem cells

It is still a matter of controversy whether hormone receptor-positive and hormone receptor-negative breast cancer are derived from the same or from different stem cells. The stochastic stem-cell model would support the hormone receptor-positive and hormone receptor-negative tumors derived from separate stem cells (Martinez-Climent, Andreu, & Prosper, 2006; Sleeman & Cremers, 2007). A more modern theory postulates that ER-positive stem cells can evolve from ER-negative ones. Liu et al. (2008) recently showed that BRCA1 regulates human mammary stem/progenitor cell fate. By using in vitro systems and a humanized NOD/SCID mouse model, they demonstrated that BRCA1 expression is required for the differentiation of ER-negative stem/progenitor cells to ER-positive luminal cells. Furthermore, clinical studies of the effect of neoadjuvant hormonal therapy on breast cancer have shown that breast cancer cells that survive after hormonal therapy have molecular signatures that recapitulate the cellular hierarchy present in the normal mouse and human breast in which ER-negative stem cells lead to ER-positive luminal cells. It is postulated that in these tumors, estrogen may indirectly affect ER-negative cancer stem-cell populations through the production of paracrine factors by ER-positive breast cancer cells (Asselin-Labat et al., 2006; Dobrescu et al., 2011; Liu & Wicha, 2010). The latter hypothesis would also support clinical data derived from a number of chemoprevention studies, which have demonstrated chemoprevention decreasing the incidence of most ER-positive breast cancer and also to a lesser extent decreasing the incidence also of ER-negative breast cancer (EBCTCG, 2005). Estrogen has also been shown to reduce the proportion of stem cells in breast cancer and thus decrease aggressiveness (Simoes et al., 2011).

7.2. Estrogen as treatment of breast cancer: Role of apoptosis

Estrogen is a well-recognized stimulator of breast cancer growth, but recent analysis from the Women's Health Initiative trial showed that estrogen-replacement therapy (ERT) given to hysterectomized women decreased invasive cancer for up to 5 years after ERT was stopped (LaCroix et al., 2011). While high-dose estrogen was successfully used to treat breast cancer in the 1940s (Haddow et al., 1944; Jordan, 2008), the underlying mechanism behind antitumor action of physiologic estrogen is now being understood as estrogen-induced apoptosis (Lewis et al., 2005; Lewis-Wambi & Jordan, 2009; Osipo et al., 2003). Estrogen deprivation induced by long-term SERM therapy results in selection of a SERM-resistant phenotype of breast cancer cells that have adapted by activation of cell survival pathways. When reexposed to pharmacologic or physiologic estrogen, these cells undergo natural cell death (Jordan & Ford, 2011). This important scientific paradigm is being actively evaluated in a phase 3 clinical trial, the Breast International group (BIG1-07) Study Of Letrozole Extension (SOLE), which is evaluating the role of continuous letrozole versus intermittent letrozole following 4–6 years of prior adjuvant endocrine therapy for postmenopausal women with hormone receptor-positive, node-positive early-stage breast cancer. The hypothesis is that letrozole deprivation for up to 3 months will trigger physiologic estrogen-stimulated apoptosis during the drug holiday and thus resensitize tumor cells to letrozole upon reintroduction (Clarke et al., 1997; Colleoni, 2011).

7.3. The role of ERβ in breast cancer

ERβ is widely expressed in the normal breast epithelium in contrast to ERα, but appears to be less important in normal development and function (Roger et al., 2001). ERβ expression is also commonly found to be decreased in breast tumors compared to normal tissue (Paruthiyil et al., 2004). While ERβ is commonly thought to be antiproliferative and proapoptotic, an interesting observation is that overexpression of ERβ in cell lines that are ERα negative, however, is associated with proliferation, invasiveness, and metastasis (Hou et al., 2004; Lazennec, Bresson, Lucas, Chauveau, & Vignon, 2001; Tonetti et al., 2003). While classic ERβ (ERβ1) is the most widely studied, ERβ2/cx, a terminally truncated variant, has also been shown to inhibit ERα activity via heterodimerization and subsequent proteosome-mediated ERα degradation (Ogawa et al., 1998; Zhao et al., 2007). Multiple studies have revealed that high ERβ1 expression, in general, is associated with a better prognosis and increased likelihood of responsiveness to endocrine therapies, but these have mainly focused on tumors that coexpress ERα and ERβ. ERα-negative tumors, however, are not uniformly hormone sensitive, and identifying the nature of ERβ isoforms and its downstream signaling pathways as well as specific response elements is key to differentially targeting ERβ1 (Murphy & Leygue, 2012). ERβ is expressed in at least 20% of triple negative breast cancers, and in these patients, tamoxifen has been shown to improve survival (Gruvberger-Saal et al., 2007). An ongoing single-arm phase 2 clinical trial is evaluating tamoxifen in triple negative, ERβ1-positive women with metastatic breast cancer (Phillips et al., 2012).

7.4. The estrogen-related receptor alpha

The estrogen-related receptor alpha (ERRα) is a member of the orphan nuclear receptor family, which has no known endogenous ligands. ERRα shares a high degree of homology with classic ERα, but does not bind E2 or other natural agonists (Giguere, Yang, Segui, & Evans, 1988). ERRα has a well-recognized role in cellular energy metabolism and other physiological processes (Ranhotra, 2010). ERRα, which is the major isoform in human breast cancer cells, and ERα can bind to similar DNA response elements and can modulate ERα signaling via receptor cross talk. Both receptors can regulate common target genes, such as ps2, which is prognostic marker in breast cancer. The ps2 gene promoter has been found to contain functional ERRE in addition to ERE (Lu, Kiriyama, Lee, & Giguere, 2001; Stein &

McDonnell, 2006). While ERRα expression in breast cancer is associated with poorer outcomes, overexpression of another isoform, ERRγ, is a good prognostic indicator (Ariazi, Clark, & Mertz, 2002). ERRα can induce expression of aromatase gene expression, thus increasing local estrogen production, which may increase the risk of malignant transformation of breast epithelium (Ranhotra, 2010). ERRα has recently been shown to be a downstream target of two tyrosine kinase growth factor receptors: human EGFR2 and the type I insulin-like growth factor receptor. ERRα is thus an appropriate target for pharmacological intervention, and identifying its functional mechanisms can lead to development of targeted therapeutic strategies (Ochnik & Yee, 2012).

REFERENCES

Ali, S., Buluwela, L., & Coombes, R. C. (2011). Antiestrogens and their therapeutic applications in breast cancer and other diseases. *Annual Review of Medicine*, *62*, 217–232.

Ali, S., & Coombes, R. C. (2002). Endocrine-responsive breast cancer and strategies for combating resistance. *Nature Reviews. Cancer*, *2*(2), 101–112.

Allen, E., & Doisy, E. A. (1983). Landmark article Sept 8, 1923. An ovarian hormone. Preliminary report on its localization, extraction and partial purification, and action in test animals. By Edgar Allen and Edward A. Doisy. *Journal of the American Medical Association*, *250*(19), 2681–2683.

Ariazi, E. A., Clark, G. M., & Mertz, J. E. (2002). Estrogen-related receptor alpha and estrogen-related receptor gamma associate with unfavorable and favorable biomarkers, respectively, in human breast cancer. *Cancer Research*, *62*(22), 6510–6518.

Aronica, S. M., Kraus, W. L., & Katzenellenbogen, B. S. (1994). Estrogen action via the cAMP signaling pathway: Stimulation of adenylate cyclase and cAMP-regulated gene transcription. *Proceedings of the National Academy of Sciences of the United States of America*, *91*(18), 8517–8521.

Asselin-Labat, M. L., Shackleton, M., Stingl, J., Vaillant, F., Forrest, N. C., Eaves, C. J., et al. (2006). Steroid hormone receptor status of mouse mammary stem cells. *Journal of the National Cancer Institute*, *98*(14), 1011–1014.

Bannister, A. J., & Kouzarides, T. (1996). The CBP co-activator is a histone acetyltransferase. *Nature*, *384*(6610), 641–643.

Bardou, V. J., Arpino, G., Elledge, R. M., Osborne, C. K., & Clark, G. M. (2003). Progesterone receptor status significantly improves outcome prediction over estrogen receptor status alone for adjuvant endocrine therapy in two large breast cancer databases. *Journal of Clinical Oncology*, *21*(10), 1973–1979.

Baselga, J., Campone, M., Piccart, M., Burris, H. A., 3rd., Rugo, H. S., Sahmoud, T., et al. (2012). Everolimus in postmenopausal hormone-receptor-positive advanced breast cancer. *The New England Journal of Medicine*, *366*(6), 520–529.

Baselga, J., Semiglazov, V., van Dam, P., Manikhas, A., Bellet, M., Mayordomo, J., et al. (2009). Phase II randomized study of neoadjuvant everolimus plus letrozole compared with placebo plus letrozole in patients with estrogen receptor-positive breast cancer. *Journal of Clinical Oncology*, *27*(16), 2630–2637.

Beato, M. (1989). Gene regulation by steroid hormones. *Cell*, *56*(3), 335–344.

Beatson, C. T. (1896a). On treatment of inoperable cases of the mamma: Suggestions for a new method of treatment with illustrative cases. *The Lancet*, *2*, 104–107.

Beatson, C. T. (1896b). On treatment of inoperable cases of the mamma: Suggestions for a new method of treatment with illustrative cases. *The Lancet, 2*, 162–165.

Beekman, J. M., Allan, G. F., Tsai, S. Y., Tsai, M. J., & O'Malley, B. W. (1993). Transcriptional activation by the estrogen receptor requires a conformational change in the ligand binding domain. *Molecular Endocrinology, 7*(10), 1266–1274.

Beeram, M., Tan, Q. T., Tekmal, R. R., Russell, D., Middleton, A., & DeGraffenried, L. A. (2007). Akt-induced endocrine therapy resistance is reversed by inhibition of mTOR signaling. *Annals of Oncology, 18*(8), 1323–1328.

Benhar, M., Engelberg, D., & Levitzki, A. (2002). ROS, stress-activated kinases and stress signaling in cancer. *EMBO Reports, 3*(5), 420–425.

Berstein, L. M., Wang, J. P., Zheng, H., Yue, W., Conaway, M., & Santen, R. J. (2004). Long-term exposure to tamoxifen induces hypersensitivity to estradiol. *Clinical Cancer Research, 10*(4), 1530–1534.

Bjornstrom, L., Kilic, E., Norman, M., Parker, M. G., & Sjoberg, M. (2001). Cross-talk between Stat5b and estrogen receptor-alpha and -beta in mammary epithelial cells. *Journal of Molecular Endocrinology, 27*(1), 93–106.

Bjornstrom, L., & Sjoberg, M. (2005). Mechanisms of estrogen receptor signaling: Convergence of genomic and nongenomic actions on target genes. *Molecular Endocrinology, 19*(4), 833–842.

Blobel, G. A., Sieff, C. A., & Orkin, S. H. (1995). Ligand-dependent repression of the erythroid transcription factor GATA-1 by the estrogen receptor. *Molecular and Cellular Biology, 15*(6), 3147–3153.

Boyd, S. (1897). On Oophorectomy in the treatment of cancer. *British Medical Journal, 2*(1918), 890–896.

Boyd, S. (1899). Remarks on Oophorectomy in the treatment of cancer of the breast. *British Medical Journal, 1*(1988), 257–262.

Boyd, S. (1900). On Oophorectomy in cancer of the breast. *British Medical Journal, 2*, 1161–1167.

Campbell, R. A., Bhat-Nakshatri, P., Patel, N. M., Constantinidou, D., Ali, S., & Nakshatri, H. (2001). Phosphatidylinositol 3-kinase/AKT-mediated activation of estrogen receptor alpha: A new model for anti-estrogen resistance. *Journal of Biological Chemistry, 276*(13), 9817–9824.

Chambliss, K. L., Yuhanna, I. S., Mineo, C., Liu, P., German, Z., Sherman, T. S., et al. (2000). Estrogen receptor alpha and endothelial nitric oxide synthase are organized into a functional signaling module in caveolae. *Circulation Research, 87*(11), E44–E52.

Chung, Y. L., Sheu, M. L., Yang, S. C., Lin, C. H., & Yen, S. H. (2002). Resistance to tamoxifen-induced apoptosis is associated with direct interaction between Her2/neu and cell membrane estrogen receptor in breast cancer. *International Journal of Cancer, 97*(3), 306–312.

Clarke, R. B., Howell, A., Potten, C. S., & Anderson, E. (1997). Dissociation between steroid receptor expression and cell proliferation in the human breast. *Cancer Research, 57*(22), 4987–4991.

Colditz, G. A. (1998). Relationship between estrogen levels, use of hormone replacement therapy, and breast cancer. *Journal of the National Cancer Institute, 90*(11), 814–823.

Cole, M. P., Jones, C. T., & Todd, I. D. (1971). A new anti-oestrogenic agent in late breast cancer. An early clinical appraisal of ICI46474. *British Journal of Cancer, 25*(2), 270–275.

Colleoni, M. (2011). OT2-02-01: The SOLE Trial: International Breast Cancer Study Group (IBCSG 35–07) and Breast International Group (BIG 1–07) Study of Letrozole Extension. *Cancer Research, 71*(Suppl. 24), 610s–611s.

Conneely, O. M., Jericevic, B. M., & Lydon, J. P. (2003). Progesterone receptors in mammary gland development and tumorigenesis. *Journal of Mammary Gland Biology and Neoplasia, 8*(2), 205–214.

Couse, J. F., & Korach, K. S. (1999). Estrogen receptor null mice: What have we learned and where will they lead us? *Endocrine Reviews, 20*(3), 358–417.

Cowley, S. M., Hoare, S., Mosselman, S., & Parker, M. G. (1997). Estrogen receptors alpha and beta form heterodimers on DNA. *Journal of Biological Chemistry, 272*(32), 19858–19862.

Cui, X., Schiff, R., Arpino, G., Osborne, C. K., & Lee, A. V. (2005). Biology of progesterone receptor loss in breast cancer and its implications for endocrine therapy. *Journal of Clinical Oncology, 23*(30), 7721–7735.

Cuzick, J., Sestak, I., Baum, M., Buzdar, A., Howell, A., Dowsett, M., et al. (2010). Effect of anastrozole and tamoxifen as adjuvant treatment for early-stage breast cancer: 10-year analysis of the ATAC trial. *The Lancet Oncology, 11*(12), 1135–1141.

Davies, C., Pan, H., Godwin, J., Gray, R., Arriagada, R., Raina, V., et al. (2013). Long-term effects of continuing adjuvant tamoxifen to 10 years versus stopping at 5 years after diagnosis of oestrogen receptor-positive breast cancer: ATLAS, a randomised trial. *The Lancet, 381*(9869), 805–816.

de Leeuw, R., Neefjes, J., & Michalides, R. (2011). A role for estrogen receptor phosphorylation in the resistance to tamoxifen. *International Journal of Breast Cancer, 2011*, 232435.

deGraffenried, L. A., Friedrichs, W. E., Russell, D. H., Donzis, E. J., Middleton, A. K., Silva, J. M., et al. (2004). Inhibition of mTOR activity restores tamoxifen response in breast cancer cells with aberrant Akt activity. *Clinical Cancer Research, 10*(23), 8059–8067.

Dobrescu, A., Chang, M., Kirtani, V., Turi, G. K., Hennawy, R., & Hindenburg, A. A. (2011). Study of estrogen receptor and progesterone receptor expression in breast ductal carcinoma in situ by immunohistochemical staining in ER/PgR-negative invasive breast cancer. *ISRN Oncology, 2011*, 673790.

EBCTCG (1998). Tamoxifen for early breast cancer: An overview of the randomised trials. Early Breast Cancer Trialists' Collaborative Group. *The Lancet, 351*(9114), 1451–1467.

EBCTCG (2005). Effects of chemotherapy and hormonal therapy for early breast cancer on recurrence and 15-year survival: An overview of the randomised trials. *The Lancet, 365*(9472), 1687–1717.

Enmark, E., Pelto-Huikko, M., Grandien, K., Lagercrantz, S., Lagercrantz, J., Fried, G., et al. (1997). Human estrogen receptor beta-gene structure, chromosomal localization, and expression pattern. *Journal of Clinical Endocrinology and Metabolism, 82*(12), 4258–4265.

Evans, R. M. (1998). The steroid and thyroid superhormone family. *Science, 240*, 889–895.

Fisher, B., Costantino, J. P., Wickerham, D. L., Redmond, C. K., Kavanah, M., Cronin, W. M., et al. (1998). Tamoxifen for prevention of breast cancer: Report of the National Surgical Adjuvant Breast and Bowel Project P-1 Study. *Journal of the National Cancer Institute, 90*(18), 1371–1388.

Flouriot, G., Brand, H., Denger, S., Metivier, R., Kos, M., Reid, G., et al. (2000). Identification of a new isoform of the human estrogen receptor-alpha (hER-alpha) that is encoded by distinct transcripts and that is able to repress hER-alpha activation function 1. *EMBO Journal, 19*(17), 4688–4700.

Forster, C., Makela, S., Warri, A., Kietz, S., Becker, D., Hultenby, K., et al. (2002). Involvement of estrogen receptor beta in terminal differentiation of mammary gland epithelium. *Proceedings of the National Academy of Sciences of the United States of America, 99*(24), 15578–15583.

Gee, A. C., Carlson, K. E., Martini, P. G., Katzenellenbogen, B. S., & Katzenellenbogen, J. A. (1999). Coactivator peptides have a differential stabilizing effect on the binding of estrogens and antiestrogens with the estrogen receptor. *Molecular Endocrinology, 13*(11), 1912–1923.

Giguere, V., Yang, N., Segui, P., & Evans, R. M. (1988). Identification of a new class of steroid hormone receptors. *Nature, 331*(6151), 91–94.

Goss, P. E. (2007). Letrozole in the extended adjuvant setting: MA.17. *Breast Cancer Research and Treatment, 105*(Suppl. 1), 45–53.

Gottardis, M. M., Robinson, S. P., Satyaswaroop, P. G., & Jordan, V. C. (1988). Contrasting actions of tamoxifen on endometrial and breast tumor growth in the athymic mouse. *Cancer Research, 48*(4), 812–815.

Gottlicher, M., Heck, S., & Herrlich, P. (1998). Transcriptional cross-talk, the second mode of steroid hormone receptor action. *Journal of Molecular Medicine (Berlin), 76*(7), 480–489.

Gradishar, W. J. (2004). Tamoxifen—What next? *The Oncologist, 9*(4), 378–384.

Gross, G. E., Clark, G. M., Chamness, G. C., & McGuire, W. L. (1984). Multiple progesterone receptor assays in human breast cancer. *Cancer Research, 44*(2), 836–840.

Gruvberger-Saal, S. K., Bendahl, P. O., Saal, L. H., Laakso, M., Hegardt, C., Eden, P., et al. (2007). Estrogen receptor beta expression is associated with tamoxifen response in ERalpha-negative breast carcinoma. *Clinical Cancer Research, 13*(7), 1987–1994.

Haddow, A., Watkinson, J. M., Paterson, E., & Koller, P. C. (1944). Influence of synthetic oestrogens on advanced malignant disease. *British Medical Journal, 2*(4368), 393–398.

Harper, M. J., & Walpole, A. L. (1967). A new derivative of triphenylethylene: Effect on implantation and mode of action in rats. *Journal of Reproduction and Fertility, 13*(1), 101–119.

Heldring, N., Pike, A., Andersson, S., Matthews, J., Cheng, G., Hartman, J., et al. (2007). Estrogen receptors: How do they signal and what are their targets. *Physiological Reviews, 87*(3), 905–931.

Hewitt, S. C., Harrell, J. C., & Korach, K. S. (2005). Lessons in estrogen biology from knockout and transgenic animals. *Annual Review of Physiology, 67*, 285–308.

Hopp, T. A., Weiss, H. L., Hilsenbeck, S. G., Cui, Y., Allred, D. C., Horwitz, K. B., et al. (2004). Breast cancer patients with progesterone receptor PR-A-rich tumors have poorer disease-free survival rates. *Clinical Cancer Research, 10*(8), 2751–2760.

Horwitz, K. B., & McGuire, W. L. (1975). Predicting response to endocrine therapy in human breast cancer: A hypothesis. *Science, 189*(4204), 726–727.

Hou, Y. F., Yuan, S. T., Li, H. C., Wu, J., Lu, J. S., Liu, G., et al. (2004). ERbeta exerts multiple stimulative effects on human breast carcinoma cells. *Oncogene, 23*(34), 5799–5806.

Huggins, C., & Dao, T. L. (1953). Adrenalectomy and oophorectomy in treatment of advanced carcinoma of the breast. *Journal of the American Medical Association, 151*(16), 1388–1394.

Hyder, S. M., Chiappetta, C., & Stancel, G. M. (1999). Interaction of human estrogen receptors alpha and beta with the same naturally occurring estrogen response elements. *Biochemical Pharmacology, 57*(6), 597–601.

Jeng, M. H., Yue, W., Eischeid, A., Wang, J. P., & Santen, R. J. (2000). Role of MAP kinase in the enhanced cell proliferation of long term estrogen deprived human breast cancer cells. *Breast Cancer Research and Treatment, 62*(3), 167–175.

Jensen, E. V. (1996). Steroid hormones, receptors, and antagonists. *Annals of the New York Academy of Sciences, 784*, 1–17.

Jensen, E. V., & Jacobson, H. I. (1960). Fate of steroid estrogens in target tissues. In G. Pincus & E. P. Vollmer (Eds.), *Biological Activities of Steroids in Relation to Cancer* (pp. 61–174). New York: Academic Press.

Johnston, S. R., Lu, B., Scott, G. K., Kushner, P. J., Smith, I. E., Dowsett, M., et al. (1999). Increased activator protein-1 DNA binding and c-Jun NH2-terminal kinase activity in human breast tumors with acquired tamoxifen resistance. *Clinical Cancer Research, 5*(2), 251–256.

Jordan, V. C. (2003). Tamoxifen: A most unlikely pioneering medicine. *Nature Reviews. Drug Discovery, 2*(3), 205–213.

Jordan, V. C. (2008). The 38th David A. Karnofsky lecture: The paradoxical actions of estrogen in breast cancer—Survival or death? *Journal of Clinical Oncology, 26*(18), 3073–3082.

Jordan, V. C. (2009). A century of deciphering the control mechanisms of sex steroid action in breast and prostate cancer: The origins of targeted therapy and chemoprevention. *Cancer Research, 69*(4), 1243–1254.

Jordan, V. C., Dix, C. J., & Allen, K. E. (1979). The effectiveness of long-term tamoxifen treatment in a laboratory model for adjuvant hormone therapy of breast cancer. *Adjuvant Therapy of Cancer, 2,* 19–26.

Jordan, V. C., & Ford, L. G. (2011). Paradoxical clinical effect of estrogen on breast cancer risk: A "new" biology of estrogen-induced apoptosis. *Cancer Prevention Research (Philadelphia, PA), 4*(5), 633–637.

Jordan, V. C., & O'Malley, B. W. (2007). Selective estrogen-receptor modulators and antihormonal resistance in breast cancer. *Journal of Clinical Oncology, 25*(36), 5815–5824.

Jordan, V. C., Phelps, E., & Lindgren, J. U. (1987). Effects of anti-estrogens on bone in castrated and intact female rats. *Breast Cancer Research and Treatment, 10*(1), 31–35.

Kahlert, S., Nuedling, S., van Eickels, M., Vetter, H., Meyer, R., & Grohe, C. (2000). Estrogen receptor alpha rapidly activates the IGF-1 receptor pathway. *Journal of Biological Chemistry, 275*(24), 18447–18453.

Katzenellenbogen, B. S., & Katzenellenbogen, J. A. (2000). Estrogen receptor transcription and transactivation: Estrogen receptor alpha and estrogen receptor beta: Regulation by selective estrogen receptor modulators and importance in breast cancer. *Breast Cancer Research, 2*(5), 335–344.

Kelsey, J. L., Gammon, M. D., & John, E. M. (1993). Reproductive factors and breast cancer. *Epidemiologic Reviews, 15*(1), 36–47.

Khan, S. A., Rogers, M. A., Khurana, K. K., Meguid, M. M., & Numann, P. J. (1998). Estrogen receptor expression in benign breast epithelium and breast cancer risk. *Journal of the National Cancer Institute, 90*(1), 37–42.

Kirkegaard, T., McGlynn, L. M., Campbell, F. M., Muller, S., Tovey, S. M., Dunne, B., et al. (2007). Amplified in breast cancer 1 in human epidermal growth factor receptor—Positive tumors of tamoxifen-treated breast cancer patients. *Clinical Cancer Research, 13*(5), 1405–1411.

Klinge, C. M., Riggs, K. A., Wickramasinghe, N. S., Emberts, C. G., McConda, D. B., Barry, P. N., et al. (2010). Estrogen receptor alpha 46 is reduced in tamoxifen resistant breast cancer cells and re-expression inhibits cell proliferation and estrogen receptor alpha 66-regulated target gene transcription. *Molecular and Cellular Endocrinology, 323*(2), 268–276.

Kos, M., Reid, G., Denger, S., & Gannon, F. (2001). Minireview: Genomic organization of the human ERalpha gene promoter region. *Molecular Endocrinology, 15*(12), 2057–2063.

Kraus, W. L., Montano, M. M., & Katzenellenbogen, B. S. (1993). Cloning of the rat progesterone receptor gene 5'-region and identification of two functionally distinct promoters. *Molecular Endocrinology, 7*(12), 1603–1616.

Kuiper, G. G., Enmark, E., Pelto-Huikko, M., Nilsson, S., & Gustafsson, J. A. (1996). Cloning of a novel receptor expressed in rat prostate and ovary. *Proceedings of the National Academy of Sciences of the United States of America, 93*(12), 5925–5930.

Kuiper, G. G., Lemmen, J. G., Carlsson, B., Corton, J. C., Safe, S. H., van der Saag, P. T., et al. (1998). Interaction of estrogenic chemicals and phytoestrogens with estrogen receptor beta. *Endocrinology, 139*(10), 4252–4263.

Kumar, P., Wu, Q., Chambliss, K. L., Yuhanna, I. S., Mumby, S. M., Mineo, C., et al. (2007). Direct interactions with G alpha i and G betagamma mediate nongenomic signaling by estrogen receptor alpha. *Molecular Endocrinology, 21*(6), 1370–1380.

Kurokawa, H., & Arteaga, C. L. (2003). ErbB (HER) receptors can abrogate antiestrogen action in human breast cancer by multiple signaling mechanisms. *Clinical Cancer Research*, *9*(1 Pt. 2), 511S–515S.

Kushner, P. J., Agard, D. A., Greene, G. L., Scanlan, T. S., Shiau, A. K., Uht, R. M., et al. (2000). Estrogen receptor pathways to AP-1. *The Journal of Steroid Biochemistry and Molecular Biology*, *74*(5), 311–317.

LaCroix, A. Z., Chlebowski, R. T., Manson, J. E., Aragaki, A. K., Johnson, K. C., Martin, L., et al. (2011). Health outcomes after stopping conjugated equine estrogens among postmenopausal women with prior hysterectomy: A randomized controlled trial. *Journal of the American Medical Association*, *305*(13), 1305–1314.

Lavinsky, R. M., Jepsen, K., Heinzel, T., Torchia, J., Mullen, T. M., Schiff, R., et al. (1998). Diverse signaling pathways modulate nuclear receptor recruitment of N-CoR and SMRT complexes. *Proceedings of the National Academy of Sciences of the United States of America*, *95*(6), 2920–2925.

Lazennec, G., Bresson, D., Lucas, A., Chauveau, C., & Vignon, F. (2001). ER beta inhibits proliferation and invasion of breast cancer cells. *Endocrinology*, *142*(9), 4120–4130.

Le Romancer, M., Poulard, C., Cohen, P., Sentis, S., Renoir, J. M., & Corbo, L. (2011). Cracking the estrogen receptor's posttranslational code in breast tumors. *Endocrine Reviews*, *32*(5), 597–622.

Lee, H., & Bai, W. (2002). Regulation of estrogen receptor nuclear export by ligand-induced and p38-mediated receptor phosphorylation. *Molecular and Cellular Biology*, *22*(16), 5835–5845.

Lemonick, M. D., & Park, A. (2001). New hope for cancer. *Time*, *157*(21), 62–69.

Lerner, L. J., Holthaus, F. J., Jr., & Thompson, C. R. (1958). A non-steroidal estrogen antiagonist 1-(p-2-diethylaminoethoxyphenyl)-1-phenyl-2-p-methoxyphenyl ethanol. *Endocrinology*, *63*(3), 295–318.

Levin, E. R. (2009). Membrane oestrogen receptor alpha signalling to cell functions. *The Journal of Physiology*, *587*(Pt. 21), 5019–5023.

Levin, E. R., & Pietras, R. J. (2008). Estrogen receptors outside the nucleus in breast cancer. *Breast Cancer Research and Treatment*, *108*(3), 351–361.

Levy, N., Tatomer, D., Herber, C. B., Zhao, X., Tang, H., Sargeant, T., et al. (2008). Differential regulation of native estrogen receptor-regulatory elements by estradiol, tamoxifen, and raloxifene. *Molecular Endocrinology*, *22*(2), 287–303.

Lewis, J. S., Osipo, C., Meeke, K., & Jordan, V. C. (2005). Estrogen-induced apoptosis in a breast cancer model resistant to long-term estrogen withdrawal. *The Journal of Steroid Biochemistry and Molecular Biology*, *94*(1–3), 131–141.

Lewis-Wambi, J. S., & Jordan, V. C. (2009). Estrogen regulation of apoptosis: How can one hormone stimulate and inhibit? *Breast Cancer Research*, *11*(3), 206.

Li, Y., Lambert, M. H., & Xu, H. E. (2003). Activation of nuclear receptors: A perspective from structural genomics. *Structure*, *11*(7), 741–746.

Liu, M. M., Albanese, C., Anderson, C. M., Hilty, K., Webb, P., Uht, R. M., et al. (2002). Opposing action of estrogen receptors alpha and beta on cyclin D1 gene expression. *Journal of Biological Chemistry*, *277*(27), 24353–24360.

Liu, S., Ginestier, C., Charafe-Jauffret, E., Foco, H., Kleer, C. G., Merajver, S. D., et al. (2008). BRCA1 regulates human mammary stem/progenitor cell fate. *Proceedings of the National Academy of Sciences of the United States of America*, *105*(5), 1680–1685.

Liu, S., & Wicha, M. S. (2010). Targeting breast cancer stem cells. *Journal of Clinical Oncology*, *28*(25), 4006–4012.

Long, B. J., Jelovac, D., Handratta, V., Thiantanawat, A., MacPherson, N., Ragaz, J., et al. (2004). Therapeutic strategies using the aromatase inhibitor letrozole and tamoxifen in a breast cancer model. *Journal of the National Cancer Institute*, *96*(6), 456–465.

Lorenzo, J. (2003). A new hypothesis for how sex steroid hormones regulate bone mass. *The Journal of Clinical Investigation, 111*(11), 1641–1643.

Love, R. R., & Philips, J. (2002). Oophorectomy for breast cancer: History revisited. *Journal of the National Cancer Institute, 94*(19), 1433–1434.

Lu, D., Kiriyama, Y., Lee, K. Y., & Giguere, V. (2001). Transcriptional regulation of the estrogen-inducible pS2 breast cancer marker gene by the ERR family of orphan nuclear receptors. *Cancer Research, 61*(18), 6755–6761.

Lu, Q., Pallas, D. C., Surks, H. K., Baur, W. E., Mendelsohn, M. E., & Karas, R. H. (2004). Striatin assembles a membrane signaling complex necessary for rapid, nongenomic activation of endothelial NO synthase by estrogen receptor alpha. *Proceedings of the National Academy of Sciences of the United States of America, 101*(49), 17126–17131.

Lubahn, D. B., Moyer, J. S., Golding, T. S., Couse, J. F., Korach, K. S., & Smithies, O. (1993). Alteration of reproductive function but not prenatal sexual development after insertional disruption of the mouse estrogen receptor gene. *Proceedings of the National Academy of Sciences of the United States of America, 90*(23), 11162–11166.

Magee, P. J., & Rowland, I. R. (2004). Phyto-oestrogens, their mechanism of action: Current evidence for a role in breast and prostate cancer. *British Journal of Nutrition, 91*(4), 513–531.

Mamounas, E. P. (2001). Adjuvant exemestane therapy after 5 years of tamoxifen: Rationale for the NSABP B-33 trial. *Oncology (Williston Park), 15*(5 Suppl. 7), 35–39.

Martinez-Climent, J. A., Andreu, E. J., & Prosper, F. (2006). Somatic stem cells and the origin of cancer. *Clinical and Translational Oncology, 8*(9), 647–663.

Massarweh, S., Osborne, C. K., Creighton, C. J., Qin, L., Tsimelzon, A., Huang, S., et al. (2008). Tamoxifen resistance in breast tumors is driven by growth factor receptor signaling with repression of classic estrogen receptor genomic function. *Cancer Research, 68*(3), 826–833.

Mauriac, L., Pippen, J. E., Quaresma Albano, J., Gertler, S. Z., & Osborne, C. K. (2003). Fulvestrant (Faslodex) versus anastrozole for the second-line treatment of advanced breast cancer in subgroups of postmenopausal women with visceral and non-visceral metastases: Combined results from two multicentre trials. *European Journal of Cancer, 39*(9), 1228–1233.

McDonnell, D. P., & Norris, J. D. (2002). Connections and regulation of the human estrogen receptor. *Science, 296*(5573), 1642–1644.

McGuire, W. L., Chamness, G. C., & Fuqua, S. A. (1991). Estrogen receptor variants in clinical breast cancer. *Molecular Endocrinology, 5*(11), 1571–1577.

McKenna, N. J., Lanz, R. B., & O'Malley, B. W. (1999). Nuclear receptor coregulators: Cellular and molecular biology. *Endocrine Reviews, 20*(3), 321–344.

Mehta, R. S., Barlow, W. E., Albain, K. S., Vandenberg, T. A., Dakhil, S. R., Tirumali, N. R., et al. (2012). Combination anastrozole and fulvestrant in metastatic breast cancer. *The New England Journal of Medicine, 367*(5), 435–444.

Menasce, L. P., White, G. R., Harrison, C. J., & Boyd, J. M. (1995). Localization of the estrogen receptor locus (ESR) to chromosome 6q25.1 by FISH and a simple post-FISH banding technique. *Genomics, 17*, 263–265.

Migliaccio, A., Castoria, G., Di Domenico, M., de Falco, A., Bilancio, A., Lombardi, M., et al. (2000). Steroid-induced androgen receptor-oestradiol receptor beta-Src complex triggers prostate cancer cell proliferation. *EMBO Journal, 19*(20), 5406–5417.

Migliaccio, A., Di Domenico, M., Castoria, G., de Falco, A., Bontempo, P., Nola, E., et al. (1996). Tyrosine kinase/p21ras/MAP-kinase pathway activation by estradiol-receptor complex in MCF-7 cells. *EMBO Journal, 15*(6), 1292–1300.

Migliaccio, A., Piccolo, D., Castoria, G., Di Domenico, M., Bilancio, A., Lombardi, M., et al. (1998). Activation of the Src/p21ras/Erk pathway by progesterone receptor via cross-talk with estrogen receptor. *EMBO Journal, 17*(7), 2008–2018.

Miodini, P., Fioravanti, L., Di Fronzo, G., & Cappelletti, V. (1999). The two phyto-oestrogens genistein and quercetin exert different effects on oestrogen receptor function. *British Journal of Cancer, 80*(8), 1150–1155.

Mosselman, S., Polman, J., & Dijkema, R. (1996). ER beta: Identification and characterization of a novel human estrogen receptor. *FEBS Letters, 392*(1), 49–53.

Murphy, L. C., & Leygue, E. (2012). The role of estrogen receptor-beta in breast cancer. *Seminars in Reproductive Medicine, 30*(1), 5–13.

Nilsson, S., Makela, S., Treuter, E., Tujague, M., Thomsen, J., Andersson, G., et al. (2001). Mechanisms of estrogen action. *Physiological Reviews, 81*(4), 1535–1565.

Ochnik, A. M., & Yee, D. (2012). Estrogen-related receptor alpha: An orphan finds a family. *Breast Cancer Research, 14*(3), 309.

Ogawa, S., Inoue, S., Watanabe, T., Orimo, A., Hosoi, T., Ouchi, Y., et al. (1998). Molecular cloning and characterization of human estrogen receptor betacx: A potential inhibitor of estrogen action in human. *Nucleic Acids Research, 26*(15), 3505–3512.

Ordonez-Moran, P., & Munoz, A. (2009). Nuclear receptors: Genomic and non-genomic effects converge. *Cell Cycle, 8*(11), 1675–1680.

Osborne, M. P. (1996). Hormonal intervention in breast cancer. Past, present, and future. *Annals of the New York Academy of Sciences, 784*, 427–432.

Osborne, C. K., Bardou, V., Hopp, T. A., Chamness, G. C., Hilsenbeck, S. G., Fuqua, S. A., et al. (2003). Role of the estrogen receptor coactivator AIB1 (SRC-3) and HER-2/neu in tamoxifen resistance in breast cancer. *Journal of the National Cancer Institute, 95*(5), 353–361.

Osborne, C. K., Coronado-Heinsohn, E. B., Hilsenbeck, S. G., McCue, B. L., Wakeling, A. E., McClelland, R. A., et al. (1995). Comparison of the effects of a pure steroidal antiestrogen with those of tamoxifen in a model of human breast cancer. *Journal of the National Cancer Institute, 87*(10), 746–750.

Osborne, C. K., & Schiff, R. (2011). Mechanisms of endocrine resistance in breast cancer. *Annual Review of Medicine, 62*, 233–247.

Osipo, C., Gajdos, C., Liu, H., Chen, B., & Jordan, V. C. (2003). Paradoxical action of fulvestrant in estradiol-induced regression of tamoxifen-stimulated breast cancer. *Journal of the National Cancer Institute, 95*(21), 1597–1608.

Paech, K., Webb, P., Kuiper, G. G., Nilsson, S., Gustafsson, J., Kushner, P. J., et al. (1997). Differential ligand activation of estrogen receptors ERalpha and ERbeta at AP1 sites. *Science, 277*(5331), 1508–1510.

Pappas, T. C., Gametchu, B., & Watson, C. S. (1995). Membrane estrogen receptors identified by multiple antibody labeling and impeded-ligand binding. *The FASEB Journal, 9*(5), 404–410.

Paruthiyil, S., Parmar, H., Kerekatte, V., Cunha, G. R., Firestone, G. L., & Leitman, D. C. (2004). Estrogen receptor beta inhibits human breast cancer cell proliferation and tumor formation by causing a G2 cell cycle arrest. *Cancer Research, 64*(1), 423–428.

Pedram, A., Razandi, M., Wallace, D. C., & Levin, E. R. (2006). Functional estrogen receptors in the mitochondria of breast cancer cells. *Molecular Biology of the Cell, 17*(5), 2125–2137.

Peter, M. E., & Krammer, P. H. (2003). The CD95(APO-1/Fas) DISC and beyond. *Cell Death and Differentiation, 10*(1), 26–35.

Pettersson, K., Delaunay, F., & Gustafsson, J. A. (2000). Estrogen receptor beta acts as a dominant regulator of estrogen signaling. *Oncogene, 19*(43), 4970–4978.

Phillips, K., Kiely, B. E., Francis, P. A., Boyle, F. M., Fox, S. B., Murphy, L., et al. (2012). ANZ1001 SORBET: Study of estrogen receptor beta and efficacy of tamoxifen, a single arm, phase II study of the efficacy of tamoxifen in triple-negative but estrogen receptor beta-positive metastatic breast cancer. *Journal of Clinical Oncology, 30*(Suppl.), abstr TPS1136.

Prossnitz, E. R., Arterburn, J. B., & Sklar, L. A. (2007). GPR30: A G protein-coupled receptor for estrogen. *Molecular and Cellular Endocrinology, 265–266*, 138–142.

Quaedackers, M. E., van den Brink, C. E., van der Saag, P. T., & Tertoolen, L. G. (2007). Direct interaction between estrogen receptor alpha and NF-kappaB in the nucleus of living cells. *Molecular and Cellular Endocrinology, 273*(1–2), 42–50.

Ranhotra, H. S. (2010). The estrogen-related receptor alpha: The oldest, yet an energetic orphan with robust biological functions. *Journal of Receptor and Signal Transduction Research, 30*(4), 193–205.

Ravdin, P. M., Green, S., Dorr, T. M., McGuire, W. L., Fabian, C., Pugh, R. P., et al. (1992). Prognostic significance of progesterone receptor levels in estrogen receptor-positive patients with metastatic breast cancer treated with tamoxifen: Results of a prospective Southwest Oncology Group study. *Journal of Clinical Oncology, 10*(8), 1284–1291.

Ray, A., Prefontaine, K. E., & Ray, P. (1994). Down-modulation of interleukin-6 gene expression by 17 beta-estradiol in the absence of high affinity DNA binding by the estrogen receptor. *Journal of Biological Chemistry, 269*(17), 12940–12946.

Razandi, M., Oh, P., Pedram, A., Schnitzer, J., & Levin, E. R. (2002). ERs associate with and regulate the production of caveolin: Implications for signaling and cellular actions. *Molecular Endocrinology, 16*(1), 100–115.

Robyr, D., Wolffe, A. P., & Wahli, W. (2000). Nuclear hormone receptor coregulators in action: Diversity for shared tasks. *Molecular Endocrinology, 14*(3), 329–347.

Roger, P., Sahla, M. E., Makela, S., Gustafsson, J. A., Baldet, P., & Rochefort, H. (2001). Decreased expression of estrogen receptor beta protein in proliferative preinvasive mammary tumors. *Cancer Research, 61*(6), 2537–2541.

Russo, J., Ao, X., Grill, C., & Russo, I. H. (1999). Pattern of distribution of cells positive for estrogen receptor alpha and progesterone receptor in relation to proliferating cells in the mammary gland. *Breast Cancer Research and Treatment, 53*(3), 217–227.

Saphner, T., Tormey, D. C., & Gray, R. (1996). Annual hazard rates of recurrence for breast cancer after primary therapy. *Journal of Clinical Oncology, 14*(10), 2738–2746.

Saville, B., Wormke, M., Wang, F., Nguyen, T., Enmark, E., Kuiper, G., et al. (2000). Ligand-, cell-, and estrogen receptor subtype (alpha/beta)-dependent activation at GC-rich (Sp1) promoter elements. *Journal of Biological Chemistry, 275*(8), 5379–5387.

Schiff, R., Massarweh, S. A., Shou, J., Bharwani, L., Mohsin, S. K., & Osborne, C. K. (2004). Cross-talk between estrogen receptor and growth factor pathways as a molecular target for overcoming endocrine resistance. *Clinical Cancer Research, 10*(1 Pt. 2), 331S–336S.

Schinzinger, A. (1889). Über Carcinoma Mammae. *Verhandlungen der Deutschen Gesellschaft für Chirurgie, 18*, 28–29.

Shang, Y., & Brown, M. (2002). Molecular determinants for the tissue specificity of SERMs. *Science, 295*(5564), 2465–2468.

Shoker, B. S., Jarvis, C., Clarke, R. B., Anderson, E., Hewlett, J., Davies, M. P., et al. (1999). Estrogen receptor-positive proliferating cells in the normal and precancerous breast. *American Journal of Pathology, 155*(6), 1811–1815.

Simoes, B. M., Piva, M., Iriondo, O., Comaills, V., Lopez-Ruiz, J. A., Zabalza, I., et al. (2011). Effects of estrogen on the proportion of stem cells in the breast. *Breast Cancer Research and Treatment, 129*(1), 23–35.

Simoncini, T., & Genazzani, A. R. (2003). Non-genomic actions of sex steroid hormones. *European Journal of Endocrinology, 148*(3), 281–292.

Simoncini, T., Hafezi-Moghadam, A., Brazil, D. P., Ley, K., Chin, W. W., & Liao, J. K. (2000). Interaction of oestrogen receptor with the regulatory subunit of phosphatidylinositol-3-OH kinase. *Nature, 407*(6803), 538–541.

Simoncini, T., Rabkin, E., & Liao, J. K. (2003). Molecular basis of cell membrane estrogen receptor interaction with phosphatidylinositol 3-kinase in endothelial cells. *Arteriosclerosis, Thrombosis, and Vascular Biology, 23*(2), 198–203.

Sleeman, J. P., & Cremers, N. (2007). New concepts in breast cancer metastasis: Tumor initiating cells and the microenvironment. *Clinical and Experimental Metastasis, 24*(8), 707–715.

Smith, C. L., & O'Malley, B. W. (2004). Coregulator function: A key to understanding tissue specificity of selective receptor modulators. *Endocrine Reviews, 25*(1), 45–71.

Song, R. X., McPherson, R. A., Adam, L., Bao, Y., Shupnik, M., Kumar, R., et al. (2002). Linkage of rapid estrogen action to MAPK activation by ERalpha-Shc association and Shc pathway activation. *Molecular Endocrinology, 16*(1), 116–127.

Song, R. X., Zhang, Z., & Santen, R. J. (2005). Estrogen rapid action via protein complex formation involving ERalpha and Src. *Trends in Endocrinology and Metabolism, 16*(8), 347–353.

Speirs, V., Skliris, G. P., Burdall, S. E., & Carder, P. J. (2002). Distinct expression patterns of ER alpha and ER beta in normal human mammary gland. *Journal of Clinical Pathology, 55*(5), 371–374.

Stein, R. A., & McDonnell, D. P. (2006). Estrogen-related receptor alpha as a therapeutic target in cancer. *Endocrine-Related Cancer, 13*(Suppl. 1), S25–S32.

Stein, B., & Yang, M. X. (1995). Repression of the interleukin-6 promoter by estrogen receptor is mediated by NF-kappa B and C/EBP beta. *Molecular and Cellular Biology, 15*(9), 4971–4979.

Stoica, G. E., Franke, T. F., Wellstein, A., Czubayko, F., List, H. J., Reiter, R., et al. (2003). Estradiol rapidly activates Akt via the ErbB2 signaling pathway. *Molecular Endocrinology, 17*(5), 818–830.

Tee, M. K., Rogatsky, I., Tzagarakis-Foster, C., Cvoro, A., An, J., Christy, R. J., et al. (2004). Estradiol and selective estrogen receptor modulators differentially regulate target genes with estrogen receptors alpha and beta. *Molecular Biology of the Cell, 15*(3), 1262–1272.

Teyssier, C., Belguise, K., Galtier, F., & Chalbos, D. (2001). Characterization of the physical interaction between estrogen receptor alpha and JUN proteins. *Journal of Biological Chemistry, 276*(39), 36361–36369.

Thurlimann, B., Keshaviah, A., Coates, A. S., Mouridsen, H., Mauriac, L., Forbes, J. F., et al. (2005). A comparison of letrozole and tamoxifen in postmenopausal women with early breast cancer. *The New England Journal of Medicine, 353*(26), 2747–2757.

Toft, D., & Gorski, J. (1966). A receptor molecule for estrogens: Isolation from the rat uterus and preliminary characterization. *Proceedings of the National Academy of Sciences of the United States of America, 55*(6), 1574–1581.

Tonetti, D. A., Rubenstein, R., DeLeon, M., Zhao, H., Pappas, S. G., Bentrem, D. J., et al. (2003). Stable transfection of an estrogen receptor beta cDNA isoform into MDA-MB-231 breast cancer cells. *The Journal of Steroid Biochemistry and Molecular Biology, 87*(1), 47–55.

Torres-Arzayus, M. I., Font de Mora, J., Yuan, J., Vazquez, F., Bronson, R., Rue, M., et al. (2004). High tumor incidence and activation of the PI3K/AKT pathway in transgenic mice define AIB1 as an oncogene. *Cancer Cell, 6*(3), 263–274.

Tremblay, A., Tremblay, G. B., Labrie, F., & Giguere, V. (1999). Ligand-independent recruitment of SRC-1 to estrogen receptor beta through phosphorylation of activation function AF-1. *Molecular Cell, 3*(4), 513–519.

Tsai, M. J., & O'Malley, B. W. (1994). Molecular mechanisms of action of steroid/thyroid receptor superfamily members. *Annual Review of Biochemistry, 63*, 451–486.

Vyhlidal, C., Samudio, I., Kladde, M. P., & Safe, S. (2000). Transcriptional activation of transforming growth factor alpha by estradiol: Requirement for both a GC-rich site and an estrogen response element half-site. *Journal of Molecular Endocrinology, 24*(3), 329–338.

Wakeling, A. E., Dukes, M., & Bowler, J. (1991). A potent specific pure antiestrogen with clinical potential. *Cancer Research, 51*(15), 3867–3873.

Wang, Z., Zhang, X., Shen, P., Loggie, B. W., Chang, Y., & Deuel, T. F. (2005). Identification, cloning, and expression of human estrogen receptor-alpha36, a novel variant of human estrogen receptor-alpha66. *Biochemical and Biophysical Research Communications, 336*(4), 1023–1027.

Webb, P., Lopez, G. N., Uht, R. M., & Kushner, P. J. (1995). Tamoxifen activation of the estrogen receptor/AP-1 pathway: Potential origin for the cell-specific estrogen-like effects of antiestrogens. *Molecular Endocrinology, 9*(4), 443–456.

Webb, P., Nguyen, P., & Kushner, P. J. (2003). Differential SERM effects on corepressor binding dictate ERalpha activity in vivo. *Journal of Biological Chemistry, 278*(9), 6912–6920.

Webb, P., Nguyen, P., Valentine, C., Lopez, G. N., Kwok, G. R., McInerney, E., et al. (1999). The estrogen receptor enhances AP-1 activity by two distinct mechanisms with different requirements for receptor transactivation functions. *Molecular Endocrinology, 13*(10), 1672–1685.

White, R., & Parker, M. G. (1998). Molecular mechanisms of steroid hormone action. *Endocrine-Related Cancer, 5*, 1–14.

Wong, C. W., McNally, C., Nickbarg, E., Komm, B. S., & Cheskis, B. J. (2002). Estrogen receptor-interacting protein that modulates its nongenomic activity-crosstalk with Src/Erk phosphorylation cascade. *Proceedings of the National Academy of Sciences of the United States of America, 99*(23), 14783–14788.

Yamnik, R. L., Digilova, A., Davis, D. C., Brodt, Z. N., Murphy, C. J., & Holz, M. K. (2009). S6 kinase 1 regulates estrogen receptor alpha in control of breast cancer cell proliferation. *Journal of Biological Chemistry, 284*(10), 6361–6369.

Zhang, X. T., Kang, L. G., Ding, L., Vranic, S., Gatalica, Z., & Wang, Z. Y. (2011). A positive feedback loop of ER-alpha36/EGFR promotes malignant growth of ER-negative breast cancer cells. *Oncogene, 30*(7), 770–780.

Zhao, C., Matthews, J., Tujague, M., Wan, J., Strom, A., Toresson, G., et al. (2007). Estrogen receptor beta2 negatively regulates the transactivation of estrogen receptor alpha in human breast cancer cells. *Cancer Research, 67*(8), 3955–3962.

Zhou, Y., Yau, C., Gray, J. W., Chew, K., Dairkee, S. H., Moore, D. H., et al. (2007). Enhanced NF kappa B and AP-1 transcriptional activity associated with antiestrogen resistant breast cancer. *BMC Cancer, 7*, 59.

Zwart, W., de Leeuw, R., Rondaij, M., Neefjes, J., Mancini, M. A., & Michalides, R. (2010). The hinge region of the human estrogen receptor determines functional synergy between AF-1 and AF-2 in the quantitative response to estradiol and tamoxifen. *Journal of Cell Science, 123*(Pt. 8), 1253–1261.

Zwart, W., Griekspoor, A., Berno, V., Lakeman, K., Jalink, K., Mancini, M., et al. (2007). PKA-induced resistance to tamoxifen is associated with an altered orientation of ERalpha towards co-activator SRC-1. *EMBO Journal, 26*(15), 3534–3544.

CHAPTER FOUR

Modulation of Estrogen Receptor Alpha Activity and Expression During Breast Cancer Progression

Gwenneg Kerdivel, Gilles Flouriot, Farzad Pakdel[1]

Institut de Recherche en Santé-Environnement-Travail (IRSET), University of Rennes 1, INSERM U1085, Team TREC, Biosit, Rennes, France

[1]Corresponding author: e-mail address: farzad.pakdel@univ-rennes1.fr

Contents

Abstract

Seventy percent of breast tumors express the estrogen receptor (ER), which is generally considered to predict a better outcome relative to ER-negative tumors, as they often respond to antiestrogen therapies. During cancer progression, mammary tumors can escape from estrogen control, resulting in the acquisition of invasive properties and resistance to treatment. ER expression is a dynamic phenomenon and is finely regulated at numerous levels, including the gene, mRNA, and protein levels. As a consequence, many molecular mechanisms have been implicated in modulating ER activity and estrogen signaling in mammary cancer. In fact, one-third of ER-positive breast cancer cells do not respond to first-line endocrine therapies, and a large subset of relapsing tumors retain ER expression. Increased knowledge of these mechanisms has led to the development of better prognostic methods and targeted therapies for patients; however,

Vitamins and Hormones, Volume 93
ISSN 0083-6729
http://dx.doi.org/10.1016/B978-0-12-416673-8.00004-6

additional research is still needed to improve patient survival. In this chapter, we focus
on the signaling pathways leading to changes in or loss of ER activity in breast cancer
progression.

1. INTRODUCTION

Estrogens, especially estradiol (E2), are essential for mammary gland
development and function. E2 has pleiotropic effects on a wide variety of
physiological pathways, including the growth and differentiation of estrogen
receptor (ER)-expressing epithelial cells. The effects of E2 are mainly mediated through the ER, which is a nuclear receptor that regulates the expression of numerous genes. Two isoforms of ER exist, ERα and ERβ, but ERα
has higher expression in the mammary gland and appears to be the principal
mediator of estrogen action in this tissue. In fact, studies in knockout mice
have highlighted the predominant role of ERα in breast cells. Mature ERα
knockout (ERαKO) mice exhibit a rudimentary structured mammary gland
with no pubertal development, while knockout of ERβ does not have a significant effect on breast development and growth (Couse & Korach, 1999).

Similar to other nuclear receptors, the ER consists of functional and
structural domains. The N-terminal region (domain A/B) includes the
transactivation domain, AF1. The central region (domain C/D) contains
the well-conserved zinc finger DNA-binding domain (DBD) and the
nuclear localization signal. The C-terminal region (domain E/F) contains
the ligand-binding domain (LBD), dimerization sites, the AF2 ligand-
dependent transactivation domain, and cofactor interaction surfaces
(Fig. 4.1). Classically, ligand binding induces dimerization and activation
of the receptor, which then binds to estrogen-responsive elements
(EREs) contained in the promoters of target genes. The conformational
changes in the receptor induced by ligand binding allow the recruitment
of transcriptional coactivators or corepressors, such as CBP/p300, SRC,
and NCOA1, via its AF1 and AF2 domains. However, there is growing evidence suggesting that ERα actions are not just mediated by direct binding to
DNA. In fact, the receptor can also interact with transcription factors, such
as specific protein 1 (Sp1), activator protein 1 (Ap1), or nuclear factor-kappa
B (NFκB), already bound to DNA. These interactions partially explain
why ERα is capable of interacting with gene promoters that do not contain
EREs, which represent one-third of E2-target genes (Stender et al., 2010).

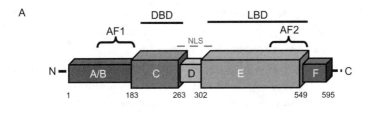

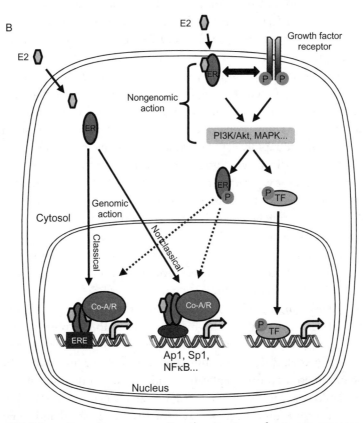

Figure 4.1 Schematic cartoon representing the structure of estrogen receptor alpha and its genomic and nongenomic actions. (A) Schematic structure–activity of human ER alpha. Domains involved in DNA/ligand binding, nuclear localization, ligand-independent transactivation (AF1), and ligand-dependent transactivation (AF2) are shown. (B) The hormone enters the cell and binds to the inactive receptor, either in the cytoplasm or directly in the nucleus. In the nucleus, the activated hormone–receptor complex forms a dimer that binds tightly to DNA directly at the ERE sites or indirectly at the Sp1, Ap1, or NFκB sites. The activated ER is then able to recruit cofactors and RNA polymerase II (pol. II), which allow the transcription of target genes. In addition, ERα can also have nongenomic actions; membrane-bound or cytosolic subsets of the receptor can mediate the activation of intracellular signaling pathways through interactions with

Recently developed technologies, such as chromatin immunoprecipitation followed by high-throughput sequencing, have allowed the identification of thousands of ERα recruitment sites across the genome, which defines its cistrome. Genome-wide studies of ERα binding have led to the conclusion that most ERα-mediated gene regulation is the result of long-range binding of the receptor to distal *cis*-regulatory elements (Carroll et al., 2005). In addition, ERα recruitment patterns are cell-type specific and can differ upon various stimuli. In fact, the ERα cistrome is controlled by the activity of the so-called pioneer factors, such as FOXA1 or GATA3, which are transcription factors capable of interacting with compacted chromatin, thereby modulating chromatin accessibility for other proteins. In addition, both E2 and ERα are able to mediate nongenomic actions that participate in estrogenic effects, which influence the physiology of many target cells and tissues. Indeed, an ER subpopulation is localized to the cytosol or the plasma membrane and is able to rapidly activate intracellular signaling pathways, including MAPK and PI3K, via interactions with adaptor proteins, such as MNAR, or with growth factor receptors, such as IGFR, epidermal growth factor receptor (EGFR), and human epidermal growth factor receptor 2 (HER2). These nongenomic effects modulate the activities of several transcription factors, including ERα itself and its cofactors (Levin & Pietras, 2008; Fig. 4.1). As discussed later in this chapter, these nongenomic actions and cross talk with growth factor receptors are speculated to be involved in resistance to endocrine therapies.

Regardless, binding of E2 to its receptor promotes the proliferation and survival of ER-expressing cells by stimulating the expression of anti-apoptotic and promitotic genes (Boudot, Kerdivel, et al., 2011; Kerdivel, Boudot, & Pakdel, 2013). The mitogenic action of E2 also favors the generation of mutations during replication and, consequently, can participate in tumor transformation (Platet, Cathiard, Gleizes, & Garcia, 2004). More than 70% of mammary tumors are positive for ERα expression and respond to estrogen signals. Moreover, it has been reported that the ERα gene (ESR1) can be amplified in breast cancers, but the frequency of this event is still under debate (Burkhardt et al., 2010; Holst et al., 2008; Moelans

---

adaptor proteins or cross talk with growth factor signaling. This results in the phosphorylation and activation of several transcription factors, including ER itself, and the modulation of the estrogenic response. Abbreviations: DBD, DNA-binding domain; LBD, ligand-binding domain; NLS, nuclear localization signal; P, phosphorylation; ERE, estrogen responsive element; TF, transcription factor; Co-A/R, coactivators or repressors.

et al., 2010). In addition, amplification of ESR1 is often correlated with high ERα expression levels and better responses to endocrine therapies (Holst et al., 2007). On the other hand, ERα also has a role in maintaining a well-differentiated epithelial phenotype that contributes to making ERα-positive tumors less aggressive than ERα-negative tumors. ERα-positive tumors are generally separated from adjacent tissues by a basal layer and grow locally under estrogen stimulation. As a consequence, these tumors are frequently less invasive and metastatic than ERα-negative cancers.

Despite its implications in breast cancer development and progression, expression of ERα is generally a good prognostic marker. Indeed, ERα-expressing tumors are mostly sensitive to endocrine therapies. Currently, most endocrine therapies are targeted at blocking the ER signaling pathway at different levels; one strategy consists of depriving the receptor of estrogen by inhibiting aromatase or by ovarian ablation, while another strategy directly targets the ER with either selective ER modulators, such as tamoxifen, or selective ER downregulators, such as fulvestrant (also known as Faslodex or ICI$_{182,780}$). Endocrine therapies have been shown to be effective for patients with ER-positive tumors and are at least partially responsible for the constant decrease observed in breast cancer mortality over the last few decades (Early Breast Cancer Trialists' Collaborative Group (EBCTCG), 2005; Siegel, Naishadham, & Jemal, 2012). In addition, endocrine therapies are selective and less toxic relative to other anticancer therapies. Unfortunately, patients treated with endocrine therapies will frequently relapse within 15 years and develop endocrine resistance.

Hormonal escape is generally associated with loss of the epithelial phenotype and acquisition of an invasive and migratory phenotype (Bandyopadhyay, Wang, Chin, & Sun, 2007). Tumor cells undergo an epithelial–mesenchymal transition (EMT), followed by local invasion of surrounding tissues. In a second time, cells can enter into the general circulation and migrate to form metastasis. Several components of growth factor pathways are generally overexpressed or overactivated in hormone-resistant breast cancer cells, explaining at least in part the E2-independent proliferation of these cells (Massarweh & Schiff, 2006). The progesterone receptor is also often downregulated in hormone-resistant tumors. One explanation for endocrine therapy resistance is the loss or downregulation of ER, as demonstrated by histology (Allred, Brown, & Medina, 2004). ERα expression, in normal or pathological breast epithelial cells, is finely regulated at numerous stages, including the gene, mRNA, and protein levels. Consequently, many molecular mechanisms may be implicated in the decrease or loss of ERα in mammary cancer. However, approximately 30% of ERα-positive breast cancer cells do not respond to first-line endocrine therapies, and a majority of relapsing tumors still expresses ERα (Gutierrez et al., 2005; Johnston et al., 1995). Thus, it is only logical to postulate the existence of mechanisms that enhance or fully bypass the classical estrogenic response and that result in antiestrogen resistance.

Modulation of estrogen signaling and ERα expression can occur through a variety of both direct and indirect mechanisms, including altered expression, breast cancer stem cells, and cross talk with growth factor signaling pathways. Mechanisms such as these, which can influence ERα activity and response to endocrine therapies during breast cancer tumorigenesis and progression, will be discussed in this chapter (Fig. 4.2).

2. DNA METHYLATION

DNA hypermethylation of cytosine-rich areas, termed "CpG islands," is a common mechanism implicated in the downregulation or misexpression of nuclear receptors. It is now clear that this phenomenon can be involved in the loss of ERα. In fact, the first investigations in this area produced contradictory information on the subject (Falette et al., 1990; Piva et al., 1990). However, with improved understanding and techniques to study epigenetics, increasing evidence suggests that silencing of the ERα gene through methylation can result in *de novo* or acquired loss of ERα expression. Using a DNA methyltransferase assay, Ottaviano et al. (1994) showed increased methyltransferase activity in ERα-negative breast cancer cell lines relative to ERα-positive cell lines. Moreover, they established that ERα negativity was associated with hypermethylation of the proximal promoter of the ERα gene, at least in cell lines. This finding was rapidly confirmed by other studies in a significant fraction of breast tumors (Chen, Ko, Yang, & Jordan, 1998; Ferguson, Lapidus, Baylin, & Davidson, 1995; Lapidus et al., 1996), and CpG island methylation was also observed in the distal promoter and exon 1 of the ERα gene (Iwase et al., 1999; Yoshida et al., 2000). In addition, a recent study suggests that aberrant methylation of the ERα gene could arise predominantly in triple-negative breast tumors (ER-, PR-, and HER2-), but this needs to be confirmed with additional studies (Prabhu et al., 2012). Overall, hypermethylation of the ERα gene is observed in approximately 25% of ER-negative mammary tumors and could serve as

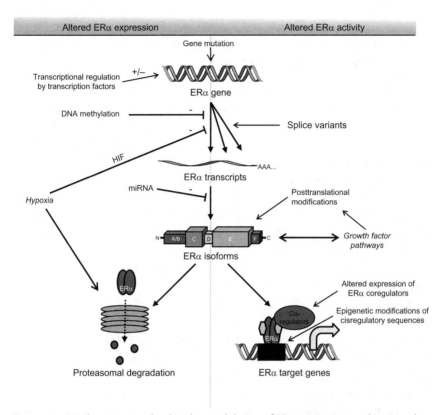

Figure 4.2 Mechanisms involved in the modulation of ERα expression and activity during cancer progression. Control of ERα activity is a dynamic phenomenon that can be influenced by many mechanisms. During cancer progression, gene expression can be silenced by methylation of the ERα promoter, by miRNAs, or by different transcription factors, including HIF. The ERα gene can undergo mutations inside the coding sequences that can either repress or modulate ERα activity. Moreover, splicing variants and posttranslational modifications, which can be mediated by growth factor signaling, can modulate ERα genomic and nongenomic actions. Finally, the estrogen response can also be altered by mechanisms that do not directly target the receptor but are mediated through its coregulators or target genes, such as epigenetic modifications of *cis*-regulatory elements in the promoters or enhancers of these genes.

a marker for poor diagnosis (Yan, Yang, & Davidson, 2001). Interestingly, demethylating drugs, such as 5-aza and deoxyC, induce the reexpression of ERα in the ER-negative MDA-MB-231 cell line. Experiments are already in progress to determine whether demethylating agents or HDAC inhibitors could be used for clinical purposes.

3. ERα TRANSCRIPTIONAL REGULATION BY *cis-* AND *trans-*ACTING ELEMENTS

ERα transcription is regulated by several cell-specific promoters and enhancers that bind a plethora of transcription factors that are differentially expressed in a tissue-specific manner. In breast cancer cells, a major enhancer element at position −3.7 kb is necessary for the increased ERα expression observed in ERα-positive cell lines. Moreover, this sequence, which has been shown to bind the Ap1 transcription factor, is essential for the differential expression of the receptor between ERα-positive and -negative breast cancer cells (Tang, Treilleux, & Brown, 1997). In addition, overexpression of c-jun in MCF-7 cells is accompanied by a downregulation of other fos and jun family members and induces loss of ERα expression and estrogen independence (Smith et al., 1999; Stossi, Madak-Erdoğan, & Katzenellenbogen, 2012).

Other transcription factors have been suggested to induce the loss of estrogen responsiveness by regulating ERα transcription, including ERα itself (Castles, Oesterreich, Hansen, & Fuqua, 1997). Snail, a transcriptional repressor related to the EMT, has been shown to repress ERα expression by directly binding regulatory sequences within the ESR1 locus (Dhasarathy, Kajita, & Wade, 2007). Moreover, the loss of ERα induces the expression of TGF-β, which upregulates Snail and can lead to a self-reinforcing feed-back loop. Another recent study described TWIST1 upregulation during cancer progression as a mechanism of hormonal escape and loss of ERα expression (Vesuna et al., 2011). Indeed, this group demonstrated that TWIST1, after binding to the ERα promoter, induces *de novo* methylation of the ERα gene promoter via recruitment of DNA methyltransferase 3B, which leads to ERα loss and hormone resistance in breast cancer cells. Interestingly, TWIST1 expression is inversely correlated with ERα expression in tumors (Mironchik et al., 2005). Our team has also identified the myocardin-related transcription factor MKL1 (megakaryoblastic leukemia 1, also termed MRTF-A, MAL, or BSAC) as a potential contributor to endocrine resistance. An initial study demonstrated that MKL1 activation results in decreased ERα transcriptional activity (Huet et al., 2008, 2009). Our latest results showed that MKL1 activation could also participate in estrogen independence by repressing ERα at both the mRNA and protein levels and, consequently, allowing breast cancer cells to proliferate without estrogen stimulation.

As described, the transcriptional regulation of ERα is complex and suggests that many factors may contribute to ERα loss if they are deregulated during cancer progression. Molecular identification of these factors could potentially lead to new targeted therapies that may result in ERα reexpression and concomitant antiestrogen responsiveness.

4. ERα GENE MUTATIONS AND SPLICE VARIANTS

The ERα gene is located on chromosome 6q25.1 and consists of eight coding exons. Loss of ERα expression could result from the homologous deletion of this region, but there is currently no evidence corroborating this hypothesis in breast cancer. The regions surrounding the ER gene often exhibit a loss of heterozygosity (LOH), but LOH at the ER gene was only seen in 20% of breast cancers (Iwase et al., 1995). Moreover, no association between LOH at 6q and ERα expression has been reported. To date, only 19 different point mutations have been observed in ERα, including a stop mutation at AA437 (Karnik, Kulkarni, Liu, Budd, & Bukowski, 1994); however, only the K303R and Y537N mutations have been clearly linked with endocrine resistance (Conway et al., 2005; Skliris, Nugent, Rowan, et al., 2010). Overall, approximately 1% of breast tumors exhibit missense mutations within the ERα gene, but the impact of these mutations on ERα expression is still unclear (Murphy, Wang, Coutt, & Dotzlaw, 1996; Roodi et al., 1995). Regardless, mutations in the ER gene do not seem to be a major cause of hormone resistance.

Several ERα mRNA splice variants have been identified in various normal tissues and in tumors, including breast cancer (Herynk & Fuqua, 2004). However, the expression of wild-type ERα was shown to be greater than that of the other spliced variants in 109 breast tumors analyzed (Zhang, Hilsenbeck, Fuqua, & Borg, 1996). Several studies have reported a role for certain splice variants in endocrine therapy resistance. The ERα46 splice variant lacking the AF1 transactivation domain was first described as a dominant-negative variant of ERα in osteoblasts and MCF-7 cells (Denger et al., 2001; Flouriot et al., 2000; Penot et al., 2005). Recently, it has been demonstrated that this variant is downregulated in resistant breast cancer lines. Moreover, overexpression of ERα46 restores the sensitivity of MCF-7 cells to tamoxifen treatment by selectively interfering with several ERα66-mediated transcriptional responses (Klinge et al., 2010). More recently, another splicing variant, ERα36, was identified and quickly correlated with endocrine resistance. This variant lacks the AF1 and AF2 transactivation domains but retains the DBD, the partial dimerization domain, and the LBD (Wang et al., 2005). A dominant-negative activity for this receptor upon ERα66 genomic actions was naturally postulated and rapidly confirmed by the same team (Wang et al., 2006). In addition, they showed that this receptor was predominantly expressed at the plasma membrane and was able to stimulate both E2-dependent and -independent activation of MAPK signaling pathways, resulting in increased cell proliferation. Furthermore, they demonstrated that high ERα36 expression levels in ERα66-positive tumors correlated with poor response to tamoxifen treatment in a cohort of 896 women (Shi et al., 2009).

5. MICRORNA DEREGULATION

The role of miRNA-mediated regulation of ERα is still unclear; however, emerging evidence highlights the role miRNA-specific regulation of protein expression in breast cancers and its impact on estrogen dependence. Indeed, ERα mRNA is characterized by a very long 3′UTR that is more than twice the length of the coding region. The 3′UTR was shown to exert a destabilizing role and mediate the rapid turnover of ERα mRNA (Kenealy et al., 2000), potentially in association with regulatory factors. In 2005, a microarray study revealed aberrant miRNA expression in breast cancer compared with normal breast tissue (Iorio et al., 2005). Moreover, this work also showed significant differences in the expression of a small group of miRNAs in ERα-positive versus ERα-negative tumors. Thus, several *in vitro* studies were performed to define the role of miRNAs in regulating ERα expression. For instance, miR-206, which was shown to be downregulated in ERα-negative cancers, is capable of targeting the 3′UTR of ERα mRNA and thereby decreasing mRNA and protein levels in ERα-positive MCF-7 breast cancer cells (Adams, Cowee, & White, 2009; Adams, Furneaux, & White, 2007; Kondo, Toyama, Sugiura, Fujii, & Yamashita, 2008). Additionally, other studies have shown that miR-22 (Xiong et al., 2010) and miR-221/222 (Di Leva et al., 2010; Zhao et al., 2008) are also involved in the regulation of ERα and have potential roles in ER-positive breast cancer (Xiong, 2012).

The ability of these miRNAs, in addition to miR-18a, miR-18b, miR-193b, and miR-302c, to target the ERα 3′UTR was confirmed by 3′UTR reporter assays in cell lines (Leivonen et al., 2009), but the significance of these findings in tumors have not yet been clearly established. Indeed, a recent report from Yoshimoto et al. only found miR-18a and miR-206 to be upregulated in ERα-negative tumors compared to ERα-positive ones. In this study, miR-193b and miR-221 were downregulated in ERα-negative tumors, and miR-22 and miR-302c expression levels showed no significant differences between ERα-positive and ERα-negative tumors (Yoshimoto et al., 2011). The literature suggests that miRNAs targeting ERα could be responsible for endocrine resistance in some subsets of breast tumors, but additional studies need to be performed to accurately evaluate the importance of specific miRNAs in mediating ER loss in breast tumors.

6. CROSS TALK WITH GROWTH FACTOR RECEPTOR SIGNALING

Control of expression through hyperactive growth factor signaling is another interesting mechanism that could contribute to the loss of ERα. Indeed, ERα-negative tumors generally exhibit high expression of growth factor receptors, and it is now obvious that the expression levels of growth factor receptors, especially HER1/2, and ERα are inversely correlated (Konecny et al., 2003; Lal, Tan, & Chen, 2005). Moreover, it has been shown that overexpression of HER1, HER2 or a constitutively active form of Raf or MEK (MAP/extracellular signal-regulated kinase kinase) in MCF-7 cells leads to estrogen resistance due to the loss of ERα expression (Oh et al., 2001). The same team showed that this loss of ERα was not due to ligand-independent activation of the receptor. The exact mechanism is still unclear but may involve MAPK-dependent activation of NFκB (Holloway, Murthy, & El-Ashry, 2004). In addition, their study and others demonstrated that this process was reversible upon treatment with growth factor receptor or MAPK inhibitors, resulting in ERα reexpression and antiestrogen sensitivity in a subset of ERα-negative breast cancers (Bayliss, Hilger, Vishnu, Diehl, & El-Ashry, 2007). From this observation arose the idea to develop therapeutic strategies targeting the inhibition of both ERα and growth factor signaling for the treatment of estrogen-resistant tumors. Several clinical reports have already demonstrated evidence that treatment with an anti-HER2 agent, such as trastuzumab, induced reexpression of ERα in some patients (Munzone et al., 2006; Xia et al., 2006). Unfortunately, the number of patients was limited, and this observation has to be confirmed in larger cohorts.

Cross talk between ERα and growth factor receptors has also been reported in ERα-positive breast cancer (Gee et al., 2005). This cross talk results in the modulation of ER signaling, which leads to hormone-independent tumor growth, and is considered a major mechanism for resistance to antiestrogen treatments. Overexpression of the EGFR (also known as HER1), the HER2 (also known as ERBB2), and the insulin–like growth factor 1 receptor have also been associated with endocrine resistance (Massarweh et al., 2008). In addition, direct activation of downstream signaling pathways, such as the MAPK or PI3K pathways, has been linked with resistance as well (Kurokawa & Arteaga, 2003). This cross talk between growth factor receptors and ERα can result in ligand-independent activation of ERα signaling pathways, including genomic and nongenomic pathways. Moreover, this cross talk could increase both the sensitivity of ERα to estrogens and its association with coregulators or reduce corepressor recruitment upon antiestrogen treatment.

The best-characterized interaction is that between ERα and the HER2/neu pathway, and it seems to play an important role in mechanisms involved in *de novo* and acquired resistance. HER2 is overexpressed in approximately 20% of patients, and it is coexpressed with ERα in half of these patients (Rexer & Arteaga, 2012).

7. ER POSTTRANSLATIONAL MODIFICATIONS

ERα can be subjected to many posttranslational modifications that can modulate both its activity and its stability (Le Romancer et al., 2011; Fig. 4.3). Indeed, phosphorylation of ERα on various residues is an important

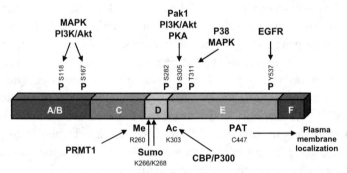

Figure 4.3 Schematic representation of posttranslational modifications involved or suspected to be involved in endocrine resistance. ERα activity can be modulated by different posttranslational modifications at various sites that can result in enhanced activity, ligand-independent activation, or altered stability of the receptor. Modified residues and pathways involved in these modifications are represented, and a palmitoylation site that is involved in anchorage to the plasma membrane is also depicted. Not all of the posttranslational modifications of ERα are listed but only those with known or suspected implications in breast cancer. Abbreviations: P, phosphorylation; Me, methylation; PAT, palmitoylation; Ac, acetylation; Sumo, sumoylation.

mechanism of ligand-independent receptor activation that can result in estrogen independence in breast cancer (Murphy, Seekallu, & Watson, 2011). These phosphorylations and the resulting receptor activation often derive from growth factor receptor-dependent signals, as discussed earlier.

Phosphorylation of S118 and S167, which may result from MAPK and PI3K/Akt pathway activation, is considered good prognostic markers due to their association with low-grade tumors (Bergqvist et al., 2006; Jiang et al., 2007). Although phosphorylation on S167 (P-S167) is accepted as an indicator of a good response to endocrine therapies, conflicting results have associated P-S118 with either good or bad responses to antiestrogen treatment (Murphy, Niu, Snell, & Watson, 2004; Zoubir et al., 2008). Earlier experiments performed in our laboratory identified the orphan nuclear receptor COUP-TF1 as a factor interacting with ERα and enhancing the phosphorylation of ERα on S118 (Métivier et al., 2002). Furthermore, immunochemical assays targeting COUP-TF1 have shown that breast tumor cells express higher levels of COUP-TF1 than normal breast epithelium. Interestingly, overexpression of COUP-TF1 in breast cancer cells leads to estrogen-independent activation of ERα, concomitant with a COUP-TF1-mediated selective modulation of multiple E2-regulated genes that results in E2-independent cell growth, a more invasive breast cancer phenotype and a partial loss of tamoxifen responsiveness (Le Dily et al., 2008). We have recently reviewed other studies that suggest a potential role for the COUP-TF family in cancer progression (Boudot, Le Dily, & Pakdel, 2011). A recent report has identified P-S282 and P-T311 on ERα as markers of good and bad responses to antiestrogens, respectively, but how these phosphorylations function in endocrine resistance is still unclear (Skliris, Nugent, Watson, & Murphy, 2010). In contrast, there are abundant *in vitro* and clinical studies describing a link between the PKA-induced phosphorylation of ERα on S305 and resistance to tamoxifen due to hypersensitivity of the receptor to estrogens (Kok et al., 2011; Zwart et al., 2007). Finally, phosphorylation of ERα on Y537 has recently been associated with a poor clinical outcome in tamoxifen-treated breast cancer patients, but the exact mechanisms are currently unknown (Skliris, Nugent, Rowan, et al., 2010).

Phosphorylation is not the only posttranslational modification of ERα. Le Romancer et al. have recently reported that ERα can be methylated at R260 by arginine N-methyltransferase 1 PRMT1, an ERα coregulator of the PRMT family. This methylation allows ERα to interact with PI3K, SRC, and focal adhesion kinase in the cytosol, leading to activation of Akt (Le Romancer et al., 2008). Overexpression of methylated ERα, in addition to PRMT1 and PRMT9 (FBXO11), was observed in breast tumors, while PRMT2, 5, and 10 were downregulated (Teyssier et al., 2010). This methylation seems to be crucial for kinase recruitment, and because kinase signaling is involved in hormone independence, it is tempting to speculate a role for it in endocrine resistance (Le Romancer, Treilleux, Bouchekioua-Bouzaghou, Sentis, & Corbo, 2010). However, further investigations will be required to evaluate the impact of ERα methylation in cancer progression. Acetylation of ERα K303 involves interactions with histone acetyltransferase activity-containing coregulators, such as CBP/p300 (Wang et al., 2001). Impaired acetylation of this residue, by mutation of the lysine to arginine, for example, triggers S305 phosphorylation and subsequent tamoxifen resistance (Fuqua et al., 2000; Wang et al., 2001). K303R mutations are suspected to be common in breast cancer, as it has been identified in approximately 6% of breast cancers and in up to 70% of samples in certain subgroups (Conway et al., 2005; Herynk et al., 2007). Concerning ERα sumoylation, little is known about its involvement in ERα activity during breast cancer progression, but two sumoylation sites have been identified in the D domain. These sumoylations are ligand dependent and result in an increased transcription of ERα target genes (Sentis, Le Romancer, Bianchin, Rostan, & Corbo, 2005). However, these modifications are triggered by the SUMO-E3 ligase PIAS1 (protein inhibitor of activated STAT) and PIAS3, which are overexpressed in breast cancer (Karamouzis, Konstantinopoulos, Badra, & Papavassiliou, 2008; Wang & Banerjee, 2004).

8. HYPOXIA

Solid tumors, including breast tumors, often exhibit a defective vasculature during disease progression that results in low oxygen levels in the tumor environment. These hypoxic conditions result in the stabilization of HIF-1α, which has been shown to be overexpressed in invasive breast cancers (Bos et al., 2001). Moreover, many reports have established an inverse correlation between ERα and HIF-1α expression (Koda, Kanczuga-Koda, Sulkowska, Surmacz, & Sulkowski, 2010; Yamamoto et al., 2008).

Interestingly, ERα expression is repressed by hypoxia due to the induction of proteasomal degradation of the receptor (Cooper et al., 2004; Kurebayashi, Otsuki, Moriya, & Sonoo, 2001; Stoner et al., 2002). HIF-1α is involved in this mechanism, but it is not yet clear how this effect is mediated. All that is currently known is that hypoxia-induced degradation of ERα does not seem to involve the MAPK or PI3K signaling pathways and that a direct interaction between ERα and HIF-1α is necessary (Cho, Kim, Lee, & Lee, 2005). In addition, a recent study has reported that hypoxia also regulates ERα at the transcriptional level by a mechanism distinct from the one resulting in receptor degradation (Ryu, Park, & Lee, 2011). Thus, the hypoxic environment generated during cancer progression could be responsible for the loss of ERα expression, allowing tumors to become more aggressive.

9. ER COREGULATORS

Increasing evidence suggests that alterations in the expression or activity of coregulators or other signaling factors with which ER interacts contribute to the loss of estrogen responsiveness and tumor progression (Kurebayashi et al., 2000; Murphy et al., 2000). For example, ERα transcriptional activity results from its direct interaction with DNA on ERE or by interaction with other transcription factors that are already bound to DNA, such as Ap1, Sp1, or NFκB. Furthermore, enhanced activity of Ap1 and NFκB has been observed in endocrine-resistant breast cancer cells (Daschner, Ciolino, Plouzek, & Yeh, 1999; Dumont et al., 1996; Zhou, Eppenberger-Castori, Eppenberger, & Benz, 2005; Zhou et al., 2007).

Moreover, increasing evidence has linked the SRC family of ERα coregulators with early relapse and endocrine resistance in ERα-negative and -positive breast cancers (Spears et al., 2012). Overexpression and phosphorylation of the ERα coactivator SRC3, also named AIB1 or NCOA1, have been reported in several breast cancer cell lines and in tumor biopsies (Anzick et al., 1997). These actions result in constitutive ERα-mediating transcription, estrogen-independent growth, and tamoxifen resistance both *in vitro* and in patients (Louie, Zou, Rabinovich, & Chen, 2004). Additionally, proline-, glutamic acid-, and leucine-rich protein 1 (PELP1) has also been shown to be upregulated in breast cancers, especially in estrogen-resistant breast cancers (Vadlamudi & Kumar, 2007). Data suggest that PELP1 acts as a scaffolding protein that mediates ERα interaction with Src kinases, leading to excessive activation of the MAPK pathway and to therapy resistance (Vallabhaneni et al., 2011).

Chan, Lykkesfeldt, Parker, and Dowsett (1999) postulated a downregulation of corepressors in hormonal resistance but failed to provide evidence for dysregulated expression of coregulator genes as a tamoxifen-resistance mechanism. Actually, only NCOR1 has been shown to be associated with tamoxifen resistance in a nude mouse model in which tamoxifen-resistant tumors exhibited lower NCOR1 levels than the tamoxifen-sensitive tumors (Lavinsky et al., 1998). More recently, an analysis of approximately 100 patients demonstrated that NCOR1 expression was necessary for full tamoxifen efficacy in ERα-positive tumors (Girault et al., 2003).

10. BREAST CANCER STEM-LIKE CELLS

Tumors generally contain heterogeneous cellular subpopulations, and there are several lines of evidence that tumors, including breast tumors, contain cancer stem-like cells (CSCs). CSCs are speculated to be responsible for tumorigenesis and can be identified by expression of tissue-specific cell surface markers. In breast tissue, CSCs have been described as enriched in cells with a $CD44^+/CD24^{-/lo}$/epithelial-specific antigen$^+$ surface markers (Al-Hajj, Wicha, Benito-Hernandez, Morrison, & Clarke, 2003). Breast CSCs are believed to be mostly ERα negative and to express mesenchymal genes. As a consequence, these CSCs could exhibit resistance to ERα-targeting therapies and be selected for by these treatments, explaining the resurgence of ERα-negative cancer cells from an initially ERα-positive tumor (Fillmore & Kuperwasser, 2008; Shipitsin et al., 2007). Moreover, there is evidence that the EGFR/HER2 pathways are upregulated in breast CSCs, thus providing a potential explanation for the observed over-expression of these pathways in treatment-resistant cancer (Korkaya, Paulson, Iovino, & Wicha, 2008; Yan et al., 2012). For a detailed discussion on this subject, see the recent review from O'Brien, Farnie, Howell, and Clarke (2011). Hence, the stem cell theory has given new insights into the tumorigenesis and progression of breast cancers by providing an additional potential mechanism for endocrine resistance.

11. PIONEER FACTORS AND ENDOCRINE-RESISTANT SPECIFIC CISTROMES

As previously described, ERα-binding events depend on the action of pioneer factors that modulate chromatin compaction to permit ERα recruitment to specifics sites (Carroll et al., 2005). Considering the newly discovered importance of these factors, especially FOXA1, in hormone-dependent cancer and in epithelial differentiation of breast cancer, a role for these factors in tumor progression and endocrine resistance has been speculated.

In fact, evidence corroborating this hypothesis has recently been reported; Hurtado and colleagues demonstrated that FOXA1 was required for estrogen–ER function and for tamoxifen–ER function (Hurtado, Holmes, Ross-Innes, Schmidt, & Carroll, 2011). Thus, an ERα-positive tumor expressing low levels of FOXA1 could have low ERα activity and, consequently, exhibit a poor response to tamoxifen. Until recently, all of the genome-wide studies of ERα-binding events were conducted in cell lines, mainly in the ERα-positive MCF-7 cell line, but Carroll's team at Cambridge University conducted the first ERα mapping study in tumors from patients (Ross-Innes et al., 2012). They showed that tumors with differential clinical outcomes display distinct ERα-recruitment patterns. These patterns were dependent on FOXA1 recruitment, but there is currently no explanation for the mechanisms regulating FOXA1 binding during cancer progression.

FOXA1 permits the recruitment of ERα to nearly 50% of its cistrome. However, ERα is also recruited to a large number of FOXA1-independent sites, and a role for other pioneer factors in guiding ERα recruitment to these locations was speculated. One such candidate is PBX1, which has also been described as essential for the estrogen response in ERα-positive breast cancers. In addition, high PBX1 expression levels were correlated with poor metastasis-free survival compared to tumors with low PBX1 expression (Magnani, Ballantyne, Zhang, & Lupien, 2011). As patients with metastatic ERα-positive breast cancer develop endocrine resistance, the authors speculated that there was a role for PBX1 in the resistance to hormonal therapies as well.

12. CONCLUSIONS AND FUTURE DIRECTIONS

ERα expression and activity are dynamic phenomena during cancer progression. Considering the importance of this factor in driving estrogen responsiveness, ERα is a critical determinant of breast cancer progression and a key target for breast cancer treatments. Endocrine therapies targeting ERα have certainly improved the clinical outcome for a large proportion of ERα-positive cancer patients, but the existence of innate or *de novo* estrogen resistance is a major clinical problem. Considering that resistance to endocrine therapies is the most common cause of breast cancer death, endocrine resistance has been and still is the focus of much research.

As reviewed in this chapter, the regulation of ERα can occur at many levels, and consequently, hormonal resistance can result from a vast variety of mechanisms. Improving the knowledge regarding these mechanisms will lead to the development of better prognostic methods and targeted therapies with greater efficacy for patients with phenotypically different tumors. New emerging tests will allow for the characterization of tumor phenotypes before the beginning of treatment so that the therapeutic protocols can be adjusted as necessary. Moreover, cancer cells are heterogeneous, and the presence of estrogen-dependent and -independent cells in some patients can be responsible for relapse, highlighting the necessity to adapt the treatment protocols during therapy to affect all of the subpopulations of cancer cells inside the tumor, including breast cancer stem cells.

There is no doubt that the recent identification of breast cancer stem cells will lead to new concepts in breast tumorigenesis and new approaches for therapy. Furthermore, drugs targeting epigenetic modifications, such as DNA methylation and histone methylation or acetylation, have been shown to be effective in differentiating cells, including CSCs, resulting in ERα reexpression and sensitivity to endocrine therapy. Clinical trials using such combinations are currently in progress and provide promising hope for patients with ERα-positive and -negative tumors.

ACKNOWLEDGMENTS

This work was supported by fellowships from Région Bretagne, INSERM and CNRS, La Ligue Contre le Cancer, the University of Rennes 1, and the European University of Brittany.

REFERENCES

Adams, B. D., Cowee, D. M., & White, B. A. (2009). The role of miR-206 in the epidermal growth factor (EGF) induced repression of estrogen receptor-alpha (ERalpha) signaling and a luminal phenotype in MCF-7 breast cancer cells. *Molecular Endocrinology, 23,* 1215–1230.

Adams, B. D., Furneaux, H., & White, B. A. (2007). The micro-ribonucleic acid (miRNA) miR-206 targets the human estrogen receptor-alpha (ERalpha) and represses ERalpha messenger RNA and protein expression in breast cancer cell lines. *Molecular Endocrinology, 21,* 1132–1147.

Al-Hajj, M., Wicha, M. S., Benito-Hernandez, A., Morrison, S. J., & Clarke, M. F. (2003). Prospective identification of tumorigenic breast cancer cells. *Proceedings of the National Academy of Sciences of the United States of America, 100,* 3983–3988.

Allred, D. C., Brown, P., & Medina, D. (2004). The origins of estrogen receptor alpha-positive and estrogen receptor alpha-negative human breast cancer. *Breast Cancer Research, 6,* 240–245.

Anzick, S. L., Kononen, J., Walker, R. L., Azorsa, D. O., Tanner, M. M., Guan, X. Y., et al. (1997). AIB1, a steroid receptor coactivator amplified in breast and ovarian cancer. *Science, 277,* 965–968.

Bandyopadhyay, A., Wang, L., Chin, S. H., & Sun, L.-Z. (2007). Inhibition of skeletal metastasis by ectopic ERalpha expression in ERalpha-negative human breast cancer cell lines. *Neoplasia*, 9, 113–118.

Bayliss, J., Hilger, A., Vishnu, P., Diehl, K., & El-Ashry, D. (2007). Reversal of the estrogen receptor negative phenotype in breast cancer and restoration of antiestrogen response. *Clinical Cancer Research*, 13, 7029–7036.

Bergqvist, J., Elmberger, G., Ohd, J., Linderholm, B., Bjohle, J., Hellborg, H., et al. (2006). Activated ERK1/2 and phosphorylated oestrogen receptor alpha are associated with improved breast cancer survival in women treated with tamoxifen. *European Journal of Cancer*, 42, 1104–1112.

Bos, R., Zhong, H., Hanrahan, C. F., Mommers, E. C., Semenza, G. L., Pinedo, H. M., et al. (2001). Levels of hypoxia-inducible factor-1 alpha during breast carcinogenesis. *Journal of the National Cancer Institute*, 93, 309–314.

Boudot, A., Kerdivel, G., Habauzit, D., Eeckhoute, J., Le Dily, F., Flouriot, G., et al. (2011). Differential estrogen-regulation of CXCL12 chemokine receptors, CXCR4 and CXCR7, contributes to the growth effect of estrogens in breast cancer cells. *PLoS One*, 6, e20898.

Boudot, A., Le Dily, F., & Pakdel, F. (2011). Involvement of COUP-TFs in cancer progression. *Cancers*, 3, 700–715.

Burkhardt, L., Grob, T. J., Hermann, I., Burandt, E., Choschzick, M., Jänicke, F., et al. (2010). Gene amplification in ductal carcinoma in situ of the breast. *Breast Cancer Research and Treatment*, 123, 757–765.

Carroll, J. S., Liu, X. S., Brodsky, A. S., Li, W., Meyer, C. A., Szary, A. J., et al. (2005). Chromosome-wide mapping of estrogen receptor binding reveals long-range regulation requiring the forkhead protein FoxA1. *Cell*, 122, 33–43.

Castles, C. G., Oesterreich, S., Hansen, R., & Fuqua, S. A. (1997). Auto-regulation of the estrogen receptor promoter. *The Journal of Steroid Biochemistry and Molecular Biology*, 62, 155–163.

Chan, C. M., Lykkesfeldt, A. E., Parker, M. G., & Dowsett, M. (1999). Expression of nuclear receptor interacting proteins TIF-1, SUG-1, receptor interacting protein 140, and corepressor SMRT in tamoxifen-resistant breast cancer. *Clinical Cancer Research*, 5, 3460–3467.

Chen, Z., Ko, A., Yang, J., & Jordan, V. C. (1998). Methylation of CpG island is not a ubiquitous mechanism for the loss of oestrogen receptor in breast cancer cells. *British Journal of Cancer*, 77, 181–185.

Cho, J., Kim, D., Lee, S., & Lee, Y. (2005). Cobalt chloride-induced estrogen receptor A down-regulation involves hypoxia-inducible factor-1α in MCF-7 human breast cancer cells. *Molecular Endocrinology*, 19, 1191–1199.

Conway, K., Parrish, E., Edmiston, S. N., Tolbert, D., Tse, C.-K. , Geradts, J., et al. (2005). The estrogen receptor-alpha A908G (K303R) mutation occurs at a low frequency in invasive breast tumors: Results from a population-based study. *Breast Cancer Research*, 7, R871–R880.

Cooper, C., Liu, G.-Y. , Niu, Y.-L. , Santos, S., Murphy, L. C., & Watson, P. H. (2004). Intermittent hypoxia induces proteasome-dependent down-regulation of estrogen receptor alpha in human breast carcinoma. *Clinical Cancer Research*, 10, 8720–8727.

Couse, J. F., & Korach, K. S. (1999). Reproductive phenotypes in the estrogen receptor-alpha knockout mouse. *Annales d'Endocrinologie*, 60, 143–148.

Daschner, P. J., Ciolino, H. P., Plouzek, C. A., & Yeh, G. C. (1999). Increased AP-1 activity in drug resistant human breast cancer MCF-7 cells. *Breast Cancer Research and Treatment*, 53, 229–240.

Denger, S., Reid, G., Kos, M., Flouriot, G., Parsch, D., Brand, H., et al. (2001). ERalpha gene expression in human primary osteoblasts: Evidence for the expression of two receptor proteins. *Molecular Endocrinology*, 15, 2064–2077.

Dhasarathy, A., Kajita, M., & Wade, P. A. (2007). The transcription factor snail mediates epithelial to mesenchymal transitions by repression of estrogen receptor-alpha. *Molecular Endocrinology, 21*, 2907–2918.

Di Leva, G., Gasparini, P., Piovan, C., Ngankeu, A., Garofalo, M., Taccioli, C., et al. (2010). MicroRNA cluster 221-222 and estrogen receptor alpha interactions in breast cancer. *Journal of the National Cancer Institute, 102*, 706–721.

Dumont, J. A., Bitonti, A. J., Wallace, C. D., Baumann, R. J., Cashman, E. A., & Cross-Doersen, D. E. (1996). Progression of MCF-7 breast cancer cells to antiestrogen-resistant phenotype is accompanied by elevated levels of AP-1 DNA-binding activity. *Cell Growth & Differentiation, 7*, 351–359.

Early Breast Cancer Trialists' Collaborative Group (EBCTCG), (2005). Effects of chemotherapy and hormonal therapy for early breast cancer on recurrence and 15-year survival: An overview of the randomised trials, 14. *Lancet, 365*, 1687–1717.

Falette, N. S., Fuqua, S. A., Chamness, G. C., Cheah, M. S., Greene, G. L., & McGuire, W. L. (1990). Estrogen receptor gene methylation in human breast tumors. *Cancer Research, 50*, 3974–3978.

Ferguson, A. T., Lapidus, R. G., Baylin, S. B., & Davidson, N. E. (1995). Demethylation of the estrogen receptor gene in estrogen receptor-negative breast cancer cells can reactivate estrogen receptor gene expression. *Cancer Research, 55*, 2279–2283.

Fillmore, C. M., & Kuperwasser, C. (2008). Human breast cancer cell lines contain stem-like cells that self-renew, give rise to phenotypically diverse progeny and survive chemotherapy. *Breast Cancer Research, 10*, R25.

Flouriot, G., Brand, H., Denger, S., Metivier, R., Kos, M., Reid, G., et al. (2000). Identification of a new isoform of the human estrogen receptor-alpha (hER-alpha) that is encoded by distinct transcripts and that is able to repress hER-alpha activation function 1. *The EMBO Journal, 19*, 4688–4700.

Fuqua, S. A., Wiltschke, C., Zhang, Q. X., Borg, A., Castles, C. G., Friedrichs, W. E., et al. (2000). A hypersensitive estrogen receptor-alpha mutation in premalignant breast lesions. *Cancer Research, 60*, 4026–4029.

Gee, J. M., Robertson, J. F., Gutteridge, E., Ellis, I. O., Pinder, S. E., Rubini, M., et al. (2005). Epidermal growth factor receptor/HER2/insulin-like growth factor receptor signalling and oestrogen receptor activity in clinical breast cancer. *Endocrine-Related Cancer, 12*(Suppl. 1), S99–S111.

Girault, I., Lerebours, F., Amarir, S., Tozlu, S., Tubiana-Hulin, M., Lidereau, R., et al. (2003). Expression analysis of estrogen receptor alpha coregulators in breast carcinoma: Evidence that NCOR1 expression is predictive of the response to tamoxifen. *Clinical Cancer Research, 9*, 1259–1266.

Gutierrez, M. C., Detre, S., Johnston, S., Mohsin, S. K., Shou, J., Allred, D. C., et al. (2005). Molecular changes in tamoxifen-resistant breast cancer: Relationship between estrogen receptor, HER-2, and p38 mitogen-activated protein kinase. *Journal of Clinical Oncology, 23*, 2469–2476.

Herynk, M. H., & Fuqua, S. A. W. (2004). Estrogen receptor mutations in human disease. *Endocrine Reviews, 25*, 869–898.

Herynk, M. H., Parra, I., Cui, Y., Beyer, A., Wu, M.-F. , Hilsenbeck, S. G., et al. (2007). Association between the estrogen receptor alpha A908G mutation and outcomes in invasive breast cancer. *Clinical Cancer Research, 13*, 3235–3243.

Holloway, J. N., Murthy, S., & El-Ashry, D. (2004). A cytoplasmic substrate of mitogen-activated protein kinase is responsible for estrogen receptor-alpha down-regulation in breast cancer cells: The role of nuclear factor-kappaB. *Molecular Endocrinology, 18*, 1396–1410.

Holst, F., Stahl, P., Hellwinkel, O., Dancau, A.-M. , Krohn, A., Wuth, L., et al. (2008). Reply to "ESR1 gene amplification in breast cancer: A common phenomenon?". *Nature Genetics, 40*, 810–812

Holst, F., Stahl, P. R., Ruiz, C., Hellwinkel, O., Jehan, Z., Wendland, M., et al. (2007). Estrogen receptor alpha (ESR1) gene amplification is frequent in breast cancer. *Nature Genetics*, *39*, 655–660.

Huet, G., Mérot, Y., Le Dily, F., Kern, L., Ferrière, F., Saligaut, C., et al. (2008). Loss of E-cadherin-mediated cell contacts reduces estrogen receptor alpha (ER alpha) transcriptional efficiency by affecting the respective contribution exerted by AF1 and AF2 transactivation functions. *Biochemical and Biophysical Research Communications*, *365*, 304–309.

Huet, G., Mérot, Y., Percevault, F., Tiffoche, C., Arnal, J.-F. , Boujrad, N., et al. (2009). Repression of the estrogen receptor-alpha transcriptional activity by the Rho/ megakaryoblastic leukemia 1 signaling pathway. *The Journal of Biological Chemistry*, *284*, 33729–33739.

Hurtado, A., Holmes, K. A., Ross-Innes, C. S., Schmidt, D., & Carroll, J. S. (2011). FOXA1 is a key determinant of estrogen receptor function and endocrine response. *Nature Genetics*, *43*, 27–33.

Iorio, M. V., Ferracin, M., Liu, C.-G. , Veronese, A., Spizzo, R., Sabbioni, S., et al. (2005). MicroRNA gene expression deregulation in human breast cancer. *Cancer Research*, *65*, 7065–7070.

Iwase, H., Greenman, J. M., Barnes, D. M., Bobrow, L., Hodgson, S., & Mathew, C. G. (1995). Loss of heterozygosity of the oestrogen receptor gene in breast cancer. *British Journal of Cancer*, *71*, 448–450.

Iwase, H., Omoto, Y., Iwata, H., Toyama, T., Hara, Y., Ando, Y., et al. (1999). DNA methylation analysis at distal and proximal promoter regions of the oestrogen receptor gene in breast cancers. *British Journal of Cancer*, *80*, 1982–1986.

Jiang, J., Sarwar, N., Peston, D., Kulinskaya, E., Shousha, S., Coombes, R. C., et al. (2007). Phosphorylation of estrogen receptor-alpha at Ser167 is indicative of longer disease-free and overall survival in breast cancer patients. *Clinical Cancer Research*, *13*, 5769–5776.

Johnston, S. R. D., Saccani-Jotti, G., Smith, I. E., Salter, J., Newby, J., Coppen, M., et al. (1995). Changes in estrogen receptor, progesterone receptor, and pS2 expression in tamoxifen-resistant human breast cancer. *Cancer Research*, *55*, 3331–3338.

Karamouzis, M. V., Konstantinopoulos, P. A., Badra, F. A., & Papavassiliou, A. G. (2008). SUMO and estrogen receptors in breast cancer. *Breast Cancer Research and Treatment*, *107*, 195–210.

Karnik, P. S., Kulkarni, S., Liu, X. P., Budd, G. T., & Bukowski, R. M. (1994). Estrogen receptor mutations in tamoxifen-resistant breast cancer. *Cancer Research*, *54*, 349–353.

Kenealy, M.-R. , Flouriot, G., Sonntag-Buck, V., Dandekar, T., Brand, H., & Gannon, F. (2000). The 3′-untranslated region of the human estrogen receptor A gene mediates rapid messenger ribonucleic acid turnover. *Endocrinology*, *141*, 2805–2813.

Kerdivel, G., Boudot, A., & Pakdel, F. (2013). Estrogen represses CXCR7 gene expression by inhibiting the recruitment of NFκB transcription factor at the CXCR7 promoter in breast cancer cells. *Biochemical and Biophysical Research Communications*, *431*, 729–733.

Klinge, C. M., Riggs, K. A., Wickramasinghe, N. S., Emberts, C. G., McConda, D. B., Barry, P. N., et al. (2010). Estrogen receptor alpha 46 is reduced in tamoxifen resistant breast cancer cells and re-expression inhibits cell proliferation and estrogen receptor alpha 66-regulated target gene transcription. *Molecular and Cellular Endocrinology*, *323*, 268–276.

Koda, M., Kanczuga-Koda, L., Sulkowska, M., Surmacz, E., & Sulkowski, S. (2010). Relationships between hypoxia markers and the leptin system, estrogen receptors in human primary and metastatic breast cancer: Effects of preoperative chemotherapy. *BMC Cancer*, *10*, 320.

Kok, M., Zwart, W., Holm, C., Fles, R., Hauptmann, M., Van't Veer, L. J., et al. (2011). PKA-induced phosphorylation of ERα at serine 305 and high PAK1 levels is associated with sensitivity to tamoxifen in ER-positive breast cancer. *Breast Cancer Research and Treatment*, *125*, 1–12.

Kondo, N., Toyama, T., Sugiura, H., Fujii, Y., & Yamashita, H. (2008). miR-206 expression is down-regulated in estrogen receptor alpha-positive human breast cancer. *Cancer Research*, *68*, 5004–5008.

Konecny, G., Pauletti, G., Pegram, M., Untch, M., Dandekar, S., Aguilar, Z., et al. (2003). Quantitative association between HER-2/neu and steroid hormone receptors in hormone receptor-positive primary breast cancer. *Journal of the National Cancer Institute*, *95*, 142–153.

Korkaya, H., Paulson, A., Iovino, F., & Wicha, M. S. (2008). HER2 regulates the mammary stem/progenitor cell population driving tumorigenesis and invasion. *Oncogene*, *27*, 6120–6130.

Kurebayashi, J., Otsuki, T., Kunisue, H., Tanaka, K., Yamamoto, S., & Sonoo, H. (2000). Expression levels of estrogen receptor-alpha, estrogen receptor-beta, coactivators, and corepressors in breast cancer. *Clinical Cancer Research*, *6*, 512–518.

Kurebayashi, J., Otsuki, T., Moriya, T., & Sonoo, H. (2001). Hypoxia reduces hormone responsiveness of human breast cancer cells. *Japanese Journal of Cancer Research*, *92*, 1093–1101.

Kurokawa, H., & Arteaga, C. L. (2003). ErbB (HER) receptors can abrogate antiestrogen action in human breast cancer by multiple signaling mechanisms. *Clinical Cancer Research*, *9*, 511S–515S.

Lal, P., Tan, L. K., & Chen, B. (2005). Correlation of HER-2 status with estrogen and progesterone receptors and histologic features in 3,655 invasive breast carcinomas. *American Journal of Clinical Pathology*, *123*, 541–546.

Lapidus, R. G., Ferguson, A. T., Ottaviano, Y. L., Parl, F. F., Smith, H. S., Weitzman, S. A., et al. (1996). Methylation of estrogen and progesterone receptor gene 5′ CpG islands correlates with lack of estrogen and progesterone receptor gene expression in breast tumors. *Clinical Cancer Research*, *2*, 805–810.

Lavinsky, R. M., Jepsen, K., Heinzel, T., Torchia, J., Mullen, T.-M. , Schiff, R., et al. (1998). Diverse signaling pathways modulate nuclear receptor recruitment of N-CoR and SMRT complexes. *PNAS*, *95*, 2920–2925.

Le Dily, F., Métivier, R., Guéguen, M.-M. , Le Péron, C., Flouriot, G., Tas, P., et al. (2008). COUP-TFI modulates estrogen signaling and influences proliferation, survival and migration of breast cancer cells. *Breast Cancer Research and Treatment*, *110*, 69–83.

Le Romancer, M., Poulard, C., Cohen, P., Sentis, S., Renoir, J.-M. , & Corbo, L. (2011). Cracking the estrogen receptor's posttranslational code in breast tumors. *Endocrine Reviews*, *32*, 597–622.

Le Romancer, M., Treilleux, I., Bouchekioua-Bouzaghou, K., Sentis, S., & Corbo, L. (2010). Methylation, a key step for nongenomic estrogen signaling in breast tumors. *Steroids*, *75*, 560–564.

Le Romancer, M., Treilleux, I., Leconte, N., Robin-Lespinasse, Y., Sentis, S., Bouchekioua-Bouzaghou, K., et al. (2008). Regulation of estrogen rapid signaling through arginine methylation by PRMT1. *Molecular Cell*, *31*, 212–221.

Leivonen, S.-K. , Mäkelä, R., Ostling, P., Kohonen, P., Haapa-Paananen, S., Kleivi, K., et al. (2009). Protein lysate microarray analysis to identify microRNAs regulating estrogen receptor signaling in breast cancer cell lines. *Oncogene*, *28*, 3926–3936.

Levin, E., & Pietras, R. (2008). Estrogen receptors outside the nucleus in breast cancer. *Breast Cancer Research and Treatment*, *108*, 351–361.

Louie, M. C., Zou, J. X., Rabinovich, A., & Chen, H.-W. (2004). ACTR/AIB1 functions as an E2F1 coactivator to promote breast cancer cell proliferation and antiestrogen resistance. *Molecular and Cellular Biology*, *24*, 5157–5171.

Magnani, L., Ballantyne, E. B., Zhang, X., & Lupien, M. (2011). PBX1 genomic pioneer function drives ERα signaling underlying progression in breast cancer. *PLoS Genetics*, *7*, e1002368.

Massarweh, S., Osborne, C. K., Creighton, C. J., Qin, L., Tsimelzon, A., Huang, S., et al. (2008). Tamoxifen resistance in breast tumors is driven by growth factor receptor signaling with repression of classic estrogen receptor genomic function. *Cancer Research, 68,* 826–833.

Massarweh, S., & Schiff, R. (2006). Resistance to endocrine therapy in breast cancer: Exploiting estrogen receptor/growth factor signaling crosstalk. *Endocrine-Related Cancer, 13*(Suppl. 1), S15–S24.

Métivier, R., Gay, F. A., Hübner, M. R., Flouriot, G., Salbert, G., Gannon, F., et al. (2002). Formation of an hER alpha-COUP-TFI complex enhances hER alpha AF-1 through Ser118 phosphorylation by MAPK. *The EMBO Journal, 21,* 3443–3453.

Mironchik, Y., Winnard, P. T., Jr., Vesuna, F., Kato, Y., Wildes, F., Pathak, A. P., et al. (2005). Twist overexpression induces in vivo angiogenesis and correlates with chromosomal instability in breast cancer. *Cancer Research, 65,* 10801–10809.

Moelans, C. B., Monsuur, H. N., de Pinth, J. H., Radersma, R. D., de Weger, R. A., & van Diest, P. J. (2010). ESR1 amplification is rare in breast cancer and is associated with high grade and high proliferation: A multiplex ligation-dependent probe amplification study. *Analytical Cellular Pathology (Amsterdam), 33,* 13–18.

Munzone, E., Curigliano, G., Rocca, A., Bonizzi, G., Renne, G., Goldhirsch, A., et al. (2006). Reverting estrogen-receptor-negative phenotype in HER-2-overexpressing advanced breast cancer patients exposed to trastuzumab plus chemotherapy. *Breast Cancer Research, 8,* R4.

Murphy, L. C., Niu, Y., Snell, L., & Watson, P. (2004). Phospho-serine-118 estrogen receptor-alpha expression is associated with better disease outcome in women treated with tamoxifen. *Clinical Cancer Research, 10,* 5902–5906.

Murphy, L. C., Seekallu, S. V., & Watson, P. H. (2011). Clinical significance of estrogen receptor phosphorylation. *Endocrine-Related Cancer, 18,* R1–R14.

Murphy, L. C., Simon, S. L., Parkes, A., Leygue, E., Dotzlaw, H., Snell, L., et al. (2000). Altered expression of estrogen receptor coregulators during human breast tumorigenesis. *Cancer Research, 60,* 6266–6271.

Murphy, L. C., Wang, M., Coutt, A., & Dotzlaw, H. (1996). Novel mutations in the estrogen receptor messenger RNA in human breast cancers. *The Journal of Clinical Endocrinology and Metabolism, 81,* 1420–1427.

O'Brien, C. S., Farnie, G., Howell, S. J., & Clarke, R. B. (2011). Breast cancer stem cells and their role in resistance to endocrine therapy. *Hormones & Cancer, 2,* 91–103.

Oh, A. S., Lorant, L. A., Holloway, J. N., Miller, D. L., Kern, F. G., & El-Ashry, D. (2001). Hyperactivation of MAPK induces loss of ERα expression in breast cancer cells. *Molecular Endocrinology, 15,* 1344–1359.

Ottaviano, Y. L., Issa, J. P., Parl, F. F., Smith, H. S., Baylin, S. B., & Davidson, N. E. (1994). Methylation of the estrogen receptor gene CpG island marks loss of estrogen receptor expression in human breast cancer cells. *Cancer Research, 54,* 2552–2555.

Penot, G., Le Péron, C., Mérot, Y., Grimaud-Fanouillère, E., Ferrière, F., Boujrad, N., et al. (2005). The human estrogen receptor-alpha isoform hERalpha46 antagonizes the proliferative influence of hERalpha66 in MCF7 breast cancer cells. *Endocrinology, 146,* 5474–5484.

Piva, R., Rimondi, A. P., Hanau, S., Maestri, I., Alvisi, A., Kumar, V. L., et al. (1990). Different methylation of oestrogen receptor DNA in human breast carcinomas with and without oestrogen receptor. *British Journal of Cancer, 61,* 270–275.

Platet, N., Cathiard, A. M., Gleizes, M., & Garcia, M. (2004). Estrogens and their receptors in breast cancer progression: A dual role in cancer proliferation and invasion. *Critical Reviews in Oncology/Hematology, 51,* 55–67.

Prabhu, J. S., Wahi, K., Korlimarla, A., Correa, M., Manjunath, S., Raman, N., et al. (2012). The epigenetic silencing of the estrogen receptor (ER) by hypermethylation of the ESR1 promoter is seen predominantly in triple-negative breast cancers in Indian women. *Tumour Biology*, *33*, 315–323.

Rexer, B. N., & Arteaga, C. L. (2012). Intrinsic and acquired resistance to HER2-targeted therapies in HER2 gene-amplified breast cancer: Mechanisms and clinical implications. *Critical Reviews in Oncogenesis*, *17*, 1–16.

Roodi, N., Bailey, L. R., Kao, W.-Y. , Verrier, C. S., Yee, C. J., Dupont, W. D., et al. (1995). Estrogen receptor gene analysis in estrogen receptor-positive and receptor-negative primary breast cancer. *Journal of the National Cancer Institute*, *87*, 446–451.

Ross-Innes, C. S., Stark, R., Teschendorff, A. E., Holmes, K. A., Ali, H. R., Dunning, M. J., et al. (2012). Differential oestrogen receptor binding is associated with clinical outcome in breast cancer. *Nature*, *481*, 389–393.

Ryu, K., Park, C., & Lee, Y. (2011). Hypoxia-inducible factor 1 alpha represses the transcription of the estrogen receptor alpha gene in human breast cancer cells. *Biochemical and Biophysical Research Communications*, *407*, 831–836.

Sentis, S., Le Romancer, M., Bianchin, C., Rostan, M.-C. , & Corbo, L. (2005). Sumoylation of the estrogen receptor alpha hinge region regulates its transcriptional activity. *Molecular Endocrinology*, *19*, 2671–2684.

Shi, L., Dong, B., Li, Z., Lu, Y., Ouyang, T., Li, J., et al. (2009). Expression of ER-α36, a novel variant of estrogen receptor α, and resistance to tamoxifen treatment in breast cancer. *Journal of Clinical Oncology*, *27*, 3423–3429.

Shipitsin, M., Campbell, L. L., Argani, P., Weremowicz, S., Bloushtain-Qimron, N., Yao, J., et al. (2007). Molecular definition of breast tumor heterogeneity. *Cancer Cell*, *11*, 259–273.

Siegel, R., Naishadham, D., & Jemal, A. (2012). Cancer statistics, 2012. *CA: A Cancer Journal for Clinicians*, *62*, 10–29.

Skliris, G. P., Nugent, Z. J., Rowan, B. G., Penner, C. R., Watson, P. H., & Murphy, L. C. (2010). A phosphorylation code for oestrogen receptor-A predicts clinical outcome to endocrine therapy in breast cancer. *Endocrine-Related Cancer*, *17*, 589–597.

Skliris, G. P., Nugent, Z., Watson, P. H., & Murphy, L. C. (2010). Estrogen receptor alpha phosphorylated at tyrosine 537 is associated with poor clinical outcome in breast cancer patients treated with tamoxifen. *Hormones & Cancer*, *1*, 215–221.

Smith, L. M., Wise, S. C., Hendricks, D. T., Sabichi, A. L., Bos, T., Reddy, P., et al. (1999). cJun overexpression in MCF-7 breast cancer cells produces a tumorigenic, invasive and hormone resistant phenotype. *Oncogene*, *18*, 6063–6070.

Spears, M., Oesterreich, S., Migliaccio, I., Guiterrez, C., Hilsenbeck, S., Quintayo, M. A., et al. (2012). The p160 ER co-regulators predict outcome in ER negative breast cancer. *Breast Cancer Research and Treatment*, *131*, 463–472.

Stender, J. D., Kim, K., Charn, T. H., Komm, B., Chang, K. C. N., Kraus, W. L., et al. (2010). Genome-wide analysis of estrogen receptor α DNA binding and tethering mechanisms identifies Runx1 as a novel tethering factor in receptor-mediated transcriptional activation. *Molecular and Cellular Biology*, *30*, 3943–3955.

Stoner, M., Saville, B., Wormke, M., Dean, D., Burghardt, R., & Safe, S. (2002). Hypoxia induces proteasome-dependent degradation of estrogen receptor alpha in ZR-75 breast cancer cells. *Molecular Endocrinology*, *16*, 2231–2242.

Stossi, F., Madak-Erdoğan, Z., & Katzenellenbogen, B. S. (2012). Macrophage-elicited loss of estrogen receptor-α in breast cancer cells via involvement of MAPK and c-Jun at the ESR1 genomic locus. *Oncogene*, *31*, 1825–1834.

Tang, Z., Treilleux, I., & Brown, M. (1997). A transcriptional enhancer required for the differential expression of the human estrogen receptor in breast cancers. *Molecular and Cellular Biology*, *17*, 1274–1280.

Teyssier, C., Le Romancer, M., Sentis, S., Jalaguier, S., Corbo, L., & Cavaillès, V. (2010). Protein arginine methylation in estrogen signaling and estrogen-related cancers. *Trends in Endocrinology and Metabolism*, *21*, 181–189.

Vadlamudi, R. K., & Kumar, R. (2007). Functional and biological properties of the nuclear receptor coregulator PELP1/MNAR. *Nuclear Receptor Signaling, 5*, e004.

Vallabhaneni, S., Nair, B. C., Cortez, V., Challa, R., Chakravarty, D., Tekmal, R. R., et al. (2011). Significance of ER-Src axis in hormonal therapy resistance. *Breast Cancer Research and Treatment, 130*, 377–385.

Vesuna, F., Lisok, A., Kimble, B., Domek, J., Kato, Y., van der Groep, P., et al. (2011). Twist contributes to hormone resistance in breast cancer by downregulating estrogen receptor-α. *Oncogene, 31*, 3223–3234.

Wang, L., & Banerjee, S. (2004). Differential PIAS3 expression in human malignancy. *Oncology Reports, 11*, 1319–1324.

Wang, C., Fu, M., Angeletti, R. H., Siconolfi-Baez, L., Reutens, A. T., Albanese, C., et al. (2001). Direct acetylation of the estrogen receptor alpha hinge region by p300 regulates transactivation and hormone sensitivity. *The Journal of Biological Chemistry, 276*, 18375–18383.

Wang, Z., Zhang, X., Shen, P., Loggie, B. W., Chang, Y., & Deuel, T. F. (2005). Identification, cloning, and expression of human estrogen receptor-alpha36, a novel variant of human estrogen receptor-alpha66. *Biochemical and Biophysical Research Communications, 336*, 1023–1027.

Wang, Z., Zhang, X., Shen, P., Loggie, B. W., Chang, Y., & Deuel, T. F. (2006). A variant of estrogen receptor-{alpha}, hER-{alpha}36: Transduction of estrogen- and antiestrogen-dependent membrane-initiated mitogenic signaling. *Proceedings of the National Academy of Sciences of the United States of America, 103*, 9063–9068.

Xia, W., Bacus, S., Hegde, P., Husain, I., Strum, J., Liu, L., et al. (2006). A model of acquired autoresistance to a potent ErbB2 tyrosine kinase inhibitor and a therapeutic strategy to prevent its onset in breast cancer. *Proceedings of the National Academy of Sciences of the United States of America, 103*, 7795–7800.

Xiong, J. (2012). Emerging roles of microRNA-22 in human disease and normal physiology. *Current Molecular Medicine, 12*, 247–258.

Xiong, J., Yu, D., Wei, N., Fu, H., Cai, T., Huang, Y., et al. (2010). An estrogen receptor alpha suppressor, microRNA-22, is downregulated in estrogen receptor alpha-positive human breast cancer cell lines and clinical samples. *The FEBS Journal, 277*, 1684–1694.

Yamamoto, Y., Ibusuki, M., Okumura, Y., Kawasoe, T., Kai, K., Iyama, K., et al. (2008). Hypoxia-inducible factor 1alpha is closely linked to an aggressive phenotype in breast cancer. *Breast Cancer Research and Treatment, 110*, 465–475.

Yan, X., Fu, C., Chen, L., Qin, J., Zeng, Q., Yuan, H., et al. (2012). Mesenchymal stem cells from primary breast cancer tissue promote cancer proliferation and enhance mammosphere formation partially via EGF/EGFR/Akt pathway. *Breast Cancer Research and Treatment, 132*, 153–164.

Yan, L., Yang, X., & Davidson, N. E. (2001). Role of DNA methylation and histone acetylation in steroid receptor expression in breast cancer. *Journal of Mammary Gland Biology and Neoplasia, 6*, 183–192.

Yoshida, T., Eguchi, H., Nakachi, K., Tanimoto, K., Higashi, Y., Suemasu, K., et al. (2000). Distinct mechanisms of loss of estrogen receptor alpha gene expression in human breast cancer: Methylation of the gene and alteration of trans-acting factors. *Carcinogenesis, 21*, 2193–2201.

Yoshimoto, N., Toyama, T., Takahashi, S., Sugiura, H., Endo, Y., Iwasa, M., et al. (2011). Distinct expressions of microRNAs that directly target estrogen receptor α in human breast cancer. *Breast Cancer Research and Treatment, 130*, 331–339.

Zhang, Q. X., Hilsenbeck, S. G., Fuqua, S. A., & Borg, A. (1996). Multiple splicing variants of the estrogen receptor are present in individual human breast tumors. *The Journal of Steroid Biochemistry and Molecular Biology, 59*, 251–260.

Zhao, J.-J. , Lin, J., Yang, H., Kong, W., He, L., Ma, X., et al. (2008). MicroRNA-221/222 negatively regulates estrogen receptor alpha and is associated with tamoxifen resistance in breast cancer. *The Journal of Biological Chemistry, 283,* 31079–31086.

Zhou, Y., Eppenberger-Castori, S., Eppenberger, U., & Benz, C. C. (2005). The NFkappaB pathway and endocrine-resistant breast cancer. *Endocrine-Related Cancer, 12*(Suppl. 1), S37–S46.

Zhou, Y., Yau, C., Gray, J. W., Chew, K., Dairkee, S. H., Moore, D. H., et al. (2007). Enhanced NF kappa B and AP-1 transcriptional activity associated with antiestrogen resistant breast cancer. *BMC Cancer, 7,* 59.

Zoubir, M., Mathieu, M. C., Mazouni, C., Liedtke, C., Corley, L., Geha, S., et al. (2008). Modulation of ER phosphorylation on serine 118 by endocrine therapy: A new surrogate marker for efficacy. *Annals of Oncology, 19,* 1402–1406.

Zwart, W., Griekspoor, A., Berno, V., Lakeman, K., Jalink, K., Mancini, M., et al. (2007). PKA-induced resistance to tamoxifen is associated with an altered orientation of ERalpha towards co-activator SRC-1. *The EMBO Journal, 26,* 3534–3544.

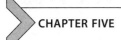

CHAPTER FIVE

Targeting Progesterone Receptors in Breast Cancer

Sebastián Giulianelli*, Alfredo Molinolo†, Claudia Lanari*,[1]

*Laboratory of Hormonal Carcinogenesis, Institute of Experimental Biology and Medicine (IBYME), Consejo Nacional de Investigaciones Científicas y Técnicas (CONICET), Buenos Aires, Argentina
†Oral and Pharyngeal Cancer Branch, National Institute of Dental and Craniofacial Research, NIDCR, NIH, Bethesda, Maryland, USA
[1]Corresponding author: e-mail address: lanari.claudia@gmail.com

Contents

Abstract

Hormone receptors represent the earliest biomarkers used in breast cancer not only as prognosis markers but, in addition, to decide treatment. However, mostly estrogen receptors have been used as therapeutic targets. There is compelling evidence indicating that progesterone receptors (PRs) play a hierarchical role in breast cancer growth and that they might be potentially used to improve the success of endocrine treatments. The two PR isoforms, PR-A and PR-B, play differential roles in regulating gene expression. Tumors overexpressing one or other PR isoform may respond different to endocrine treatment. In this chapter, we highlight the evidence regarding progestins as promoters or inhibitors of cell proliferation in order to understand the dual role of PR in regulating tumor growth, underscoring thus the need of biomarkers to identify which patients may benefit with an antiprogestin/progestin treatment.

Vitamins and Hormones, Volume 93
ISSN 0083-6729
http://dx.doi.org/10.1016/B978-0-12-416673-8.00009-5

1. INTRODUCTION

In this chapter, we review the available information about the roles of progestin and the progesterone receptors (PRs) in modulating breast cancer growth in different experimental models that we believe provide evidence supporting PRs as possible targets for breast cancer treatment.

2. PROGESTINS AND BREAST CANCER RISK

The association of estrogen and progestin in hormone replacement therapy (HRT) has been linked to an increased risk of developing breast cancer by several large prospective cohort studies, such as those from the Women's Health Initiative (WHI) and the Million Women Study. Until then, most observational studies had suggested that estrogen alone and estrogen plus progestin were associated with an increased risk of developing breast cancer. The WHI designed and ran two randomized hormone therapy trials, placebo-controlled, to evaluate the effects of estrogen alone and estrogen plus progestin HRT. In the WHI trial in postmenopausal women with an intact uterus, in which estrogen plus progestin was evaluated, combined hormone therapy significantly increased the risk of breast cancer. The combined therapy was also associated with delayed diagnosis and a significant increase in breast cancer mortality. Surprisingly, a decreased risk of breast cancer was found in the group of postmenopausal women with prior hysterectomy using estrogen alone. No significant delay in breast cancer diagnosis was observed (Chlebowski et al., 2003; Women's Health Initiative, 2002). These results have been confirmed by the Million Women Study, which concluded that "current use of HRT is associated with an increased risk of incident and fatal breast cancer; the effect is substantially greater for oestrogen-progestogen combinations than for other types of HRT" (Beral, 2003). However, the different effects of estrogen plus progestin versus estrogen alone on breast cancer incidence are not yet completely understood. These results, further confirmed by other studies, have been recently reviewed by Chlebowski and Anderson (2012).

3. PROGESTINS STIMULATING BREAST CANCER GROWTH IN ANIMAL MODELS

Loeb and Moskop Kirtz (1939), and later, Muhlbock and Boot (1959), showed that pituitary implants were associated with the development of mammary carcinomas in BALB/c mice, and they suggested that increased levels of progesterone (Pg) played a role mediating these effects. During the 1960s and 1970s, most mouse models of breast cancer relied on the use of strains carrying the mouse mammary tumor virus (MMTV). In these pregnancy-dependent tumors, progestins alone (Nagasawa, Aoki, Sakagami, & Ishida, 1988) or combined with estrogens (Nie, 1964; Sluyser & Van Nie, 1974; Van Nie & Thung, 1965; Yanai & Nagasawa, 1976) stimulated growth. In 1986, we showed that the continuous administration of medroxyprogesterone acetate (MPA) to female BALB/c mice induced the development of ductal mammary carcinomas with an average incidence of 80% (Lanari, Molinolo, & Pasqualini, 1986). In the same year, Kiss et al. demonstrated in the MXT mouse mammary cancer that the intraperitoneal administration of Pg induced increased cell proliferation in the tumors but not in the uterus, thus underlining the differential effects that progestins exert in both organs (Kiss, Paridaens, Heuson, & Danguy, 1986).

All the ductal MPA-induced mammary carcinomas of our model that were maintained in vivo by subcutaneous transplantation into BALB/c female mice expressed high levels of estrogen receptors (ERs) and PRs (Lanari, Kordon, Molinolo, Pasqualini, & Charreau, 1989; Molinolo, Lanari, Charreau, Sanjuan, & Pasqualini, 1987). The tumors were initially progestin-dependent in vivo, but occasionally, they would grow in untreated mice, although maintaining the expression of hormone receptors (Giulianelli et al., 2008; Helguero et al., 2003; Montecchia et al., 1999). Pg, as MPA, was able to induce mammary carcinomas in BALB/c mice, but most of these carcinomas were lobular rather than ductal and rapidly lost hormone receptors expression after successive syngeneic transplantation (Kordon et al., 1993). Although this is an important difference between the natural and the synthetic hormone, both agents were able to stimulate mammary cancer progression (Kordon, Lanari, Meiss, Charreau, & Pasqualini, 1990). Similar results were observed in the MXT model (Formelli, Ronchi, & Di Fronzo, 1985; Kiss et al., 1986). Tumor growth in several transplanted carcinomas from the MPA-induced tumor model was completely blocked by three different antiprogestins or antisense oligonucleotides to PR (asPR; Lamb et al., 2005; Montecchia et al., 1999). Few other mammary carcinoma models would originate tumors with functional ER and PR. One of them is the MXT mouse model, in which carcinomas were induced by urethane (Watson, Medina, & Clark, 1977), and is one of the earliest mammary tumor models in mice reported to be ER+/PR+. Other models are spontaneous mammary carcinomas maintained by transplantations (Kumar et al., 1998; Simian, Manzur, Rodriguez, Kier Joffe, &

Klein, 2009), ERα inducible models in BRCA1$^{f/f;MMTV-Cre/p53+/-/CERM}$ mice (Jones et al., 2008), and a recently described STAT1 KO model (Chan et al., 2012).

In 1992, and later in 1998, we demonstrated that MPA could promote the carcinogenic effects of N-nitrosomethylurea (MNU) to induce mammary carcinomas in BALB/c mice. The tumors were completely different from those induced by MPA alone not only histologically but also in their biology (Pazos, Lanari, Charreau, & Molinolo, 1998; Pazos, Lanari, Meiss, Charreau, & Pasqualini, 1992). Similar promoting effects of MPA were reported in a dimethylbenzanthracene (DMBA)-induced mouse model (Aldaz, Liao, LaBate, & Johnston, 1996).

In rats, starting on 1948, a series of reports showed that progestins in combination with chemical carcinogens could increase the incidence of mammary carcinomas (Bresciani, 1971; Cantarow, Stansey, & Pashkis, 1948; Diamond & Hollander, 1979; Jabara, 1967). In 1989, Robinson and Jordan (1987) showed in the DMBA rat breast cancer model that Pg prevented the inhibitory effect induced by tamoxifen, and in the same year, Russo et al. reported that MPA contraception inhibited mammary gland differentiation and increased DMBA-induced mammary carcinogenesis (Russo, Gimotty, Dupuis, & Russo, 1989). More recently, using some variations of these models, it has been shown that MPA and Pg reduced the latency and increased the incidence of ER+/PR+ DMBA-induced mammary tumors in Sprague–Dawley rats (Benakanakere et al., 2006). Other progestins, such as norethindrone acetate and norgestrel, showed the opposite effect (Benakanakere, Besch-Williford, Carroll, & Hyder, 2010). MPA was also associated with an increase in mammary adenomas and carcinomas in Beagle dogs (Concannon, Altszuler, Hampshire, Butler, & Hansel, 1980) and cats (Misdorp, 1991).

In 1998, the International Agency for Research on Cancer (IARC) changed the status of MPA (IARC Scientific Publications, 1999), and the evaluation report considered that there was sufficient evidence in experimental animals for the carcinogenicity of MPA. Further supporting a role for progestins as proproliferative agents, in 1999 Lydon and colleagues, using the PR knockout mouse model, showed that PR-mediated signaling pathways were essential for DMBA-induced mammary gland tumorigenesis (Lydon, Ge, Kittrell, Medina, & O'Malley, 1999). The work of Haslam (Fluck & Haslam, 1996; Wang, Counterman, & Haslam, 1990) and Shyamala (Shyamala, Yang, Cardiff, & Dale, 2000) that demonstrated the pivotal role of Pg in the proliferation of the mouse mammary glands also supported these findings. By that time, there were also some reports, previous than the WHI study, that reported an increased risk of breast cancer in MPA-treated women (Ross, Paganini-Hill, Wan, & Pike, 2000).

4. *IN VITRO* STUDIES

Although most of the *in vitro* studies in rat models focused on the effect of estrogens, several studies report that Pg participates in the development of alveolar architecture of mammary glands isolated from adult rats grown in organ cultures (Koyama, Sinha, & Dao, 1972) and on the proliferation of organoids of mammary glands grown in collagen (Edery, McGrath, Larson, & Nandi, 1984). Manni and colleagues, using an MNU-induced rat mammary tumor growing in soft agar, also reported a significant increase in the colonies' size by incubation with the progestin R5020 (pro-megestone) or Pg (Manni, Badger, Wright, Ahmed, & Demers, 1987). Richards et al. showed a synergic effect when Pg was combined with EGF (Richards, Edery, Osborn, Larson, & Nandi, 1986).

In mice, the papers of Nandi's lab showed that Pg exerted a synergic effect with prolactin (Imagawa, Tomooka, Hamamoto, & Nandi, 1985) or with EGF stimulating mammary cell proliferation (Imagawa et al., 1985; Nandi, Guzman, & Yang, 1995) and promoting cell transformation in the presence of MNU (Miyamoto, Guzman, Osborn, & Nandi, 1988). Our group was able to show in primary cultures of progestin-induced mouse mammary carcinomas that MPA or Pg were able to stimulate cell prolifer-ation in the presence of low levels of steroid stripped serum (Dran et al., 1995). This effect was obtained with progestin concentrations lower than 0.01 nM (Bottino et al., 2011). We proposed that, at these concentrations, progestins induced slight stimulatory effects activating nongenomic signals. At concentrations close to the K_d of the PR, the proliferative effects were stronger and involved PR-mediated classical gene activation. Electropho-retic motility shift assays confirmed that MPA only at 10 nM concentrations activated PRs able to bind PRE (Pg-responsive elements) oligonucleotides (Bottino et al., 2011). The proliferative effect of progestins was blocked with antiprogestins (10 nM; Lamb, Simian, Molinolo, Pazos, & Lanari, 1999) or asPR (Lamb et al., 2005), indicating that PRs played a pivotal role in cell proliferation *in vitro*. These tumors expressed higher levels of PR-A than PR-B isoforms. Moreover, lobular carcinomas lacking ERα or PRs were not affected by progestin treatment. There are very few reports regarding the effects of progestins in cells growing in matrigel or in three dimensions. In our laboratory, it has been shown that MPA still stimulates cell proliferation of mammary carcinomas overexpressing PR–A in 3D cultures (Polo et al., 2010).

The ER+/PR+ human breast cancer T47D (Keydar et al., 1979) and MCF-7 (Soule, Vazguez, Long, Albert, & Brennan, 1973) cell lines have extensively been used to study the action of estrogens and Pg on cell proliferation, cell signaling, or gene expression *in vitro*. Hissom and Moore (1987) were the first to report that R5020 induced stimulation of cell proliferation in T47D cells, while the antiprogestin Mifepristone (MFP, RU486) inhibited the R5020-induced growth stimulation (Hissom, Bowden, & Moore, 1989), supporting the involvement of PRs. Similarly, Manni et al. reported a significant colony-stimulatory effect induced by Pg in MCF-7 cells in soft agar (Manni, Wright, & Buck, 1991). Braunsberg and colleagues showed that MPA stimulated or inhibited cell growth in two sublines of MCF-7 cells (Braunsberg, Coldham, Leake, Cowan, & Wong, 1987). Longman and Buehring showed that progestins were able to stimulate malignant mammary epithelial cells in primary culture (Longman & Buehring, 1987). The proliferative effects induced by progestins may work through increasing proliferative signals, as well as inhibiting cell death (Moore, Conover, & Franks, 2000). In this regard, it has been shown that progestins protect from serum starvation-induced apoptosis in T47D and MCF-7 breast cancer cell lines (Moore, Spence, Kiningham, & Dillon, 2006; Ory et al., 2001), and from radiation-induced apoptosis in PR positive cells (Vares et al., 2004).

It has been suggested that a single pulse of Pg stimulates only one round of cell division, followed by growth arrest in late G1 of the next cycle (Groshong et al., 1997; Lange et al., 2008; Musgrove, Lee, & Sutherland, 1991). During the first round of cell division, there is a transient induction of cell cycle progression genes, and these changes include increased phosphorylation of RB, increased expression of cyclins (D1, D3, E, A, and B), activation of cyclin-CDKs, and induction of *FOS* and *MYC* gene expression (Musgrove et al., 2001). CDK-inhibitors, p21 and p27, rise during this proliferative phase of progestin treatment (Groshong et al., 1997). The growth arrest in late G1 phase of the second cycle, after 24–48 h of Pg treatment, is accompanied by a reversal of the above cell cycle parameters, except for p21 and p27 that are continuously increased by the treatment, reaching a peak level at 24–48 h (Lange, Richer, & Horwitz, 1999). A second dose of Pg, administered 48 h after the first, extends the growth arrest. However, if the second dose of Pg is administered 72 h after the first one, there is an increase in the percentage of cells in S/G2-phase of the cell cycle (Groshong et al., 1997). The authors proposed that transient or intermittent doses of Pg are stimulatory, while continuous or sustained doses of Pg are inhibitory. These biphasic effects of progestins inducing cell cycle progression followed by arrest in G1 were also described by other authors (Boonyaratanakornkit et al., 2007; Quiles et al., 2009). On the other hand, Moore and colleagues reported that progestins can induce cell proliferation for many rounds of cell cycles in the absence of serum. Even more, whereas control cells undergo apoptosis, progestin-treated cells show an increase in antiapoptotic proteins like BCL-XL (Moore et al., 2000). Progestins can also increase the sensitivity of breast cancer cells to other mitogens such as insulin-like growth factor-II (Elizalde et al., 1998; Goldfine, Papa, Vigneri, Siiteri, & Rosenthal, 1992), heregulin (Balana, Lupu, Labriola, Charreau, & Elizalde, 1999), vascular endothelial growth factor (VEGF— Wu, Richer, Horwitz, & Hyder, 2004), WNT-1 (Lange, Gioeli, Hammes, & Marker, 2007), PDGFA (Soares, Guerreiro, & Botelho, 2007), and FGF-4 (Lopez Perez, Liang, Besch-Williford, Mafuvadze, & Hyder, 2012), or increase the expression of growth factor receptors, such as insulin receptor (Papa et al., 1990), EGFR, ERBB2, and ERBB3 (Balana et al., 2001; Lange, Richer, Shen, & Horwitz, 1998), FGFR-2 (Giulianelli et al., 2008), FGFR-3 (Cerliani et al., 2012), or enhance the sensitivity of their downstream signaling pathways (Lange et al., 1999). Although most of the studies have been carried out using MCF-7 or T47D human breast cancer cells, progestins also proved to stimulate cell proliferation in other cells lines such as the IBH-6, IBH-7, and IBH-4 cells (Vazquez, Mladovan, Garbovesky, Baldi, & Luthy, 2004).

In xenografts, PRs affect the growth of human breast tumors. Using T47D cells which express only PR-B or PR-A isoforms (T47D-YB and T47D-YA cells, respectively), PR-A tumors grow slower than PR-B tumors in an estrogenized environment despite the absence of Pg (Sartorius, Shen, & Horwitz, 2003). It was reported that Pg or MPA did not support T47D tumor growth in estrogen-treated ovariectomized nude mice (Sartorius, Harvell, Shen, & Horwitz, 2005). However, progestins increased the expression of the myoepithelial cytokeratins (CK) 5 and 6, while decreasing the expression of luminal epithelial CK8, CK18, and CK19. The authors concluded that progestins induced a transition of the cell subpopulations from a luminal to a myoepithelial lineage, a phenotype that is associated with poor prognosis (Sartorius et al., 2005). Other authors have shown that MPA and Pg also promote the growth of human breast xenograft tumors in mice (Liang, Besch-Williford, Brekken, & Hyder, 2007).

In BT-474 and T47D breast cancer cells, Liang and colleagues showed that progestins were able to reestablish the growth of xenografted tumors regressing in an estrogenized environment in nude mice depending on the expression of VEGF (Liang et al., 2010). Meanwhile, MFP blocked the progestin-induced growth stimulation, indicating the involvement of PR. In this model, progestins also promoted the increase of lymph nodes metastasis (Liang et al., 2010) and reduced FGF-2 and FGF-8 levels, while increasing the levels of FGF-4 (Lopez Perez et al., 2012).

We have demonstrated that T47D cells expressing the constitutive active form of FGFR-2 (FGFR-2 CA) are able to grow in NOD/SCID mice in the absence of exogenous added hormones, involving the ligand-independent activation of the PR (Cerliani et al., 2011). Progestins also increased the growth of MCF-7 xenografts under certain experimental conditions (Kubota, Josui, Fukutomi, & Kitajima, 1995). In addition, increased invasive properties were reported in ZR-75 cells by Pg pretreatment in combination with EGF (Kato et al., 2005).

5. PROGESTINS INHIBITING BREAST CANCER GROWTH

Different laboratories have described Pg inhibition of breast cancer growth, an effect first described by Huggins (1967). The inhibitory effect in rat mammary carcinogenesis was then related to the timing of carcinogen administration, and the effect was associated with the differentiation state of the gland prior to the carcinogenic insult (Grubbs, Farnell, Hill, & McDonough, 1985; Inoh, Kamiya, Fujii, & Yokoro, 1985; Jabara, Toyne, & Harcourt, 1973; Kledzik, Bradley, & Meites, 1974). Nagasawa et al. also reported that MPA reduced the development of mammary hyperplasias in SHN mice (Nagasawa, Fujii, & Hagiwara, 1985). Moreover, in our experimental model, progestins (MPA or Pg) inhibited the growth of hormone-independent (HI) variants which express high levels of PR-B and almost no PR-A (unpublished results). Poulin et al. also reported an inhibitory effect for MPA that was ascribed to its androgenic of glucocorticoid properties rather than to its progestin effect (Poulin, Baker, Poirier, & Labrie, 1989). Along this line, MDA-MB-231 breast cancer cells transfected with androgen receptor were inhibited by MPA when transplanted in vivo (Buchanan et al., 2005). All this information suggests that progestins may stimulate or inhibit breast cancer growth depending on the presence of other hormone receptors in addition to PRs or on the prevailing PR isoform expressed.

High doses of MPA had been used to treat breast cancer patients with good results in some subjects (Cuna, Calciati, Strada, Bumma, & Campio, 1978). However, the mechanism of MPA action remains still elusive.

As mentioned above, some reports also show in *in vitro* studies that progestins stimulate, have no effect on, or inhibit cell proliferation (Poulin et al., 1989; Schatz, Soto, & Sonnenschein, 1985; Vignon, Bardon, Chalbos, & Rochefort, 1983). The *in vitro* studies reporting progestin inhibition of human breast cancer cell proliferation have been done under conditions in which the control cells were in a stimulatory phase, and this effect was associated with an anti-inflammatory effect of PRs regulating NFkB and COX-2 expression (Chen, Hardy, & Mendelson, 2011). Different inhibitory or stimulatory effects were reported by the same authors in varying experimental conditions (Berthois, Katzenellenbogen, & Katzenellenbogen, 1986; Gill et al., 1991; Hissom & Moore, 1987). In our MPA-induced tumor model, we demonstrated that the tumors that were inhibited by MPA *in vivo* (those expressing high PR-B levels) also showed an inhibitory effect in 2D and 3D cultures when incubated with 10-nM MPA. This inhibitory effect was due to increased cell death (Victoria Wargon, María Laura Polo, Virginia Novaro and Claudia Lanari, unpublished results).

6. THE SYSTEMIC EFFECT OF PROGESTINS

The role of progestins in tumor growth is not clear. Many attempts were made to ascribe the immunosuppressant role of Pg to its permissive role in breast cancer growth. However, the experimental evidence suggests that the indirect effects of Pg might have a secondary effect in breast cancer growth if any. Supporting this fact, there is no increase in mammary tumor incidence in immunosuppressed mice with respect to their wild-type counterparts. Hormone-dependent (HD) tumors also need a progestin to grow in immunosuppressed mice (Kordon et al., 1990). However, as Pg might change the tumor microenvironment immune milieu, and as the microenvironment participates in tumor growth, this issue deserves further consideration. A completely different picture is obtained with chemical carcinogenesis approaches. It is well known that tumors induced by chemical carcinogens are highly immunogenic since they induce mutations that may give rise to antigenic proteins (Franco et al., 1996; Prehn & Main, 1957). However, this kind of experiments should not be extrapolated to spontaneous breast cancers in which they express almost no tumor-specific antigens (Franco et al., 1996; Hewitt, Blake, & Walder, 1976). Similarly in the WHI study, MPA increased breast cancer incidence, but it significantly decreased colon cancer incidence showing once more the specific nature of each tissue regarding MPA responsiveness (Women's Health Initiative, 2002). Our group in collaboration with others have shown the presence of PRs in NK cells (Arruvito et al., 2008), and in addition, we demonstrated that MPA treatment may increase antibody production (Vermeulen et al., 2001). These indirect effects may collaborate to induce a pro-tumorigenic milieu. Other indirect effect of MPA described in mice is the increase of EGF in serum (Kordon et al., 1994). This salivary gland's EGF may participate in priming cells to the hormonal effects of progestins.

7. PRs AND GENE EXPRESSION

PRs are members of the nuclear hormone receptor family of ligand-dependent transcription factors that function by binding to specific palindromic DNA-binding sites (PRE sequences) on target genes or through interaction to other DNA-bound transcription factors (Beato, Herrlich, & Schutz, 1995; Dressing, Hagan, Knutson, Daniel, & Lange, 2009; Jacobsen & Horwitz, 2012; Mangelsdorf et al., 1995; Obr & Edwards, 2012; Olefsky, 2001). PRs have a DNA-binding domain (DBD) between an N-terminal region including activation (AF) and inhibitory functions, and a downstream C-terminal ligand-binding domain (LBD). The two PR isoforms, PR-A and PR-B, have identical DBD and LBD with an additional N-terminal region called "B-upstream segment" only present in PR-B that confers specific AF activity.

The classical view of the transcriptional action of PRs included the following concepts: (1) unliganded receptors are located in the cytosol bound to heat-shock proteins (HSPs); (2) in the presence of Pg, PRs are released from HSP, dimerize, and translocate to the nucleus; (3) they bind PRE sites in promoters of PR-regulated genes; and (4) coactivators are recruited and gene transcription starts. However, this simple model cannot explain other actions of PRs. Dimerization may not be required for PR transcription, and PRs may bind to sites other than PRE sequences: there is also strong evidence that PRs may also have a transcriptional activity when bound as nomomers in the promoters of PR-regulated genes that contain only PRE half-site elements (Giulianelli, Vaque, Soldati, et al., 2012; Giulianelli, Vaque, Wargon, et al., 2012; Jacobsen & Horwitz, 2012).

PRs also play an active role in transducing signaling pathways from the cell membrane (Bottino et al., 2011; Carnevale et al., 2007). In the cell cultures of MPA-induced mouse mammary carcinomas, the classical membrane PRs were detected using different approaches. Interestingly in T47D cells, PR is mostly nuclear, and as these cells are among the most widely used in *in vitro* studies, this has probably contributed to hamper the isolation of membrane PRs in breast cancer cells. To add another level of complexity, membrane PRs that contain seven transmembrane domains, typical of G protein-coupled receptors, interact with classical PR signaling (Zhu, Rice, Pang, Pace, & Thomas, 2003). Transcripts of these novel receptors are present in human breast cancer cell lines (Dressing, Alyea, Pang, & Thomas, 2012; Dressing & Thomas, 2007) and MPA-induced mammary carcinomas (Bottino et al., 2011). However, since synthetic progestins as R5020 or MPA or antiprogestins don't bind to these receptors (Thomas et al., 2007), we will not be reviewing them in this chapter.

Two models of classical Pg-activated cytoplasmic signaling pathways have been proposed: (1) an early interaction between ERα and PR-B necessary for c-Src/p21^{Ras}/Erk, PI3K/Akt, and JAK/STAT activation (Ballare et al., 2003; Migliaccio et al., 1998; Vicent et al., 2010); (2) PRs directly interact and activate c-Src tyrosine kinases through a polyproline motif in the amino-terminal domain of PRs (Boonyaratanakornkit et al., 2001). Interestingly, both genomic and nongenomic actions of progestins/PR can mediate gene transcription, through direct or indirect binding to DNA for genomic effects, or through other signaling pathways as the MAPK, AKT, or STAT pathways in which the PR does not have a direct participation in the transcription machinery. We still have to understand how these two pathways interact, and the specific role of each PR isoform mediating these effects.

PR-A or PR-B may regulate some overlapping genes, but most of them are isoform specific. In a first study, Richer and colleagues described 94 progestin-regulated genes: 25 regulated by both PR, 65 by PR-B only, and 4 by PR-A (Richer et al., 2002), suggesting some differences between the two PR isoforms in sequence recognition and/or interaction with other transcription factors. In a later study using larger microarrays, more than 300 Pg-regulated genes were described: 25 by both PR, 229 by PR-B, and 83 by PR-A (Tung et al., 2006). PR-B are usually stronger activators than PR-A in the presence of Pg (Jacobsen, Schittone, Richer, & Horwitz, 2005). However, in the absence of Pg, PR-A proved to be stronger transactivators (Jacobsen et al., 2005). Both heterodimers and homodimers are capable of gene regulation.

Different genes were selected to analyze the transcription activity of PRs in breast cancer models or normal mammary glands. Progestins upregulate the human CDK inhibitor, p21, in breast cancer cells. Its promoter lacks canonical PRE sites. Instead, activated PRs interact with the promoter through the transcription factor Sp1 and CBP/p300, mediating transcriptional upregulation by Pg (Owen, Richer, Tung, Takimoto, & Horwitz, 1998). The proto-oncogene *MYC* is involved in the regulation of cell proliferation, differentiation, transformation, and apoptosis (Gonzalez & Hurley, 2010), and it is upregulated by progestins (Musgrove et al., 1991) through a functional PRE-like sequence (Moore et al., 1997). The overexpression of BRCA1 in T47D cells blocked the progestin-induced *MYC* expression by interfering with the recruitment of PR and inhibited the association of coactivators (SRC-1 and AIB1), thus enhancing the binding of the corepressor (HDAC1) at the *MYC* PRE sequence (Katiyar, Ma, Riegel, Fan, & Rosen, 2009). We have recently demonstrated, using the same T47D cells, that MPA or FGF-2 regulates the expression of MYC and that PRs mediate this effect (Cerliani et al., 2011; Giulianelli, Vaque, Soldati, et al., 2012). There are several PRE half-sites at *MYC* promoter that can mediate PR binding. The expression of MYC induced by MPA was shown to be mediated by an interaction among PR, ERα, STAT5, and FGFR-2 at the *MYC* promoter (Cerliani et al., 2011; Giulianelli, Vaque, Soldati, et al., 2012).

We have shown that, in some mouse mammary carcinomas that have switched from a progestin-dependent phenotype and do not need the exogenous administration of the hormone to grow, the PR still drives tumor growth (Lamb et al., 2005; Montecchia et al., 1999). We have proposed that tumor cells recruit stromal cells that are able to provide the growth factors necessary to stimulate cell proliferation and that FGF-2 is one of them. In support of this hypothesis, we have shown that carcinoma-associated fibroblasts (CAFs) from HI tumors from the MPA–murine breast cancer model expressed increased levels of FGF-2 than those from HD tumors and that FGF-2 was able to activate the PR (Giulianelli et al., 2008). Moreover, FGFR-2 was found in the nuclei of the tumor cells interacting with STAT5 and PRs at the promoters of *MYC* (Cerliani et al., 2011). Later studies confirmed that ERα was also associated with PRs at these same sites at the cyclin D1 (*CCND1*) and *MYC* promoters (Giulianelli, Vaque, Soldati, et al., 2012). Recently, Friedl's lab has demonstrated that FGF-2 together with HB-EGF, heparanase-1, and SDF1 participate as paracrine factors produced by human CAFs inducing T47D cell proliferation

(Su, Sung, Beebe, & Friedl, 2012). Other membrane players such as ERBB2 were also found to be acting as part of multimeric complexes at the *CCND1* promoter involving PRs and STAT3 (Beguelin et al., 2010). In Fig. 5.1, we summarize our hypothesis about the proliferative loop that may be occurring in breast cancer cells by Pg/PR. In this figure, it can be noticed that there are several levels through which to regulate or inhibit gene transcription. The most effective may be the blockage of PR; however, the blockage of ERα, AKT/MAPK, or STAT5, or the blockage of paracrine factors such as FGF-2, and their receptors FGFR-2, may also decrease the effectiveness of

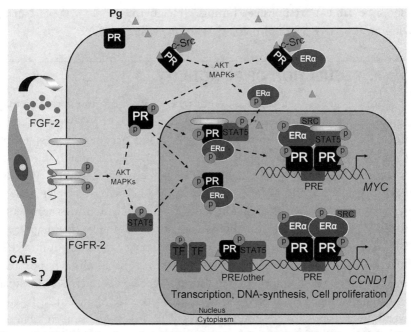

Figure 5.1 Proliferative loop involving progestin- or growth factor-induced PR activation in breast cancer cells. PRs can be activated by their specific ligands (Pg, MPA, R5020, among others) or they can be activated by ligand-independent mechanisms. Progestins induce the activation of MAPK/AKT signaling pathways by the association of the nuclear PRs found in the cell membrane with c-Src, that in turn phosphorylate PR, ERα, and transcription factors necessary for PR binding to the gene promoters and activation of cell proliferation-related genes like *CCND1* or *MYC*. In the absence of exogenous hormone supply, PRs can also be activated by growth factors such as FGF-2, secreted by carcinoma-associated fibroblasts (CAFs). FGF-2, by binding to their cognate receptors FGFR-2, induces PR activation and the interaction among activated PR, FGFR-2, STAT5, and other steroid receptor coactivators (SRC) at the promoters of proliferative target genes. (See Color Insert.)

this transcriptional machinery. In fact, we have shown that PI3K/AKT pathway inhibitors (Riggio et al., 2012), antiestrogens (Giulianelli, Vaque, Soldati, et al., 2012; Lamb et al., 2003), FGFR-2 inhibitors (Cerliani et al., 2011), and antibodies to FGF-2 that decrease CAFs-induced tumor cell proliferation (Giulianelli et al., 2008) also decrease PR-driven tumor growth. However, only antiprogestins induced complete tumor regressions in both HD and HI variants from the MPA-murine breast cancer model expressing high levels of PR-A (Cerliani et al., 2010; Montecchia et al., 1999; Vanzulli et al., 2002; Wargon et al., 2009). The *in vivo* administration of asPR inhibited tumor growth supporting the key role of PRs (Lamb et al., 2005). Since some HI tumors did not respond to antiprogestins, we reclassified this group into responsive and unresponsive tumors (Helguero et al., 2003; Lanari, Wargon, Rojas, & Molinolo, 2012; Wargon et al., 2011).

8. REGULATION OF PR ACTIVITY

It now seems clear that a different ratio of PR isoform expression may change the repertoire of transcripts/proteins expressed. PR-A overexpressing human breast cancers may show a decreased tamoxifen responsiveness (Hopp et al., 2004). Our experimental data suggest that these tumors might be sensitive to an antiprogestin treatment (Helguero et al., 2003; Wargon et al., 2011, 2009). PR isoform expression may be regulated by epigenetic mechanisms. Promoter methylation was shown in our murine experimental model (Wargon et al., 2011) and human breast cancer samples (Pathiraja et al., 2011), suggesting that treatment with demethylating agents may induce PR isoform reexpression and a change in the hormone/antihormone responsiveness. Another level of epigenetic regulation might be the microRNAs (small noncoding endogenous RNAs—Esteller, 2011; Lee & Shin, 2012). In fact, several microRNAs were found to regulate PR expression (Cochrane et al., 2012; Cui, Li, Feng, & Ding, 2011). The clinical implications of these microRNAs remain to be determined. Other posttranslational modifications such as sumoylation of PRs may also affect gene PR activity as recently demonstrated by Lange's lab (Knutson et al., 2012).

9. PRs AS THERAPEUTICAL TARGETS FOR BREAST CANCER TREATMENT

The information regarding antiprogestin treatment in breast cancer models and in patients has been recently reviewed by our group

(Lanari et al., 2012). In this chapter, we have reviewed the available data supporting the role of progestins as modulators of breast cancer growth and the possible validity of antiprogestins as an effective therapeutic approach for breast cancer treatment. So where do we stand now? At the moment, experimental data indicate that the PR isoform ratio may be predictive for this response. The next challenge is to find support for this hypothesis in breast cancer patients and to identify markers that may predict this response. It is interesting to remark from our studies that the inhibitory effects induced by antiprogestins were always stronger than those induced by progestins, suggesting that antiprogestins are better potential therapeutic agents. In addition, when analyzing all the information available, it becomes clearly evident that the therapeutic effect of progestins/antiprogestins is intrinsic to the biology of the tumors, rather than depending on indirect immune or systemic effects. However, microenvironmental factors may participate indirectly in the regulation of PR isoform expression and activation. The fact that PRs are activated by paracrine factors (Cerliani et al., 2011), or by AKT signaling (Riggio et al., 2012), and that PRs may interact with ERα at the transcriptional machinery (Giulianelli, Vaque, Soldati, et al., 2012) of target proliferative genes suggests that therapeutic approaches should include a combination of ER and PR inhibitors together with therapies aimed to block the stromal–parenchymal interactions.

ACKNOWLEDGMENTS

We wish to thank the Avon Foundation for AACR travel awards, the UICC for the ICRETT fellowships awarded to fellows from our labs, and Fundación Sales, CONICET, and Agencia de Promoción Científica y Tecnológica from Argentina for funding. Dr. Molinolo is supported by the Intramural Research Program, NIDCR, NIH.

REFERENCES

Aldaz, C. M., Liao, Q. Y., LaBate, M., & Johnston, D. A. (1996). Medroxyprogesterone acetate accelerates the development and increases the incidence of mouse mammary tumors induced by dimethylbenzanthracene. *Carcinogenesis, 17,* 2069–2072.

Arruvito, L., Giulianelli, S., Flores, A. C., Paladino, N., Barboza, M., Lanari, C., et al. (2008). NK cells expressing a progesterone receptor are susceptible to progesterone-induced apoptosis. *Journal of Immunology, 180,* 5746–5753.

Balana, M. E., Labriola, L., Salatino, M., Movsichoff, F., Peters, G., Charreau, E. H., et al. (2001). Activation of ErbB-2 via a hierarchical interaction between ErbB-2 and type I insulin-like growth factor receptor in mammary tumor cells. *Oncogene, 20,* 34–47.

Balana, M. E., Lupu, R., Labriola, L., Charreau, E. H., & Elizalde, P. V. (1999). Interactions between progestins and heregulin (HRG) signaling pathways: HRG acts as mediator of progestins proliferative effects in mouse mammary adenocarcinomas. *Oncogene, 18,* 6370–6379.

Ballare, C., Uhrig, M., Bechtold, T., Sancho, E., Di Domenico, M., Migliaccio, A., et al. (2003). Two domains of the progesterone receptor interact with the estrogen receptor and are required for progesterone activation of the c-Src/Erk pathway in mammalian cells. *Molecular and Cellular Biology, 23*, 1994–2008.

Beato, M., Herrlich, P., & Schutz, G. (1995). Steroid hormone receptors: Many actors in search of a plot. *Cell, 83*, 851–857.

Beguelin, W., Diaz Flaque, M. C., Proietti, C. J., Cayrol, F., Rivas, M. A., Tkach, M., et al. (2010). Progesterone receptor induces ErbB-2 nuclear translocation to promote breast cancer growth via a novel transcriptional effect: ErbB-2 function as a coactivator of Stat3. *Molecular and Cellular Biology, 30*, 5456–5472.

Benakanakere, I., Besch-Williford, C., Carroll, C. E., & Hyder, S. M. (2010). Synthetic progestins differentially promote or prevent 7,12-dimethylbenz(a)anthracene-induced mammary tumors in Sprague-Dawley rats. *Cancer Prevention Research (Philadelphia, PA), 3*, 1157–1167.

Benakanakere, I., Besch-Williford, C., Schnell, J., Brandt, S., Ellersieck, M. R., Molinolo, A., et al. (2006). Natural and synthetic progestins accelerate 7,12-dimethylbenz[a]anthracene-initiated mammary tumors and increase angiogenesis in Sprague-Dawley rats. *Clinical Cancer Research, 12*, 4062–4071.

Beral, V. (2003). Breast cancer and hormone-replacement therapy in the Million Women Study. *Lancet, 362*, 419–427.

Berthois, Y., Katzenellenbogen, J. A., & Katzenellenbogen, B. S. (1986). Phenol red in tissue culture media is a weak estrogen: Implications concerning the study of estrogen-responsive cells in culture. *Proceedings of the National Academy of Sciences of the United States of America, 83*, 2496–2500.

Boonyaratanakornkit, V., McGowan, E., Sherman, L., Mancini, M. A., Cheskis, B. J., & Edwards, D. P. (2007). The role of extranuclear signaling actions of progesterone receptor in mediating progesterone regulation of gene expression and the cell cycle. *Molecular Endocrinology, 21*, 359–375.

Boonyaratanakornkit, V., Scott, M. P., Ribon, V., Sherman, L., Anderson, S. M., Maller, J. L., et al. (2001). Progesterone receptor contains a proline-rich motif that directly interacts with SH3 domains and activates c-Src family tyrosine kinases. *Molecular Cell, 8*, 269–280.

Bottino, M. C., Cerliani, J. P., Rojas, P., Giulianelli, S., Soldati, R., Mondillo, C., et al. (2011). Classical membrane progesterone receptors in murine mammary carcinomas: Agonistic effects of progestins and RU-486 mediating rapid non-genomic effects. *Breast Cancer Research and Treatment, 126*, 621–636.

Braunsberg, H., Coldham, N. G., Leake, R. E., Cowan, S. K., & Wong, W. (1987). Actions of a progestogen on human breast cancer cells: Mechanisms of growth stimulation and inhibition. *European Journal of Cancer & Clinical Oncology, 23*, 563–571.

Bresciani, F. (1971). *Ovarian steroid control of cell proliferation in the mammary gland and cancer. Basic action of sex steroids on target organs.* Basel: Karger Publishing Company.

Buchanan, G., Birrell, S. N., Peters, A. A., Bianco-Miotto, T., Ramsay, K., Cops, E. J., et al. (2005). Decreased androgen receptor levels and receptor function in breast cancer contribute to the failure of response to medroxyprogesterone acetate. *Cancer Research, 65*, 8487–8496.

Cantarow, W., Stansey, J., & Pashkis, K. E. (1948). The influence of sex hormones on mammary tumors induced by 2-acetaminofluorene. *Cancer Research, 8*, 412–418.

Carnevale, R. P., Proietti, C. J., Salatino, M., Urtreger, A., Peluffo, G., Edwards, D. P., et al. (2007). Progestin effects on breast cancer cell proliferation, proteases activation, and in vivo development of metastatic phenotype all depend on progesterone receptor capacity to activate cytoplasmic signaling pathways. *Molecular Endocrinology, 21*, 1335–1358.

Cerliani, J. P., Giulianelli, S., Sahores, A., Wargon, V., Gongora, A., Baldi, A., et al. (2010). Mifepristone inhibits MPA-and FGF2-induced mammary tumor growth but not FGF2-induced mammary hyperplasia. *Medicina*, *70*, 529–532.

Cerliani, J. P., Guillardoy, T., Giulianelli, S., Vaque, J. P., Gutkind, J. S., Vanzulli, S. I., et al. (2011). Interaction between FGFR-2, STAT5, and progesterone receptors in breast cancer. *Cancer Research*, *71*, 3720–3731.

Cerliani, J. P., Vanzulli, S. I., Pinero, C. P., Bottino, M. C., Sahores, A., Nunez, M., et al. (2012). Associated expressions of FGFR-2 and FGFR-3: From mouse mammary gland physiology to human breast cancer. *Breast Cancer Research and Treatment*, *133*, 997–1008.

Chan, S. R., Vermi, W., Luo, J., Lucini, L., Rickert, C., Fowler, A. M., et al. (2012). STAT1-deficient mice spontaneously develop estrogen receptor alpha-positive luminal mammary carcinomas. *Breast Cancer Research*, *14*, R16.

Chen, C. C., Hardy, D. B., & Mendelson, C. R. (2011). Progesterone receptor inhibits proliferation of human breast cancer cells via induction of MAPK phosphatase 1 (MKP-1/DUSP1). *Journal of Biology*, *286*, 43091–43102.

Chlebowski, R. T., & Anderson, G. L. (2012). Changing concepts: Menopausal hormone therapy and breast cancer. *Journal of the National Cancer Institute*, *104*, 517–527.

Chlebowski, R. T., Hendrix, S. L., Langer, R. D., Stefanick, M. L., Gass, M., Lane, D., et al. (2003). Influence of estrogen plus progestin on breast cancer and mammography in healthy postmenopausal women: The Women's Health Initiative Randomized Trial. *Journal of the American Medical Association*, *289*, 3243–3253.

Cochrane, D. R., Jacobsen, B. M., Connaghan, K. D., Howe, E. N., Bain, D. L., & Richer, J. K. (2012). Progestin regulated miRNAs that mediate progesterone receptor action in breast cancer. *Molecular and Cellular Endocrinology*, *355*, 15–24.

Concannon, P., Altszuler, N., Hampshire, J., Butler, W. R., & Hansel, W. (1980). Growth hormone, prolactin, and cortisol in dogs developing mammary nodules and an acromegaly-like appearance during treatment with medroxyprogesterone acetate. *Endocrinology*, *106*, 1173–1177.

Cui, W., Li, Q., Feng, L., & Ding, W. (2011). MiR-126-3p regulates progesterone receptors and involves development and lactation of mouse mammary gland. *Molecular and Cellular Biochemistry*, *355*, 17–25.

Cuna, G. R., Calciati, A., Strada, M. R., Bumma, C., & Campio, L. (1978). High dose medroxyprogesterone acetate (MPA) treatment in metastatic carcinoma of the breast: A dose-response evaluation. *Tumori*, *64*, 143–149.

Diamond, E. J., & Hollander, V. P. (1979). Progesterone and breast cancer. *Mount Sinai Journal of Medicine*, *46*, 225–235.

Dran, G., Luthy, I. A., Molinolo, A. A., Charreau, E. H., Pasqualini, C. D., & Lanari, C. (1995). Effect of medroxyprogesterone acetate (MPA) and serum factors on cell proliferation in primary cultures of an MPA-induced mammary adenocarcinoma. *Breast Cancer Research and Treatment*, *35*, 173–186.

Dressing, G. E., Alyea, R., Pang, Y., & Thomas, P. (2012). Membrane progesterone receptors (mPRs) mediate progestin induced antimorbidity in breast cancer cells and are expressed in human breast tumors. *Hormones and Cancer*, *3*, 101–112.

Dressing, G. E., Hagan, C. R., Knutson, T. P., Daniel, A. R., & Lange, C. A. (2009). Progesterone receptors act as sensors for mitogenic protein kinases in breast cancer models. *Endocrine-Related Cancer*, *16*, 351–361.

Dressing, G. E., & Thomas, P. (2007). Identification of membrane progestin receptors in human breast cancer cell lines and biopsies and their potential involvement in breast cancer. *Steroids*, *72*, 111–116.

Edery, M., McGrath, M., Larson, L., & Nandi, S. (1984). Correlation between in vitro growth and regulation of estrogen and progesterone receptors in rat mammary epithelial cells. *Endocrinology*, *115*, 1691–1697.

Elizalde, P. V., Lanari, C., Molinolo, A. A., Guerra, F. K., Balana, M. E., Simian, M., et al. (1998). Involvement of insulin-like growth factors-I and -II and their receptors in medroxyprogesterone acetate-induced growth of mouse mammary adenocarcinomas. *Journal of Steroid Biochemistry and Molecular Biology, 67*, 305–317.

Esteller, M. (2011). Non-coding RNAs in human disease. *Nature Reviews. Genetics, 12*, 861–874.

Fluck, M. M., & Haslam, S. Z. (1996). Mammary tumors induced by polyomavirus. *Breast Cancer Research and Treatment, 39*, 45–56.

Formelli, F., Ronchi, E., & Di Fronzo, G. (1985). Effect of medroxyprogesterone acetate on the growth of mouse transplanted tumors: Relation with hormone sensitivity. *Anticancer Research, 5*, 313–319.

Franco, M., Bustuoabad, O. D., di Gianni, P. D., Goldman, A., Pasqualini, C. D., & Ruggiero, R. A. (1996). A serum-mediated mechanism for concomitant resistance shared by immunogenic and non-immunogenic murine tumours. *British Journal of Cancer, 74*, 178–186.

Gill, P. G., Tilley, W. D., De Young, N. J., Lensink, I. L., Dixon, P. D., & Horsfall, D. J. (1991). Inhibition of T47D human breast cancer cell growth by the synthetic progestin R5020: Effects of serum, estradiol, insulin, and EGF. *Breast Cancer Research and Treatment, 20*, 53–62.

Giulianelli, S., Cerliani, J. P., Lamb, C. A., Fabris, V. T., Bottino, M. C., Gorostiaga, M. A., et al. (2008). Carcinoma-associated fibroblasts activate progesterone receptors and induce hormone independent mammary tumor growth: A role for the FGF-2/FGFR-2 axis. *International Journal of Cancer, 123*, 2518–2531.

Giulianelli, S., Vaque, J. P., Soldati, R., Wargon, V., Vanzulli, S. I., Martins, R., et al. (2012). Estrogen receptor alpha mediates progestin-induced mammary tumor growth by interacting with progesterone receptors at the cyclin D1/MYC promoters. *Cancer Research, 72*, 2416–2427.

Giulianelli, S., Vaque, J. P., Wargon, V., Soldati, R., Vanzulli, S. I., Martins, R., et al. (2012). The role of estrogen receptor alpha in breast cancer cell proliferation mediated by progestins. *Medicina, 72*, 315–320.

Goldfine, I. D., Papa, V., Vigneri, R., Siiteri, P., & Rosenthal, S. (1992). Progestin regulation of insulin and insulin-like growth factor I receptors in cultured human breast cancer cells. *Breast Cancer Research and Treatment, 22*, 69–79.

Gonzalez, V., & Hurley, L. H. (2010). The c-MYC NHE III(1): Function and regulation. *Annual Review of Pharmacology and Toxicology, 50*, 111–129.

Groshong, S. D., Owen, G. I., Grimison, B., Schauer, I. E., Todd, M. C., Langan, T. A., et al. (1997). Biphasic regulation of breast cancer cell growth by progesterone: Role of the cyclin-dependent kinase inhibitors, p21 and p27(Kip1). *Molecular Endocrinology, 11*, 1593–1607.

Grubbs, C. J., Farnell, D. R., Hill, D. L., & McDonough, K. C. (1985). Chemoprevention of N-nitroso-N-methylurea-induced mammary cancers by pretreatment with 17 beta-estradiol and progesterone. *Journal of the National Cancer Institute, 74*, 927–931.

Helguero, L. A., Viegas, M., Asaithamby, A., Shyamala, G., Lanari, C., & Molinolo, A. A. (2003). Progesterone receptor expression in medroxyprogesterone acetate-induced murine mammary carcinomas and response to endocrine treatment. *Breast Cancer Research and Treatment, 79*, 379–390.

Hewitt, H. B., Blake, E. R., & Walder, A. S. (1976). A critique of the evidence for active host defence against cancer, based on personal studies of 27 murine tumours of spontaneous origin. *British Journal of Cancer, 33*, 241–259.

Hissom, J. R., Bowden, R. T., & Moore, M. R. (1989). Effects of progestins, estrogens, and antihormones on growth and lactate dehydrogenase in the human breast cancer cell line T47D. *Endocrinology, 125*, 418–423.

Hissom, J. R., & Moore, M. R. (1987). Progestin effects on growth in the human breast cancer cell line T-47D—Possible therapeutic implications. *Biochemical and Biophysical Research Communications, 145*, 706–711.

Hopp, T. A., Weiss, H. L., Hilsenbeck, S. G., Cui, Y., Allred, D. C., Horwitz, K. B., et al. (2004). Breast cancer patients with progesterone receptor PR-A-rich tumors have poorer disease-free survival rates. *Clinical Cancer Research, 10*, 2751–2760.

Huggins, C. (1967). Endocrine-induced regression of cancers. *Science, 156*, 1050–1054.

IARC Scientific Publications (1999). *Hormonal contraception and postmenopausal hormonal therapy (2-9 June 1998)*. Lyon, France: IARC Scientific Publications, World Health Organization.

Imagawa, W., Tomooka, Y., Hamamoto, S., & Nandi, S. (1985). Stimulation of mammary epithelial cell growth in vitro: Interaction of epidermal growth factor and mammogenic hormones. *Endocrinology, 116*, 1514–1524.

Inoh, A., Kamiya, K., Fujii, Y., & Yokoro, K. (1985). Protective effects of progesterone and tamoxifen in estrogen-induced mammary carcinogenesis in ovariectomized W/Fu rats. *Japanese Journal of Cancer Research, 76*, 699–704.

Jabara, A. G. (1967). Effects of progesterone on 9,10-dimethyl-1,2-benzanthracene-induced mammary tumours in Sprague-Dawley rats. *British Journal of Cancer, 21*, 418–429.

Jabara, A. G., Toyne, P. H., & Harcourt, A. G. (1973). Effects of time and duration of progesterone administration on mammary tumours induced by 7,12-dimethylbenz(a)anthracene in Sprague-Dawley rats. *British Journal of Cancer, 27*, 63–71.

Jacobsen, B. M., & Horwitz, K. B. (2012). Progesterone receptors, their isoforms and progesterone regulated transcription. *Molecular and Cellular Endocrinology, 357*, 18–29.

Jacobsen, B. M., Schittone, S. A., Richer, J. K., & Horwitz, K. B. (2005). Progesterone-independent effects of human progesterone receptors (PRs) in estrogen receptor-positive breast cancer: PR isoform-specific gene regulation and tumor biology. *Molecular Endocrinology, 19*, 574–587.

Jones, L. P., Tilli, M. T., Assefnia, S., Torre, K., Halama, E. D., Parrish, A., et al. (2008). Activation of estrogen signaling pathways collaborates with loss of Brca1 to promote development of ERalpha-negative and ERalpha-positive mammary preneoplasia and cancer. *Oncogene, 27*, 794–802.

Katiyar, P., Ma, Y., Riegel, A., Fan, S., & Rosen, E. M. (2009). Mechanism of BRCA1-mediated inhibition of progesterone receptor transcriptional activity. *Molecular Endocrinology, 23*, 1135–1146.

Kato, S., Pinto, M., Carvajal, A., Espinoza, N., Monso, C., Sadarangani, A., et al. (2005). Progesterone increases tissue factor gene expression, procoagulant activity, and invasion in the breast cancer cell line ZR-75-1. *Journal of Clinical Endocrinology and Metabolism, 90*, 1181–1188.

Keydar, I., Chen, L., Karby, S., Weiss, F. R., Delarea, J., Radu, M., et al. (1979). Establishment and characterization of a cell line of human breast carcinoma origin. *European Journal of Cancer, 15*, 659–670.

Kiss, R., Paridaens, R. J., Heuson, J. C., & Danguy, A. J. (1986). Effect of progesterone on cell proliferation in the MXT mouse hormone-sensitive mammary neoplasm. *Journal of the National Cancer Institute, 77*, 173–178.

Kledzik, G. S., Bradley, C. J., & Meites, J. (1974). Reduction of carcinogen-induced mammary cancer incidence in rats by early treatment with hormones or drugs. *Cancer Research, 34*, 2953–2956.

Knutson, T. P., Daniel, A. R., Fan, D., Silverstein, K. A., Covington, K. R., Fuqua, S. A., et al. (2012). Phosphorylated and sumoylation-deficient progesterone receptors drive proliferative gene signatures during breast cancer progression. *Breast Cancer Research, 14*, R95.

Kordon, E. C., Guerra, F., Molinolo, A. A., Charreau, E. H., Pasqualini, C. D., Pazos, P., et al. (1994). Effect of sialoadenectomy on medroxyprogesterone-acetate-induced mammary carcinogenesis in BALB/c mice. Correlation between histology and epidermal-growth-factor receptor content. *International Journal of Cancer, 59*, 196–203.

Kordon, E., Lanari, C., Meiss, R., Charreau, E., & Pasqualini, C. D. (1990). Hormone dependence of a mouse mammary tumor line induced in vivo by medroxyprogesterone acetate. *Breast Cancer Research and Treatment, 17*, 33–43.

Kordon, E. C., Molinolo, A. A., Pasqualini, C. D., Charreau, E. H., Pazos, P., Dran, G., et al. (1993). Progesterone induction of mammary carcinomas in BALB/c female mice. Correlation between progestin dependence and morphology. *Breast Cancer Research and Treatment, 28*, 29–39.

Koyama, H., Sinha, D., & Dao, T. L. (1972). Effects of hormones and 7,12-dimethylbenz[a] anthracene on rat mammary tissue grown in organ culture. *Journal of the National Cancer Institute, 48*, 1671–1680.

Kubota, T., Josui, K., Fukutomi, T., & Kitajima, M. (1995). Growth regulation by estradiol, progesterone and recombinant human epidermal growth factor of human breast carcinoma xenografts grown serially in nude mice. *Anticancer Research, 15*, 1275–1278.

Kumar, N. S., Richer, J., Owen, G., Litman, E., Horwitz, K. B., & Leslie, K. K. (1998). Selective down-regulation of progesterone receptor isoform B in poorly differentiated human endometrial cancer cells: Implications for unopposed estrogen action. *Cancer Research, 58*, 1860–1865.

Lamb, C. A., Helguero, L. A., Fabris, V., Lucas, C., Molinolo, A. A., & Lanari, C. (2003). Differential effects of raloxifene, tamoxifen and fulvestrant on a murine mammary carcinoma. *Breast Cancer Research and Treatment, 79*, 25–35.

Lamb, C. A., Helguero, L. A., Giulianelli, S., Soldati, R., Vanzulli, S. I., Molinolo, A., et al. (2005). Antisense oligonucleotides targeting the progesterone receptor inhibit hormone-independent breast cancer growth in mice. *Breast Cancer Research, 7*, R1111–R1121.

Lamb, C., Simian, M., Molinolo, A., Pazos, P., & Lanari, C. (1999). Regulation of cell growth of a progestin-dependent murine mammary carcinoma in vitro: Progesterone receptor involvement in serum or growth factor-induced cell proliferation. *Journal of Steroid Biochemistry and Molecular Biology, 70*, 133–142.

Lanari, C., Kordon, E., Molinolo, A., Pasqualini, C. D., & Charreau, E. H. (1989). Mammary adenocarcinomas induced by medroxyprogesterone acetate: Hormone dependence and EGF receptors of BALB/c in vivo sublines. *International Journal of Cancer, 43*, 845–850.

Lanari, C., Molinolo, A. A., & Pasqualini, C. D. (1986). Induction of mammary adenocarcinomas by medroxyprogesterone acetate in BALB/c female mice. *Cancer Letters, 33*, 215–223.

Lanari, C., Wargon, V., Rojas, P., & Molinolo, A. A. (2012). Antiprogestins in breast cancer treatment: Are we ready? *Endocrine-Related Cancer, 19*, R35–R50.

Lange, C. A., Gioeli, D., Hammes, S. R., & Marker, P. C. (2007). Integration of rapid signaling events with steroid hormone receptor action in breast and prostate cancer. *Annual Review of Physiology, 69*, 171–199.

Lange, C. A., Richer, J. K., & Horwitz, K. B. (1999). Hypothesis: Progesterone primes breast cancer cells for cross-talk with proliferative or antiproliferative signals. *Molecular Endocrinology, 13*, 829–836.

Lange, C. A., Richer, J. K., Shen, T., & Horwitz, K. B. (1998). Convergence of progesterone and epidermal growth factor signaling in breast cancer. Potentiation of mitogen-activated protein kinase pathways. *Journal of Biological Chemistry, 273*, 31308–31316.

Lange, C. A., Sartorius, C. A., Abdel-Hafiz, H., Spillman, M. A., Horwitz, K. B., & Jacobsen, B. M. (2008). Progesterone receptor action: Translating studies in breast cancer models to clinical insights. *Advances in Experimental Medicine and Biology, 630*, 94–111.

Lee, D., & Shin, C. (2012). MicroRNA-target interactions: New insights from genome-wide approaches. *Annals of the New York Academy of Sciences*, *1271*, 118–128.

Liang, Y., Benakanakere, I., Besch-Williford, C., Hyder, R. S., Ellersieck, M. R., & Hyder, S. M. (2010). Synthetic progestins induce growth and metastasis of BT-474 human breast cancer xenografts in nude mice. *Menopause*, *17*, 1040–1047.

Liang, Y., Besch-Williford, C., Brekken, R. A., & Hyder, S. M. (2007). Progestin-dependent progression of human breast tumor xenografts: A novel model for evaluating antitumor therapeutics. *Cancer Research*, *67*, 9929–9936.

Loeb, C., & Moskop Kirtz, M. M. (1939). The effect of transplants of anterior lobes of the hypophysis on the growth of the mammary gland and on the development of mammary gland carcinoma in various strains of mice. *American Journal of Cancer*, *36*, 56–82.

Longman, S. M., & Buehring, G. C. (1987). Oral contraceptives and breast cancer. In vitro effect of contraceptive steroids on human mammary cell growth. *Cancer*, *59*, 281–287.

Lopez Perez, F. R., Liang, Y., Besch-Williford, C. L., Mafuvadze, B., & Hyder, S. M. (2012). Differential expression of FGF family members in a progestin-dependent BT-474 human breast cancer xenograft model. *Histology and Histopathology*, *27*, 337–345.

Lydon, J. P., Ge, G., Kittrell, F. S., Medina, D., & O'Malley, B. W. (1999). Murine mammary gland carcinogenesis is critically dependent on progesterone receptor function. *Cancer Research*, *59*, 4276–4284.

Mangelsdorf, D. J., Thummel, C., Beato, M., Herrlich, P., Schutz, G., Umesono, K., et al. (1995). The nuclear receptor superfamily: The second decade. *Cell*, *83*, 835–839.

Manni, A., Badger, B., Wright, C., Ahmed, S. R., & Demers, L. M. (1987). Effects of progestins on growth of experimental breast cancer in culture: Interaction with estradiol and prolactin and involvement of the polyamine pathway. *Cancer Research*, *47*, 3066–3071.

Manni, A., Wright, C., & Buck, H. (1991). Growth factor involvement in the multi-hormonal regulation of MCF-7 breast cancer cell growth in soft agar. *Breast Cancer Research and Treatment*, *20*, 43–52.

Migliaccio, A., Piccolo, D., Castoria, G., Di Domenico, M., Bilancio, A., Lombardi, M., et al. (1998). Activation of the Src/p21ras/Erk pathway by progesterone receptor via cross-talk with estrogen receptor. *EMBO Journal*, *17*, 2008–2018.

Misdorp, W. (1991). Progestagens and mammary tumours in dogs and cats. *Acta Endocrinologica*, *125*(Suppl. 1), 27–31.

Miyamoto, S., Guzman, R. C., Osborn, R. C., & Nandi, S. (1988). Neoplastic transformation of mouse mammary epithelial cells by in vitro exposure to N-methyl-N-nitrosourea. *Proceedings of the National Academy of Sciences of the United States of America*, *85*, 477–481.

Molinolo, A. A., Lanari, C., Charreau, E. H., Sanjuan, N., & Pasqualini, C. D. (1987). Mouse mammary tumors induced by medroxyprogesterone acetate: Immunohisto-chemistry and hormonal receptors. *Journal of the National Cancer Institute*, *79*, 1341–1350.

Montecchia, M. F., Lamb, C., Molinolo, A. A., Luthy, I. A., Pazos, P., Charreau, E., et al. (1999). Progesterone receptor involvement in independent tumor growth in MPA-induced murine mammary adenocarcinomas. *Journal of Steroid Biochemistry and Molecular Biology*, *68*, 11–21.

Moore, M. R., Conover, J. L., & Franks, K. M. (2000). Progestin effects on long-term growth, death, and Bcl-xL in breast cancer cells. *Biochemical and Biophysical Research Communications*, *277*, 650–654.

Moore, M. R., Spence, J. B., Kiningham, K. K., & Dillon, J. L. (2006). Progestin inhibition of cell death in human breast cancer cell lines. *Journal of Steroid Biochemistry and Molecular Biology*, *98*, 218–227.

Moore, M. R., Zhou, J. L., Blankenship, K. A., Strobl, J. S., Edwards, D. P., & Gentry, R. N. (1997). A sequence in the 5' flanking region confers progestin responsiveness on the human c-myc gene. *Journal of Steroid Biochemistry and Molecular Biology*, *62*, 243–252.

Muhlbock, O., & Boot, L. M. (1959). Induction of mammary cancer in mice without the mammary tumor agent by isografts of hypophyses. *Cancer Research, 19*, 402–412.

Musgrove, E. A., Hunter, L. J., Lee, C. S., Swarbrick, A., Hui, R., & Sutherland, R. L. (2001). Cyclin D1 overexpression induces progestin resistance in T-47D breast cancer cells despite p27(Kip1) association with cyclin E-Cdk2. *Journal of Biological Chemistry, 276*, 47675–47683.

Musgrove, E. A., Lee, C. S., & Sutherland, R. L. (1991). Progestins both stimulate and inhibit breast cancer cell cycle progression while increasing expression of transforming growth factor alpha, epidermal growth factor receptor, c-fos, and c-myc genes. *Molecular and Cellular Biology, 11*, 5032–5043.

Nagasawa, H., Aoki, M., Sakagami, N., & Ishida, M. (1988). Medroxyprogesterone acetate enhances spontaneous mammary tumorigenesis and uterine adenomyosis in mice. *Breast Cancer Research and Treatment, 12*, 59–66.

Nagasawa, H., Fujii, M., & Hagiwara, K. (1985). Inhibition by medroxyprogesterone acetate of precancerous mammary hyperplastic alveolar nodule formation in mice. *Breast Cancer Research and Treatment, 5*, 31–36.

Nandi, S., Guzman, R. C., & Yang, J. (1995). Hormones and mammary carcinogenesis in mice, rats, and humans: A unifying hypothesis. *Proceedings of the National Academy of Sciences of the United States of America, 92*, 3650–3657.

Nie, R. V. (1964). Growth and regression of hormone-sensitive mammary tumors in mice. *Jaarboek van Kankeronderzoek en Kankerbestrijding in Nederland, 14*, 17–20.

Obr, A. E., & Edwards, D. P. (2012). The biology of progesterone receptor in the normal mammary gland and in breast cancer. *Molecular and Cellular Endocrinology, 357*, 4–17.

Olefsky, J. M. (2001). Nuclear receptor minireview series. *Journal of Biological Chemistry, 276*, 36863–36864.

Ory, K., Lebeau, J., Levalois, C., Bishay, K., Fouchet, P., Allemand, I., et al. (2001). Apoptosis inhibition mediated by medroxyprogesterone acetate treatment of breast cancer cell lines. *Breast Cancer Research and Treatment, 68*, 187–198.

Owen, G. I., Richer, J. K., Tung, L., Takimoto, G., & Horwitz, K. B. (1998). Progesterone regulates transcription of the p21(WAF1) cyclin-dependent kinase inhibitor gene through Sp1 and CBP/p300. *Journal of Biological Chemistry, 273*, 10696–10701.

Papa, V., Pezzino, V., Costantino, A., Belfiore, A., Giuffrida, D., Frittitta, L., et al. (1990). Elevated insulin receptor content in human breast cancer. *Journal of Clinical Investigation, 86*, 1503–1510.

Pathiraja, T. N., Shetty, P. B., Jelinek, J., He, R., Hartmaier, R., Margossian, A. L., et al. (2011). Progesterone receptor isoform-specific promoter methylation: Association of PRA promoter methylation with worse outcome in breast cancer patients. *Clinical Cancer Research, 17*, 4177–4186.

Pazos, P., Lanari, C., Charreau, E. H., & Molinolo, A. A. (1998). Promoter effect of medroxyprogesterone acetate (MPA) in N-methyl-N-nitrosourea (MNU) induced mammary tumors in BALB/c mice. *Carcinogenesis, 19*, 529–531.

Pazos, P., Lanari, C., Meiss, R., Charreau, E. H., & Pasqualini, C. D. (1992). Mammary carcinogenesis induced by N-methyl-N-nitrosourea (MNU) and medroxyprogesterone acetate (MPA) in BALB/c mice. *Breast Cancer Research and Treatment, 20*, 133–138.

Polo, M. L., Arnoni, M. V., Riggio, M., Wargon, V., Lanari, C., & Novaro, V. (2010). Responsiveness to PI3K and MEK inhibitors in breast cancer. Use of a 3D culture system to study pathways related to hormone independence in mice. *PLoS One, 5*, e10786.

Poulin, R., Baker, D., Poirier, D., & Labrie, F. (1989). Androgen and glucocorticoid receptor-mediated inhibition of cell proliferation by medroxyprogesterone acetate in ZR-75-1 human breast cancer cells. *Breast Cancer Research and Treatment, 13*, 161–172.

Prehn, R. T., & Main, J. M. (1957). Immunity to methylcholanthrene-induced sarcomas. *Journal of the National Cancer Institute, 18*, 769–778.

Quiles, I., Millan-Arino, L., Subtil-Rodriguez, A., Minana, B., Spinedi, N., Ballare, C., et al. (2009). Mutational analysis of progesterone receptor functional domains in stable cell lines delineates sets of genes regulated by different mechanisms. *Molecular Endocrinology, 23*, 809–826.

Richards, J. E., Edery, M., Osborn, R. C., Larson, L. N., & Nandi, S. (1986). Effect of hormones and epidermal growth factor on the growth of the hormone-responsive 13762NF rat mammary tumor in collagen gel culture. *Journal of the National Cancer Institute, 76*, 669–682.

Richer, J. K., Jacobsen, B. M., Manning, N. G., Abel, M. G., Wolf, D. M., & Horwitz, K. B. (2002). Differential gene regulation by the two progesterone receptor isoforms in human breast cancer cells. *Journal of Biological Chemistry, 277*, 5209–5218.

Riggio, M., Polo, M. L., Blaustein, M., Colman-Lerner, A., Luthy, I., Lanari, C., et al. (2012). PI3K/AKT pathway regulates phosphorylation of steroid receptors, hormone independence and tumor differentiation in breast cancer. *Carcinogenesis, 33*, 509–518.

Robinson, S. P., & Jordan, V. C. (1987). Reversal of the antitumor effects of tamoxifen by progesterone in the 7,12-dimethylbenzanthracene-induced rat mammary carcinoma model. *Cancer Research, 47*, 5386–5390.

Ross, R. K., Paganini-Hill, A., Wan, P. C., & Pike, M. C. (2000). Effect of hormone replacement therapy on breast cancer risk: Estrogen versus estrogen plus progestin. *Journal of the National Cancer Institute, 92*, 328–332.

Russo, I. H., Gimotty, P., Dupuis, M., & Russo, J. (1989). Effect of medroxyprogesterone acetate on the response of the rat mammary gland to carcinogenesis. *British Journal of Cancer, 59*, 210–216.

Sartorius, C. A., Harvell, D. M., Shen, T., & Horwitz, K. B. (2005). Progestins initiate a luminal to myoepithelial switch in estrogen-dependent human breast tumors without altering growth. *Cancer Research, 65*, 9779–9788.

Sartorius, C. A., Shen, T., & Horwitz, K. B. (2003). Progesterone receptors A and B differentially affect the growth of estrogen-dependent human breast tumor xenografts. *Breast Cancer Research and Treatment, 79*, 287–299.

Schatz, R. W., Soto, A. M., & Sonnenschein, C. (1985). Effects of interaction between estradiol-17 beta and progesterone on the proliferation of cloned breast tumor cells (MCF-7 and T47D). *Journal of Cellular Physiology, 124*, 386–390.

Shyamala, G., Yang, X., Cardiff, R. D., & Dale, E. (2000). Impact of progesterone receptor on cell-fate decisions during mammary gland development. *Proceedings of the National Academy of Sciences of the United States of America, 97*, 3044–3049.

Simian, M., Manzur, T., Rodriguez, V., Kier Joffe, E. B., & Klein, S. (2009). A spontaneous estrogen dependent, tamoxifen sensitive mouse mammary tumor: A new model system to study hormone-responsiveness in immune competent mice. *Breast Cancer Research and Treatment, 113*, 1–8.

Sluyser, M., & Van Nie, R. (1974). Estrogen receptor content and hormone-responsive growth of mouse mammary tumors. *Cancer Research, 34*, 3253–3257.

Soares, R., Guerreiro, S., & Botelho, M. (2007). Elucidating progesterone effects in breast cancer: Cross talk with PDGF signaling pathway in smooth muscle cell. *Journal of Cellular Biochemistry, 100*, 174–183.

Soule, H. D., Vazquez, J., Long, A., Albert, S., & Brennan, M. (1973). A human cell line from a pleural effusion derived from a breast carcinoma. *Journal of the National Cancer Institute, 51*, 1409–1416.

Su, G., Sung, K. E., Beebe, D. J., & Friedl, A. (2012). Functional screen of paracrine signals in breast carcinoma fibroblasts. *PLoS One, 7*, e46685.

Thomas, P., Pang, Y., Dong, J., Groenen, P., Kelder, J., de Vlieg, J., et al. (2007). Steroid and G protein binding characteristics of the seatrout and human progestin membrane receptor alpha subtypes and their evolutionary origins. *Endocrinology, 148*, 705–718.

Tung, L., Abdel-Hafiz, H., Shen, T., Harvell, D. M., Nitao, L. K., Richer, J. K., et al. (2006). Progesterone receptors (PR)-B and -A regulate transcription by different mechanisms: AF-3 exerts regulatory control over coactivator binding to PR-B. *Molecular Endocrinology*, *20*, 2656–2670.

Van Nie, R., & Thung, P. J. (1965). Responsiveness of mouse mammary tumours to pregnancy. *European Journal of Cancer*, *1*, 41–50.

Vanzulli, S., Efeyan, A., Benavides, F., Helguero, L. A., Peters, G., Shen, J., et al. (2002). p21, p27 and p53 in estrogen and antiprogestin-induced tumor regression of experimental mouse mammary ductal carcinomas. *Carcinogenesis*, *23*, 749–758.

Vares, G., Ory, K., Lectard, B., Levalois, C., Altmeyer-Morel, S., Chevillard, S., et al. (2004). Progesterone prevents radiation-induced apoptosis in breast cancer cells. *Oncogene*, *23*, 4603–4613.

Vazquez, S. M., Mladovan, A., Garbovesky, C., Baldi, A., & Luthy, I. A. (2004). Three novel hormone-responsive cell lines derived from primary human breast carcinomas: Functional characterization. *Journal of Cellular Physiology*, *199*, 460–469.

Vermeulen, M., Pazos, P., Lanari, C., Molinolo, A., Gamberale, R., Geffner, J. R., et al. (2001). Medroxyprogesterone acetate enhances in vivo and in vitro antibody production. *Immunology*, *104*, 80–86.

Vicent, G. P., Nacht, A. S., Zaurin, R., Ballare, C., Clausell, J., & Beato, M. (2010). Minireview: Role of kinases and chromatin remodeling in progesterone signaling to chromatin. *Molecular Endocrinology*, *24*, 2088–2098.

Vignon, F., Bardon, S., Chalbos, D., & Rochefort, H. (1983). Antiestrogenic effect of R5020, a synthetic progestin in human breast cancer cells in culture. *Journal of Clinical Endocrinology and Metabolism*, *56*, 1124–1130.

Wang, S., Counterman, L. J., & Haslam, S. Z. (1990). Progesterone action in normal mouse mammary gland. *Endocrinology*, *127*, 2183–2189.

Wargon, V., Fernandez, S. V., Goin, M., Giulianelli, S., Russo, J., & Lanari, C. (2011). Hypermethylation of the progesterone receptor A in constitutive antiprogestin-resistant mouse mammary carcinomas. *Breast Cancer Research and Treatment*, *126*, 319–332.

Wargon, V., Helguero, L. A., Bolado, J., Rojas, P., Novaro, V., Molinolo, A., et al. (2009). Reversal of antiprogestin resistance and progesterone receptor isoform ratio in acquired resistant mammary carcinomas. *Breast Cancer Research and Treatment*, *116*, 449–460.

Watson, C., Medina, D., & Clark, J. H. (1977). Estrogen receptor characterization in a transplantable mouse mammary tumor. *Cancer Research*, *37*, 3344–3348.

Women's Health Initiative (2002). Risks and benefits of estrogen plus progestin in healthy postmenopausal women: Principal results from the Women's Health Initiative randomized controlled trial. *Journal of the American Medical Association*, *288*, 321–333.

Wu, J., Richer, J., Horwitz, K. B., & Hyder, S. M. (2004). Progestin-dependent induction of vascular endothelial growth factor in human breast cancer cells: Preferential regulation by progesterone receptor B. *Cancer Research*, *64*, 2238–2244.

Yanai, R., & Nagasawa, H. (1976). Importance of progesterone in DNA synthesis of pregnancy-dependent mammary tumors in mice. *International Journal of Cancer*, *18*, 317–321.

Zhu, Y., Rice, C. D., Pang, Y., Pace, M., & Thomas, P. (2003). Cloning, expression, and characterization of a membrane progestin receptor and evidence it is an intermediary in meiotic maturation of fish oocytes. *Proceedings of the National Academy of Sciences of the United States of America*, *100*, 2231–2236.

CHAPTER SIX

The Hyperplastic Phenotype in PR-A and PR-B Transgenic Mice: Lessons on the Role of Estrogen and Progesterone Receptors in the Mouse Mammary Gland and Breast Cancer

Rocio Sampayo, Sol Recouvreux, Marina Simian[1]

Área Investigación, Instituto de Oncología "Angel H. Roffo", Avda. San Martin 5481, Buenos Aires, Argentina
[1]Corresponding author: e-mail address: marina.simian@galuzzi.com

Contents

Abstract

Progesterone receptor (PR) belongs to the superfamily of steroid receptors and mediates the action of progesterone in its target tissues. In the mammary gland, in particular, PR expression is restricted to the luminal epithelial cell compartment. The generation of estrogen receptor-α (ER) and PR knockout mice allowed the specific characterization of the roles of each of these in mammary gland development: ER is critical for ductal morphogenesis, whereas PR has a key role in lobuloalveolar differentiation. To further study the role PR isoforms have in mammary gland biology, transgenic mice overexpressing either the "A" (PR-A) or the "B" (PR-B) isoforms of PR were generated. Overexpression of

Vitamins and Hormones, Volume 93
ISSN 0083-6729
http://dx.doi.org/10.1016/B978-0-12-416673-8.00012-5

185

the A isoform of PR led to increased side branching, multilayered ducts, loss of basement membrane integrity, and alterations in matrix metalloproteinase activation in the mammary gland. Moreover, levels of TGFβ1 and p21 were diminished and those of cyclin D1 increased. Interestingly, the phenotype was counteracted by antiestrogens, suggesting that ER is essential for the manifestation of the hyperplasias. Mice overexpressing the B isoform of PR had limited ductal growth but retained the ability to differentiate during pregnancy. Levels of latent and active TGFβ1 were increased compared to PR-A transgenics.

The phenotypes of these transgenic mice are further discussed in the context of the impact of progesterone on mammary stem cells and breast cancer. We conclude that an adequate balance between the A and B isoforms of PR is critical for tissue homeostasis. Future work to further understand the biology of PR in breast biology will hopefully lead to new and effective preventive and therapeutic alternatives for patients.

1. INTRODUCTION

The ovarian steroids estrogens and progesterone are key players in mammary gland development. Through their cognate receptors, they regulate epithelial cell proliferation and differentiation. The generation of estrogen receptor-α (ER) and progesterone receptor (PR) knockout mice allowed the specific characterization of the roles of each of these receptors in mammary gland development: ER is critical for ductal morphogenesis, whereas PR has a key role in lobuloalveolar differentiation (Bocchinfuso & Korach, 1997; Lydon et al., 1995). To further study the role PR isoforms have in mammary gland biology, transgenic mice overexpressing either the "A" or the "B" isoforms of PR were generated (Shyamala, Yang, Cardiff, & Dale, 2000; Shyamala, Yang, Silberstein, Barcellos-Hoff, & Dale, 1998). Mammary gland development in both these mice strains turned out to be abnormal, with PR-A transgenic mice having a hyperplastic phenotype characterized by excessive lateral ductal branching, whereas in PR-B mice inappropriate alveolar growth was observed. These experiments clearly showed in an *in vivo* setting that an appropriate balance between the A and B isoforms of PR is critical for normal mammary development. Moreover, they suggest that the imbalance observed in human breast cancers toward an increase in the A isoform of PR may have mechanistic implications in the development of this disease (Mote, Bartow, Tran, & Clarke, 2002). In this chapter, we review our current knowledge on the functions of PRs in mammary gland development and analyze in detail the phenotype of the PR-A and PR-B transgenic mice to further understand the role of progesterone's signaling pathway in mammary gland development and breast cancer.

2. DEVELOPMENTAL STAGES IN THE MOUSE MAMMARY GLAND

The mammary gland is a particular organ given that most of its development occurs postnataly. The overall pattern of growth and differentiation is similar between rodents and humans; thus much of what we know about mammary gland biology and the mechanisms leading to breast cancer derive from experiments carried out in mice and rats. In all species, mammary glands are composed by an epithelium and a stroma, separated by the basement membrane. The epithelial compartment is composed of two cell types, luminal epithelial cells that conform the ducts and become milk secretory during lactation and myoepithelial cells that surround the luminal cells and enable the expulsion of milk from the alveoli (Nandi, 1958; Williams & Daniel, 1983). The embryonic stage of development is characterized by the formation of rudimentary epithelial structures from the mammary placodes that invades the surrounding adipose tissue. A small number of branches form from these buds giving rise to the rudimentary ductal tree that is present at birth (Cowin & Wysolmerski, 2010). Puberty enables the next stage of development. In the mouse, at week 3 the increase in circulating estrogen leads to the formation of the end buds that invade the fat pad (Daniel, Silberstein, & Strickland, 1987). The ducts elongate and give rise to secondary branches as a result of a process called bifurcation. In ERKO mice, the ducts lack terminal end buds and do not invade the fat pad reflecting the importance of signaling through ER at this stage of development (Mueller, Clark, Myers, & Korach, 2002). By puberty, the ducts reach the end of the fat pad, with large spaces remaining between them (Daniel, Silberstein, Van Horn, Strickland, & Robinson, 1989). These are filled during pregnancy when the gland reaches full lobuloalveolar development. At this stage, signaling through PR positively regulates the increase in side branching and the formation of alveolar structures which will be responsible for milk production (Shyamala, 1999). In PRKO mice, both proliferation and differentiation associated to pregnancy are hampered (Lydon et al., 1995). After weaning, the mammary gland regresses through the process of involution which is characterized by massive cell death and tissue remodeling (Talhouk, Bissell, & Werb, 1992), reaching a state similar to the one it had before pregnancy.

3. SPATIOTEMPORAL EXPRESSION OF ESTROGEN AND PROGESTERONE RECEPTORS IN THE MOUSE MAMMARY GLAND

In the embryonic mouse mammary gland, expression of ER-α has been found in the mesenchyme that is present surrounding the epithelial rudiment in 14- to16-day-old fetuses (Narbaitz, Stumpf, & Sar, 1980; Shyamala et al., 2002). As early as day 1 after birth, ER-α expression can be detected in mammary epithelial cells and in the dense stroma surrounding the epithelium (Shyamala et al., 2002). Five percent of epithelial cells are positive at day 1, and this increases to about 50% by day 7. This percentage remains practically unchanged throughout the life span of the mice. In the mammary gland of adult mice, ER-α expression is mostly found in the luminal epithelial cells. No staining has been reported for myoepithelial cells (Shyamala et al., 2002). The dense fibrous stroma around the nipple area and the primary mammary ducts are also positive for ER-α, and heterogeneous expression is detected in adipocytes of the mammary fat pad. Hormonal manipulations such as ovariectomy and treatment with estradiol do not significantly modify the percentage of ER-α-positive cells in the adult mammary gland, but they do affect the level of ER-α expression per cell (Shyamala et al., 2002). However, at the beginning of pregnancy, the percentage of ER-α-positive cells begins to decline reaching its lowest level by late pregnancy when only 3–5% of epithelial cells are ER-α positive (Shyamala et al., 2002). This is believed to be the result of sustained high levels of circulating estradiol. At the onset of lactation, ER-α levels are recovered (Shyamala et al., 2002).

PR expression can be regulated by estradiol; however, there are differences between the expression patterns of ER and PR. In 18- to 19-day-old embryos, about 8% of the epithelial cells present in the epithelial rudiment are positive for PR; there are no positive cells in the mesenchyme (Shyamala et al., 2002). A considerable decrease in the percentage of PR positive cells is observed at day 1, with only 2% of cells being positive. However, by day 7, the percentage of positive cells increases and continues to do so till puberty when approximately 55% of cells are positive (Shyamala et al., 2002). The increase in the percentage of positive cells is accompanied by an increase in the amounts of PR per cell (Shyamala et al., 2002). No PR expression has been detected in myoepithelial cells or in the stromal compartment (Shyamala et al., 2002). With the generation of lobuloalveolar structures during pregnancy, the number of PR positive cells decreases as well as the amount of PR expressed by cell. During lactation, PR positive cells are not detected. After lactational involution, PR levels are detected once again, with 20% of cells being positive (Shyamala et al., 2002). These levels are significantly lower than those found in age-matched nulliparous mice, with 40% of luminal cells being PR positive (Shyamala et al., 2002). Estradiol positively regulates PR expression levels, whereas ovariectomy has the opposite effect (Shyamala et al., 2002).

3.1. Differential expression of PR-A and PR-B during mouse mammary development

To further understand the role of progesterone signaling on mammary gland development, several authors have looked into the differential expression of PR isoforms. PR exists in two molecular forms known as the "A" and "B" isoforms. They are both transcribed from the same PR gene that presents two distinct promoters (Kastner et al., 1990). They are structurally similar except for the fact that PR-B is 164 aa longer than PR-A at the N-terminus (Kraus, Montano, & Katzenellenbogen, 1993). This additional domain accounts for the differential functional activities of both isoforms; a distinct set of transcriptional coregulators binds PR-B in this region (Giangrande, Kimbrel, Edwards, & McDonnell, 2000; Sartorius et al., 1994). *In vitro* studies suggest that PR-A is a transrepressor with the capacity of inhibiting both PR-B and ER-α actions, whereas PR-B is a strong transactivator (Vegeto et al., 1993).

Immunohistochemical studies using specific antibodies for each of PR isoform revealed that in the adult mouse mammary gland, it is very rare to find a cell that expresses both PR-A and PR-B (Aupperlee, Smith, Kariagina, & Haslam, 2005). PR-A is predominantly expressed in the virgin mammary gland, whereas PR-B levels rise during pregnancy when lobuloalveolar development takes place (Aupperlee et al., 2005). Interestingly, PR-B colocalizes extensively with BrdU and cyclin D1 in alveolar epithelial cells during pregnancy, whereas PR-A, expressed in ductal cells in the virgin gland, is seldom associated to the proliferative compartment (Aupperlee et al., 2005). Studies aimed at investigating the hormonal regulation of PR isoforms in the mouse mammary gland revealed that PR-A levels are induced by estrogen and downregulated by progesterone. On the other hand, progesterone or estrogen plus progesterone induced PR-B (Aupperlee & Haslam, 2007). Thus, PR isoforms are differentially regulated by estrogens and progesterone in the mouse mammary gland.

4. THE GENERATION OF PR-A AND PR-B TRANSGENIC MICE

Most studies aimed at studying the relative impact of the A and B isoforms of PR in the mammary gland have been carried out *in vitro* using immortalized or tumorigenic cell lines (Daniel, Hagan, & Lange, 2011). To further assess whether these observations were valid for normal developmental processes, Shyamala Harris created transgenic mice overexpressing either the A or the B isoform of PR (Shyamala et al., 1998, 2000). Her goal was to understand whether the imbalance in the ratio of the A to B isoforms of PR could have a direct impact on mammary development. This is a clinically important question given the fact that an increase in the A/B ratio is observed in certain less differentiated and aggressive human breast tumors (Mote et al., 2002). Next, we describe what we know to date regarding the impact of overexpressing either the A or the B isoform of PR in the mouse mammary gland.

4.1. Phenotype of PR-A mice

To create the PR-A transgenic mice, a binary system was used given the possibility that fertility or pregnancy could be affected by the imbalance in the PR isoforms. Mice carrying a GAL-4 gene driven by the murine cytomegalovirus (CMV) were crossed with mice carrying a PR-A gene under the control of four GAL-4 binding sited (Fig. 6.1). The result was the generation of mice carrying additional PR-A gene (Shyamala et al., 1998).

Immunofluorescence studies carried out on mammary glands of ovariectomized prepubertal and adult mice showed that in both cases, the transgenic mice expressed higher levels of PR in epithelial cells. In ovariectomized prepubertal female mice, PR expression was detected in structures resembling end buds. Moreover, in intact adult PR-A transgenics, ducts with more than one layer of cells were detected and they were positive for PR (Shyamala et al., 1998).

Morphological characterization was carried out by analysis of mammary gland whole mounts. Comparison of the mammary glands of 5- to 6-week-old prepubertal transgenic mice with their transgene negative controls revealed that there were no differences; in both cases, 50–60% of the fat pad had been filled and a similar number of end buds were detected. However, upon ovariectomy, the end buds in the mammary glands of the control mice regressed, as expected; this was not the case for the transgenic mice.

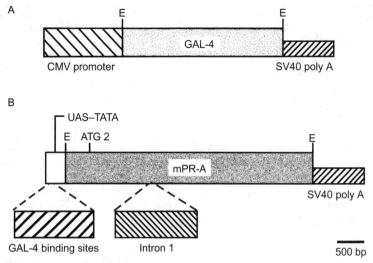

Figure 6.1 Schematic representation of plasmid construction for the binary system. (A) Insertion of the GAL-4 gene into the CMV promoter expression plasmid containing simian virus 40 splice and polyadenylylation sequences. (B) mPR cDNA (A form with only ATG 2) containing intron 1 and simian virus 40 splice and polyadenylylation sequences fused to UAS–TATA fragment containing four GAL-4 binding sites. E, *Eco*RI. *Shyamala et al. (1998), Copyright (1998) National Academy of Sciences, USA.*

End buds persisted in the PR–A transgenic mice and only disappeared after prolonged ovariectomy (Shyamala et al., 1998). Analysis of young adult mice (10–14 weeks old) revealed that the degree of ductal branching was similar in transgenic and control mice. However, once adult, mammary glands of transgenic mice showed extensive lateral branching with the presence of very thick ducts (Fig. 6.2). The degree of lateral branching in some cases resembled early pregnancy. The lateral structures in transgenics showed bulbous structures and a high number of buds were detected in areas that are normally growth-quiescent. The tips of the ducts of transgenic mice presented additional aberrant morphology in the form of clustered buds compared to the smooth ends found in normal terminal buds (Shyamala et al., 1998).

Histological analysis of the mammary glands of PR–A transgenic mice revealed that the thickening of the ducts was due to the presence of multiple layers of cells; ducts are normally composed of one layer of epithelial cells. Moreover, regions of indistinct stromal–epithelial boundaries were detected, and disorganized masses of epithelial cells were observed at the tip of some ducts (Shyamala et al., 1998).

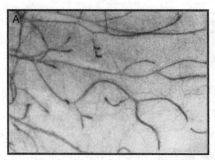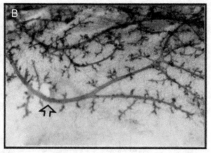

Figure 6.2 Morphological characteristics of mammary glands in adult PR-A transgenic mice. Whole mounts of mammary glands from young (10–14 weeks old) control PR-A transgene-negative (A) and PR-A transgenic mice (B) are shown. In (B), the open arrow shows thick ducts. Extensive lateral branching can be seen in the transgenic compared to the control. *Shyamala et al. (1998), Copyright (1998) National Academy of Sciences, USA.*

To further understand what was going on in the mammary glands of PR-A transgenic mice, immunofluorescence studies were carried out. E-cadherin staining revealed that the bulbous structures were characterized by a loss of organization in the epithelial cells of the duct (Shyamala et al., 1998). Given that a loss in stromal–epithelial boundaries had been observed by histological analysis, studies were carried out to investigate whether the basement membrane was affected. Immunofluorescence for laminin, laminin-5, collagen IV, and collagen III all showed a loss of basement membrane integrity in abnormal structures in mammary glands of PR-A mice (Shyamala et al., 1998; Simian, Bissell, Barcellos-Hoff, & Shyamala, 2009). This lead us to investigate whether matrix metalloproteinase levels were affected given that they play a major role in extracellular matrix remodeling in the mammary gland. Zymography assays revealed that levels of MMP-2 and MMP-9 were not significantly higher in extracts of PR-A mammary glands compared to controls (Simian et al., 2009). To further investigate whether there could be a link between the steady-state levels of PR and MMP activity, we analyzed tissues derived from PR null mutant mice and compared them to littermate controls. We found that there was a significant decrease in the total levels of MMP-2 in the PR null tissues, suggesting that PR levels impact proteolytic activity (Simian et al., 2009). The next question to be answered was whether signaling through ER or PR affected either the levels or the activation of MMP-2 and MMP-9. To answer this question, we treated ovariectomized wild-type and PR-A mice with vehicle, estrogen, progesterone, or both. Zymography of extracts derived from these mammary glands revealed that MMP-2 is activated as a result of exposure to estrogen and progesterone and that only in PR-A transgenics, where PR levels are maintained even after ovariectomy, progesterone alone leads to MMP-2 activation (Simian et al., 2009).

To further understand the aberrant features associated to the PR-A transgenic, mammary glands studies were carried out to analyze alterations in gene expression and growth potential. In areas of aberrant growth and loss of organization, epithelial cells showed a decrease in p21 expression, an increase in cyclin D1, a decrease in ER-α, and an increase in proliferation (Chou, Uehara, Lowry, & Shyamala, 2003). In areas of normal morphology, only a decrease in p21 was observed compared to control mammary glands (Chou et al., 2003). Moreover, analysis of latent and active TGFβ1 showed that they were both diminished in the mammary glands of PR-A transgenics compared to controls (Simian et al., 2009). TGFβ is regulated by estradiol and progesterone in the mammary gland and restricts the proliferative response to these steroids (Ewan et al., 2005). Whole mounts of mammary glands derived from mice subjected to ovariectomy and hormonal treatments showed that the phenotype of PR-A transgenic mice is dependent on signaling through ER and PR as the hyperplastic phenotype is recovered upon treatment with both hormones (Simian et al., 2009). Interestingly, antiprogestins like mifepristone and RU486 do not reverse the hyperplastic phenotype, whereas the antiestrogen ICI182,780 does (Simian et al., 2009). This would suggest that cross talk between PR-A and ER is essential for the manifestation of the hyperplastic phenotype.

Mammary epithelial cells are presumed immortal if they can be propagated *in vivo*, through serial transplantation, for more than five generations. Tissue fragments derived from PR-A transgenic mice were propagated up to eight generations (Shyamala et al., 2000). This fact, together with the decrease in p21 and increase in cyclin D1, concludes that the ducts contain presumptive immortalized cells indicative of early stages of transformation.

4.2. Phenotype of PR-B mice

To generate mice carrying an excess of the B form of PR, a binary system as that described for the PR-A transgenic mice was used. As explained above, a GAL-4 gene, driven by the murine cytomegalovirus promoter (CMV-GAL-4 mice), served as a transactivator of the PR-B gene, which carried four GAL-4 binding sites (UAS-PR-B mice). Crossing the CMV-GAL-4 mice with the UAS-PR-B mice generated bigenic mice carrying additional PR-B gene (Shyamala et al., 2000).

Whole mounts of young adult mice (10–14 weeks old) did not show any difference between wild-type and transgenic littermates. However, at 20 weeks of age, in 20% of PR-B transgenic mice, the fat pad was not completely filled, in contrast to wild-type controls (Shyamala et al., 2000). Also, in some of these glands, there were regions with no lateral branching. Interestingly, in these glands, no end buds could be seen, suggesting a cessation of growth (Shyamala et al., 2000). To verify that growth was compromised as a result of the increase in PR-B, serial transplantation studies were carried out. Growth was compromised in some of the first-generation transplants where the ducts did not extend to fill the fat pad. In the second generation, however, a significant number of transplants did not fill the fat pad, and in the third, growth was extremely limited (Fig. 6.3). In control mice, as previously shown by others, transplants filled the fat pad even in the third generation (Shyamala et al., 2000).

Interestingly, the limited growth recorded for the PR-B transplants was intrinsic of the epithelial tissue and not derived from host factors because the failure to grow was seen even when the tissue was transplanted into cleared

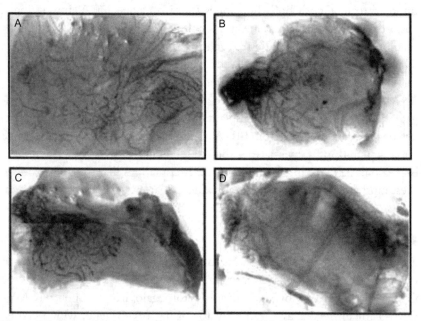

Figure 6.3 Photomicrographs of mammary tissues of PR-B transgenics. (A) Generation three outgrowth of tissue from a wild-type mouse. Outgrowths of serially transplanted mammary tissues of PR-B transgenics in the first (B), second (C), and third (D) generation. *Shyamala et al. (2000), Copyright (2000) National Academy of Sciences, USA.*

fat pads of wild-type littermates. Interestingly, when mice carrying third-generation transplants were mated, the mammary glands displayed lobuloalveolar development, suggesting that even though ductal growth is compromised, the capacity to differentiate is not affected (Shyamala et al., 2000). Histological analysis of outgrowths of PR-B transgenics revealed that the lobules were slightly abnormal. They formed compact acini and were recurrently embedded in highly cellular connective tissue; the structures were disorganized with limited secondary and tertiary ductal branching. Moreover, the alveoli were less differentiated as revealed by a lack of cytoplasmatic lipid vacuoles. A high number of mitotic figures were observed and some of these were abnormal (Shyamala et al., 2000).

To further understand what other signaling pathways could be implicated in the phenotype observed of PR-B mice, levels of latent and active TGFβ1 were measured and compared to those of PR-A transgenics. We found that both latent and active forms of TGFβ1 were present at higher levels compared to PR-A transgenics, although only the increase in LAP was statistically significant (Simian et al., 2009). We have not yet analyzed the levels of MMPs in mammary glands of PR-B transgenics or basement membrane integrity. Table 6.1 compares the phenotypes of PR-A and PR-B transgenics.

5. BREAST CANCER AND PRs

ERs have been traditionally associated to breast cancer to the point that adjuvant hormonal treatments are exclusively directed against this hormone receptor (Sengupta & Jordan, 2008). However, we know today that PR is a potent mitogen for breast cells. One of the main functions of progesterone signaling through PR is to mediate the expansion of the epithelial compartment and thus allow lobuloalveolar development in preparation for lactation (Stingl, 2011). We reviewed above the spatiotemporal expression pattern of PR in the mouse mammary gland. We also described the phenotypes found in PR-A and PR-B transgenic mice, which clearly reveal that the balance between PR isoforms is critical for mammary development. Moreover, overexpression of PR-A leads to the development of preneoplastic lesions (Chou et al., 2003). Other experimental models have strongly suggested that PRs play a key role in the development of breast cancer. In breast cancer cell lines, PR was shown to increase survival, growth, and anchorage-independent growth (Faivre & Lange, 2007; Lamb, Simian, Molinolo, Pazos, & Lanari, 1999; Moore, Conover, & Franks, 2000).

Table 6.1 Comparison between PR-A and PR-B transgenic mice

Transgenic mouse phenotype	PR-A	PR-B	References
Ductal development	Increased side branching Multilayered ducts	Incomplete ductal development	Shyamala et al. (1998) Shyamala et al. (2000)
Lobuloalveolar development	Not affected	Not affected	Shyamala et al. (1998) Shyamala et al. (2000)
Basement membrane integrity	Loss of collagen IV, laminin-5, and collagen III	ND	Shyamala et al. (1998) Simian et al. (2009)
MMPs	Activation of MMP-2 by progesterone	ND	Simian et al. (2009)
LAP/TGFβ-1	Decreased	Increased	Simian et al. (2009)
BrdU-positive cells	Increased	Not affected	Chou et al. (2003)
Cyclin D1	Increased	Not affected	Chou et al., 2003
p21	Decreased	Slightly elevated	Chou et al. (2003)

ND, not determined.

In mouse models of breast cancer, genetic disruption of the tumor suppressor *BRCA1* and tumors induced by chemical carcinogens were in both cases dependent on PR signaling for progression (Lydon, Ge, Kittrell, Medina, & O'Malley, 1999; Poole et al., 2006). On the other hand, long-term administration of medroxyprogesterone acetate induced mammary tumors in BALB/c mice (Lanari, Kordon, Molinolo, Pasqualini, & Charreau, 1989). In rats, antiprogestins inhibited the appearance of spontaneous mammary lesions and breast tumors induced by chemical carcinogenesis (Wiehle, Lantvit, Yamada, & Christov, 2011). In humans, large clinical trials have shown that in postmenopausal women, administration of progestin in hormone replacement therapy leads to an increase in the incidence and grade of breast tumors (Chlebowski et al., 2010). All these results strongly suggest that further studies oriented at understanding the role of PR isoforms in mammary gland biology and breast cancer development could lead to novel therapeutic alternatives that could target PR. In Section 6, we review recent findings related to the role of PRs and stem cells that are relevant in the context of the phenotypes described for the PR-A and PR-B transgenic mice.

6. PRs AND MAMMARY STEM CELLS

It is now widely accepted that in the mammary gland, there is a population of undifferentiated stem cells that give rise to terminally differentiated epithelial and myoepithelial cells (Visvader & Smith, 2011). Mammary stem cells are devoid of ER and PR, and until recently, we did not understand how estrogen and progesterone modulated them (Asselin-Labat et al., 2006; Visvader, 2009). Two seminal papers published in *Nature* show the important role progesterone has in regulating the stem cells in the mouse mammary gland. Asselin-Labat et al. (2010) and Joshi et al. (2010) elegantly showed that steroid hormones, in particular, progesterone, play a key role. They demonstrate that mammary stem cell numbers peak during the diestrus phase of the murine estrous cycle, when progesterone levels are highest (Joshi et al., 2010). Moreover, during pregnancy, when progesterone levels increase, so does the number of stem cells (Asselin-Labat et al., 2010; Joshi et al., 2010). In the mammary gland, paracrine factors mediate the stimulatory effect of estrogen and progesterone on cell proliferation. Both reports show that progesterone exerts its effect by regulating the levels of RANKL in the ER+/PR+ luminal cell population which then acts on the mammary stem cell population that expresses RANK receptor. Thus, the RANKL–RANK axis, downstream of PR, has a direct impact on the expansion of stem cells. These experiments were further supported by the inhibitory effect observed when mice were treated with an anti-RANKL antibody (Asselin-Labat et al., 2010). Interestingly, the authors show a peek in the amount of stem cells in mid-pregnancy (Asselin-Labat et al., 2010), which coincides with the previously reported switch in the relative amounts of PR-A:PR-B, with an increase in PR-B that accompanies the beginning of cell differentiation that culminates with lactation after birth (Aupperlee et al., 2005). We believe that this interesting observation, together with the phenotypes found in the PR-A and PR-B transgenics, suggests that the A isoform of PR would be responsible for the expansion of the stem cell population via RANKL–RANK and that PR-B would have a counter effect, leading to differentiation. Moreover, the fact that an altered ratio in PR-A:PR-B, with a decrease in PR-B, is an early event in tumor development in patients argues in favor of this hypothesis.

7. CONCLUSION AND FUTURE DIRECTIONS

The generation of the PR-A and PR-B transgenics has allowed us to have a deeper understanding of PR function, in particular, in the mouse mammary gland. The most relevant conclusion is that an adequate balance between the A and B isoforms of PR is critical for tissue homeostasis. The fact that by only increasing the relative amounts of PR-A, breast hyperplasias are generated in mice supports the idea that PR plays a key role in mammary carcinogenesis. This is reinforced by the observation that in human breast tumor samples, a relative increase in A to B isoform is an early event in tumorigenesis. The finding that progesterone signaling through PR is critical in stem cell expansion in the mammary gland may have direct implications on mammary carcinogenesis: one could hypothesize that alterations in PR signaling would lead to a loss of control in the stem cell maintenance and as a consequence generate greater susceptibility to cancer. Whether this is so is an important question which we hope to address shortly in the field. Finally, the impact of progestins on the development of breast cancer in women taking hormone replacement therapy only supports an active role of PR signaling in breast tumorigenesis. Future work to further understand the biology of PR in breast biology will hopefully lead to new and effective preventive and therapeutic alternatives for patients.

ACKNOWLEDGMENTS

This work is supported by grants from the Ministerio de Ciencia y Tecnologia (PICT 2008-0325) and the Florencia Fiorini Foundation to M. S. R. S. is a CONICET doctoral fellow, S. R. is a predoctoral student from the University of Buenos Aires, and M. S. is a CONICET Career Researcher.

REFERENCES

Asselin-Labat, M. L., Shackleton, M., Stingl, J., Vaillant, F., Forrest, N. C., Eaves, C. J., et al. (2006). Steroid hormone receptor status of mouse mammary stem cells. *Journal of the National Cancer Institute*, *98*, 1011–1014.

Asselin-Labat, M. L., Vaillant, F., Sheridan, J. M., Pal, B., Wu, D., Simpson, E. R., et al. (2010). Control of mammary stem cell function by steroid hormone signalling. *Nature*, *465*, 798–802.

Aupperlee, M. D., & Haslam, S. Z. (2007). Differential hormonal regulation and function of progesterone receptor isoforms in normal adult mouse mammary gland. *Endocrinology*, *148*, 2290–2300.

Aupperlee, M. D., Smith, K. T., Kariagina, A., & Haslam, S. Z. (2005). Progesterone receptor isoforms A and B: Temporal and spatial differences in expression during murine mammary gland development. *Endocrinology, 146*, 3577–3588.

Bocchinfuso, W. P., & Korach, K. S. (1997). Mammary gland development and tumorigenesis in estrogen receptor knockout mice. *Journal of Mammary Gland Biology and Neoplasia, 2*, 323–334.

Chlebowski, R. T., Anderson, G. L., Gass, M., Lane, D. S., Aragaki, A. K., Kuller, L. H., et al. (2010). Estrogen plus progestin and breast cancer incidence and mortality in postmenopausal women. *JAMA: The Journal of the American Medical Association, 304*, 1684–1692.

Chou, Y. C., Uehara, N., Lowry, J. R., & Shyamala, G. (2003). Mammary epithelial cells of PR-A transgenic mice exhibit distinct alterations in gene expression and growth potential associated with transformation. *Carcinogenesis, 24*, 403–409.

Cowin, P., & Wysolmerski, J. (2010). Molecular mechanisms guiding embryonic mammary gland development. *Cold Spring Harbor Perspectives in Biology, 2*, a003251.

Daniel, A. R., Hagan, C. R., & Lange, C. A. (2011). Progesterone receptor action: Defining a role in breast cancer. *Expert Review of Endocrinology and Metabolism, 6*, 359–369.

Daniel, C. W., Silberstein, G. B., & Strickland, P. (1987). Direct action of 17 beta-estradiol on mouse mammary ducts analyzed by sustained release implants and steroid autoradiography. *Cancer Research, 47*, 6052–6057.

Daniel, C. W., Silberstein, G. B., Van Horn, K., Strickland, P., & Robinson, S. (1989). TGF-beta 1-induced inhibition of mouse mammary ductal growth: Developmental specificity and characterization. *Developmental Biology, 135*, 20–30.

Ewan, K. B., Oketch-Rabah, H. A., Ravani, S. A., Shyamala, G., Moses, H. L., & Barcellos-Hoff, M. H. (2005). Proliferation of estrogen receptor-alpha-positive mammary epithelial cells is restrained by transforming growth factor-beta1 in adult mice. *The American Journal of Pathology, 167*, 409–417.

Faivre, E. J., & Lange, C. A. (2007). Progesterone receptors upregulate Wnt-1 to induce epidermal growth factor receptor transactivation and c-Src-dependent sustained activation of Erk1/2 mitogen-activated protein kinase in breast cancer cells. *Molecular and Cellular Biology, 27*, 466–480.

Giangrande, P. H., Kimbrel, E. A., Edwards, D. P., & McDonnell, D. P. (2000). The opposing transcriptional activities of the two isoforms of the human progesterone receptor are due to differential cofactor binding. *Molecular and Cellular Biology, 20*, 3102–3115.

Joshi, P. A., Jackson, H. W., Beristain, A. G., Di Grappa, M. A., Mote, P. A., Clarke, C. L., et al. (2010). Progesterone induces adult mammary stem cell expansion. *Nature, 465*, 803–807.

Kastner, P., Krust, A., Turcotte, B., Stropp, U., Tora, L., Gronemeyer, H., et al. (1990). Two distinct estrogen-regulated promoters generate transcripts encoding the two functionally different human progesterone receptor forms A and B. *The EMBO Journal, 9*, 1603–1614.

Kraus, W. L., Montano, M. M., & Katzenellenbogen, B. S. (1993). Cloning of the rat progesterone receptor gene 5'-region and identification of two functionally distinct promoters. *Molecular Endocrinology, 7*, 1603–1616.

Lamb, C., Simian, M., Molinolo, A., Pazos, P., & Lanari, C. (1999). Regulation of cell growth of a progestin-dependent murine mammary carcinoma in vitro: Progesterone receptor involvement in serum or growth factor-induced cell proliferation. *The Journal of Steroid Biochemistry and Molecular Biology, 70*, 133–142.

Lanari, C., Kordon, E., Molinolo, A., Pasqualini, C. D., & Charreau, E. H. (1989). Mammary adenocarcinomas induced by medroxyprogesterone acetate: Hormone dependence and EGF receptors of BALB/c in vivo sublines. *International Journal of Cancer, 43*, 845–850.

Lydon, J. P., DeMayo, F. J., Funk, C. R., Mani, S. K., Hughes, A. R., Montgomery, C. A., Jr., et al. (1995). Mice lacking progesterone receptor exhibit pleiotropic reproductive abnormalities. *Genes & Development, 9,* 2266–2278.

Lydon, J. P., Ge, G., Kittrell, F. S., Medina, D., & O'Malley, B. W. (1999). Murine mammary gland carcinogenesis is critically dependent on progesterone receptor function. *Cancer Research, 59,* 4276–4284.

Moore, M. R., Conover, J. L., & Franks, K. M. (2000). Progestin effects on long-term growth, death, and Bcl-xL in breast cancer cells. *Biochemical and Biophysical Research Communications, 277,* 650–654.

Mote, P. A., Bartow, S., Tran, N., & Clarke, C. L. (2002). Loss of co-ordinate expression of progesterone receptors A and B is an early event in breast carcinogenesis. *Breast Cancer Research and Treatment, 72,* 163–172.

Mueller, S. O., Clark, J. A., Myers, P. H., & Korach, K. S. (2002). Mammary gland development in adult mice requires epithelial and stromal estrogen receptor alpha. *Endocrinology, 143,* 2357–2365.

Nandi, S. (1958). Endocrine control of mammary gland development and function in C3H/Crgl mouse. *Journal of the National Cancer Institute, 21,* 1039–1063.

Narbaitz, R., Stumpf, W. E., & Sar, M. (1980). Estrogen receptors in mammary gland primordia of fetal mouse. *Anatomy and Embryology, 158,* 161–166.

Poole, A. J., Li, Y., Kim, Y., Lin, S. C., Lee, W. H., & Lee, E. Y. (2006). Prevention of Brca1-mediated mammary tumorigenesis in mice by a progesterone antagonist. *Science, 314,* 1467–1470.

Sartorius, C. A., Melville, M. Y., Hovland, A. R., Tung, L., Takimoto, G. S., & Horwitz, K. B. (1994). A third transactivation function (AF3) of human progesterone receptors located in the unique N-terminal segment of the B-isoform. *Molecular Endocrinology, 8,* 1347–1360.

Sengupta, S., & Jordan, V. C. (2008). Selective estrogen modulators as an anticancer tool: Mechanisms of efficiency and resistance. *Advances in Experimental Medicine and Biology, 630,* 206–219.

Shyamala, G. (1999). Progesterone signaling and mammary gland morphogenesis. *Journal of Mammary Gland Biology and Neoplasia, 4,* 89–104.

Shyamala, G., Chou, Y. C., Louie, S. G., Guzman, R. C., Smith, G. H., & Nandi, S. (2002). Cellular expression of estrogen and progesterone receptors in mammary glands: Regulation by hormones, development and aging. *The Journal of Steroid Biochemistry and Molecular Biology, 80,* 137–148.

Shyamala, G., Yang, X., Cardiff, R. D., & Dale, E. (2000). Impact of progesterone receptor on cell-fate decisions during mammary gland development. *Proceedings of the National Academy of Sciences of the United States of America, 97,* 3044–3049.

Shyamala, G., Yang, X., Silberstein, G., Barcellos-Hoff, M. H., & Dale, E. (1998). Transgenic mice carrying an imbalance in the native ratio of A to B forms of progesterone receptor exhibit developmental abnormalities in mammary glands. *Proceedings of the National Academy of Sciences of the United States of America, 95,* 696–701.

Simian, M., Bissell, M. J., Barcellos-Hoff, M. H., & Shyamala, G. (2009). Estrogen and progesterone receptors have distinct roles in the establishment of the hyperplastic phenotype in PR-A transgenic mice. *Breast Cancer Research, 11,* R72.

Stingl, J. (2011). Estrogen and progesterone in normal mammary gland development and in cancer. *Hormones & Cancer, 2,* 85–90.

Talhouk, R. S., Bissell, M. J., & Werb, Z. (1992). Coordinated expression of extracellular matrix-degrading proteinases and their inhibitors regulates mammary epithelial function during involution. *The Journal of Cell Biology, 118,* 1271–1282.

Vegeto, E., Shahbaz, M. M., Wen, D. X., Goldman, M. E., O'Malley, B. W., & McDonnell, D. P. (1993). Human progesterone receptor A form is a cell- and promoter-specific repressor of human progesterone receptor B function. *Molecular Endocrinology, 7,* 1244–1255.

Visvader, J. E. (2009). Keeping abreast of the mammary epithelial hierarchy and breast tumorigenesis. *Genes & Development, 23,* 2563–2577.

Visvader, J. E., & Smith, G. H. (2011). Murine mammary epithelial stem cells: Discovery, function, and current status. *Cold Spring Harbor Perspectives in Biology, 3,* a004879.

Wiehle, R., Lantvit, D., Yamada, T., & Christov, K. (2011). CDB-4124, a progesterone receptor modulator, inhibits mammary carcinogenesis by suppressing cell proliferation and inducing apoptosis. *Cancer Prevention Research (Philadelphia, PA), 4,* 414–424.

Williams, J. M., & Daniel, C. W. (1983). Mammary ductal elongation: Differentiation of myoepithelium and basal lamina during branching morphogenesis. *Developmental Biology, 97,* 274–290.

CHAPTER SEVEN

FOXP1 and Estrogen Signaling in Breast Cancer

Nobuhiro Ijichi[*], Kazuhiro Ikeda[*], Kuniko Horie-Inoue[*], Satoshi Inoue[*,†,‡,1]

[*]Division of Gene Regulation and Signal Transduction, Research Center for Genomic Medicine, Saitama Medical University, Saitama, Japan
[†]Department of Geriatric Medicine, Graduate School of Medicine, The University of Tokyo, Tokyo, Japan
[‡]Department of Anti-Aging Medicine, Graduate School of Medicine, The University of Tokyo, Tokyo, Japan
[1]Corresponding author: e-mail address: Inoue-Ger@h.u-tokyo.ac.jp

Contents

Abstract

Breast cancers are considered to be primarily regulated by estrogen signaling pathways because estrogen-dependent proliferation is observed in the majority of breast cancer cases. Thus, hormone therapy using antiestrogen drugs such as tamoxifen is effective for breast cancers expressing estrogen receptor α (ERα). However, acquired resistance during the endocrine therapy is a critical unresolved problem in breast cancer. Recently, a forkhead transcription factor FOXA1 has been reported to play an important role in the regulation of ERα-mediated transcription and proliferation of breast cancer. Interestingly, immunohistochemical analysis of breast cancer specimens has revealed that nuclear immunoreactivities of FOXP1 as well as those of FOXA1 are positively correlated with hormone receptor status, including ERα and progesterone receptor. In particular, the double-positive immunoreactivities of FOXP1 and FOXA1 are significantly associated with a favorable prognosis for survival of breast cancer patients receiving adjuvant tamoxifen therapy. The functions of FOXP1 and FOXA1 have been characterized in cultured cells; further, similar to FOXA1, FOXP1 is assumed to be a critical transcription factor for ERα signaling, and both forkhead transcription factors can serve as predictive factors for acquired endocrine resistance in breast cancer.

Vitamins and Hormones, Volume 93
ISSN 0083-6729
http://dx.doi.org/10.1016/B978-0-12-416673-8.00006-X

1. INTRODUCTION

Estrogen is a sex steroid hormone that regulates various cellular events through its cognate estrogen receptor α (ERα), which functions as a transcription factor that activates the transcription of its target genes (Platet, Cathiard, Gleizes, & Garcia, 2004). Clinically, ERα is noted as the defining feature of luminal breast cancer, which accounts for a large portion of breast cancers. Luminal breast cancer is generally treated with endocrine therapy using classical antiestrogen agents such as tamoxifen, which acts as an antagonist for ERα in breast cancer cells. Because of the sensitivity to endocrine therapy, ERα-positive luminal breast cancer is considered to have better prognosis than ERα-negative breast cancer. However, resistance to antiestrogen therapies is often acquired in a substantial fraction of recurrent breast cancers. Identification of the factors involved in the mechanisms underlying endocrine resistance, recurrence, or poor prognosis of breast cancer will be useful for understanding the exact pathophysiology of the disease and for developing alternative diagnostic methods and treatment specific to the disease.

The transcriptional activity of ERα is regulated by a number of regulatory cofactors, including chromatin-remodeling complexes, coactivators, and corepressors (Hall & McDonnell, 2005). Moreover, several transcription factors, including those belonging to the forkhead box (FOX) family, modulate the transcriptional activity of ERα. In particular, as described in detail below, FOXA1 plays a crucial role in the ERα-mediated transcription in breast cancer cells (Carroll et al., 2005; Hurtado, Holmes, Ross-Innes, Schmidt, & Carroll, 2011; Lupien et al., 2008). In addition, recent clinicopathological and *in vitro* studies have shown that another member belonging to the FOX family, FOXP1, is closely related to the biology of breast cancer (Ijichi et al., 2012; Shigekawa et al., 2011). This chapter focuses on the potential role of FOXP1 compared to that of FOXA1 in the pathophysiology of breast cancer and discusses the clinical relevance of these forkhead factors in the disease, particularly in association with hormone therapy.

2. FOXP1 AND FOXA1 IN ERα-POSITIVE BREAST CANCER CELLS

FOXP1 and FOXA1 are transcription factors, which belong to the FOX family that includes a conserved forkhead DNA-binding domain

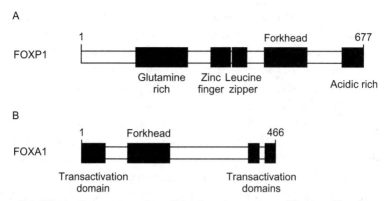

Figure 7.1 Schematic representation of the domain structure of forkhead box transcription factor FOXA1 and FOXP1 proteins. (A) FOXP1 structure. Forkhead domain is located in the C-terminal region of the FOXP1 protein. Zinc finger and leucine zipper domains, responsible for dimerization of FOXP1, are located in the central region. (B) FOXA1 structure. Forkhead domain is located in N-terminal region of FOXA1 protein. Three transactivation domains are located in both terminal regions.

(Fig. 7.1; Li, Weidenfeld, & Morrisey, 2004; Wang, Lin, Li, & Tucker, 2003). Recently, genome-wide studies with an aim of identifying ERα- and androgen receptor (AR)-binding sites have shown that FOXA1 plays a role in regulation of the nuclear receptor-mediated gene networks (Carroll et al., 2005, 2006; Lupien et al., 2008). FOXA1 is recognized as a pioneer transcription factor because binding of FOXA1 to chromatin DNA facilitates subsequent recruitment of ERα and AR to the genome (Grange, Roux, Rigaud, & Pictet, 1991; Lupien et al., 2008). Genome-wide mapping of ERα-, AR-, and FOXA1-binding events in breast and prostate cancer cells using high-throughput sequencing has further uncovered the involvement of several collaborative factors, including TLE1 and activator protein 2γ (AP-2γ), in the nuclear receptor-mediated transcription (Holmes et al., 2012; Tan et al., 2011). In breast cancer cells, several FOX family transcription factors may contribute to the ERα-mediated transcription by directly interacting with the ERα protein, as exemplified by FOXA1 and FKHR/FOXO1 (Carroll & Brown, 2006; Schuur et al., 2001).

Recent studies have shown that FOXP1 and FOXA1 play critical roles in estrogen signaling and in the biology of ERα-positive breast cancer (Ijichi et al., 2012; Shigekawa et al., 2011). These studies showed an upregulation in the expressions of *FOXP1* and *FOXA1* mRNAs induced by 17β-estradiol (E2) stimulation in ERα-positive MCF-7 cells. The upregulation of both genes was observed in the early phase (3 h) after E2 stimulation, which suggests that both FOXP1 and FOXA1 are transcriptionally regulated by the estrogen in breast cancer cells. In addition, Giguère and his colleagues reported that estrogen upregulates the levels of FOXA1 protein 4–8 h after E2 stimulation (Laganière et al., 2005). Consistent with these findings, the findings of genome-wide chromatin immunoprecipitation (ChIP) analysis based on microarrays (ChIP-chip) showed three and two functional estrogen receptor-binding sites (ERBSs) within the *FOXP1* and *FOXA1* gene loci, respectively, in the genome of MCF-7 cells (Carroll et al., 2005). Conventional ChIP assay showed more than twofold enrichments of estrogen-dependent recruitment of ERα in these ERBSs, which suggested that the recruitment of ERα in the *FOXP1* and *FOXA1* loci contributes to the estrogen-dependent transcription of both *FOX* genes.

Further, FOXP1 and FOXA1 have been shown to serve as transcription factors that directly regulate the ERα-mediated transcription. Luciferase reporter analysis using a vector containing an estrogen-responsive element (ERE, ERE-tk-*luc*) showed that overexpression of either FOXP1 or FOXA1 significantly stimulated the ERα-mediated transactivation in MCF-7 cells in response to estrogen. siRNA-mediated knockdown of FOXA1 reduced ERα-mediated transactivation in the presence or absence of estrogen in MCF-7 cells. Consistent with these observations, the results of other studies showed upregulation of known estrogen-responsive genes, including *SHP* (Lai, Harnish, & Evans, 2003) and *LRH-1* (Annicotte et al., 2005), in FOXP1-overexpressing MCF-7 cells treated with estrogen. Similarly, the contribution of FOXA1 to ERα-mediated transcription was further confirmed by the FOXA1 siRNA-dependent reduction in estrogen-induced expressions of prototypic ERα target genes, progesterone receptor (*PgR*), and growth regulation by estrogen in breast cancer 1 (*GREB1*) (Ghosh, Thompson, & Weigel, 2000; Kastner et al., 1990). These observations suggest that both FOXP1 and FOXA1 stimulate ERα transcription activity in response to estrogen.

The mutual transcriptional regulations of *ERα* and *FOX* genes indicate that both FOXA1 and FOXP1 have the potential to promote estrogen-dependent proliferation of breast cancer cells. Moreover, FOXA1 also upregulates the migration of MCF-7 cells. These findings suggest that FOXP1 and FOXA1 regulate ERα in a positive feedback manner and play crucial roles in the estrogen-dependent cellular responses of ERα-positive breast cancer cells (Fig. 7.2).

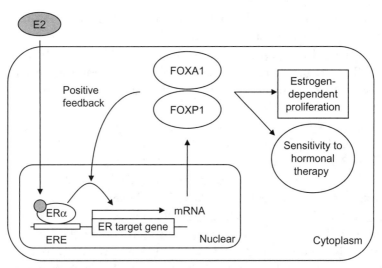

Figure 7.2 Model for cellular functions of FOXP1 and FOXA1 in estrogen signaling. *FOXP1* and *FOXA1* are primary target genes for estrogen receptor α (ERα) and regulate the ERα-mediated transcription in a positive feedback manner. FOXP1 and FOXA1 promote estrogen-dependent proliferation of breast cancer cells and contribute to the sensitivity to hormone therapy.

3. CLINICOPATHOLOGICAL SIGNIFICANCES OF FOXP1 AND FOXA1 IN ER-POSITIVE BREAST CANCER

Recent global gene expression studies on breast cancer have shown that high FOXA1 expression was positively correlated with the status of hormone receptors ERα and PgR and negatively correlated with histological grade and proliferation markers (Badve et al., 2007; Habashy et al., 2008; Thorat et al., 2008). In addition, FOXA1 expression was associated with better prognosis of cancer-specific survival, which indicated that FOXA1 can serve as a predictor for good prognosis of breast cancer (Badve et al., 2007; Habashy et al., 2008; Thorat et al., 2008; Wolf et al., 2007). On the basis of gene expression profiling studies, researchers have classified breast cancers into the following five intrinsic subtypes with unique molecular characteristics and prognostic significance (Perou et al., 2000; Sørlie et al., 2001): luminal A and B, HER2+/ERα−, basal-like, and normal-like subtypes. Luminal subtypes A and B are ERα-positive breast cancers, distinguishing subtype A from B by its higher levels of ERα and better prognosis of the patients (Sørlie et al., 2001). Among these subtypes, FOXA1 expression is best associated with luminal subtype A and FOXA1 immuno-reactivity is shown as a significant predictor of cancer-specific survival for patients with ERα-positive tumors (Badve et al., 2007; Mehta et al., 2012). The prognostic relevance of FOXA1 in the breast cancers with rel-atively low risk will be useful for the determination of therapeutic methods (Badve et al., 2007; Thorat et al., 2008).

Altered expression of FOXP1 is associated with various types of tumors, including breast cancer (Banham et al., 2001, 2007; Barrans, Fenton, Banham, Owen, & Jack, 2004; Bates et al., 2008; Craig et al., 2011; Fox et al., 2004; Goatly et al., 2008; Hoeller, Schneider, Haralambieva, Dirnhofer, & Tzankov, 2010; Prown et al., 2008; Sagaert et al., 2006; Takayama et al., 2008; Wang et al., 2004; Zhang et al., 2010). FOXP1 immunoreactivity may be associated with the immunoreac-tivity of ERα and PgR in breast cancer, which may predict favorable prog-nosis in patients (Banham et al., 2005; Rayoo et al., 2009). A recent study showed that FOXP1 immunoreactivity was significantly enhanced in breast cancer samples for tamoxifen-treated patients without relapse, compared with samples for those with relapse within 5 years after surgery (Shigekawa et al., 2011). It was also demonstrated that a positive immuno-reactivity for either FOXP1 or FOXA1 significantly correlated with better relapse-free and overall survivals for breast cancer patients with adjuvant tamoxifen therapy, compared with either FOXP1- or FOXA1-negative immunoreactivity (Ijichi et al., 2012). Univariate and multivariate propor-tional analyses showed that the relapse-free and overall survival rates were associated with FOXA1 and FOXP1 immunoreactivities. For the relapse-free survival, either FOXP1 or FOXA1 immunoreactivity was found to be a significant prognostic predictor through univariate analysis ($P=0.001$ and 0.002, respectively), whereas only FOXP1 immunore-activity was a better prognostic predictor based on multivariate analysis ($P=0.026$). On the other hand, neither FOXP1 nor FOXA1 was signifi-cantly associated with overall survival by multivariate analysis. Notably, double-positive FOXP1 and FOXA1 immunoreactivities were significantly associated with more favorable prognosis for the relapse-free and overall survivals compared with either FOXP1- or FOXA1-negative immuno-reactivity based on multivariate analyses ($P=0.002$ and 0.002, respectively). These findings suggest that the combined analyses of the FOXA1 and FOXP1 immunoreactivities provide powerful prognostic indicators for the patients with ERα-positive breast cancers treated with adjuvant tamoxifen therapy.

Carroll and his colleagues showed that FOXA1 also plays a role in the differential ER-binding events in the tumors with a poor outcome (Ross-Innes et al., 2012). Notably, an siRNA-mediated knockdown study showed that ERα signals, including ERα occupancy and estrogen-dependent cell growth, are FOXA1 dependent in both tamoxifen-sensitive and tamoxifen-refractory MCF-7 cells (Hurtado et al., 2011). Further studies are required to answer the question whether the ER/FOXA1-driven growth is associated with tumor recurrence in various stages of the disease.

4. CONCLUSIONS AND FUTURE DIRECTIONS

A recent genome-wide study using ChIP analysis with high-throughput sequencing revealed that FOXA1 is a critical transcription factor that contributes to most of the ERα-chromatin interactions and estrogen-dependent changes of gene expression (Hurtado et al., 2011). FOXA1 influences genome-wide chromatin accessibility of ERα in response to different ligands, including both estrogen and tamoxifen (Hurtado et al., 2011). Thus, FOXA1 is considered as a major determinant for estrogen–ERα activity and endocrine response in breast cancer cells. Since FOXP1 exhibits functions analogous to those of FOXA1 in the ER-mediated transcription and its immunoreactivity has a clinicopathological significance along with FOXA1 immunoreactivity in breast cancer, it is assumed that FOXP1 also plays an important role in the regulation of ERα activity and tamoxifen responsiveness in breast cancer, functioning cooperatively with FOXA1. Future genome-wide studies of FOXP1 binding as well as ERα and FOXA1 occupancy will elucidate the precise interactions of these transcription factors in the ERα-mediated signaling pathways.

In summary, *FOXP1* and *FOXA1* are primary ERα target genes and critical transcription factors that regulate the ERα activity. Both FOX proteins will be potential biomarkers for the prediction of breast cancer prognosis. Pharmacological modulation of FOXP1 and FOXA1 activities may be clinically useful in the prevention and/or treatment of breast cancer.

ACKNOWLEDGMENTS

We thank the support by grants from MHLW; the Program for Promotion of Fundamental Studies in Health Science of the NIBIO; grants from JSPS, grants of the Cell Innovation Program, P-DIRECT and the Support Project of Strategic Research Center in Private Universities from the MEXT; Institutional Grant from the Medical Research Center, Saitama Medical University (#23-1-1-09, NI).

REFERENCES

Annicotte, J. S., Chavey, C., Servant, N., Teyssier, J., Bardin, A., Licznar, A., et al. (2005). The nuclear receptor liver receptor homolog-1 is an estrogen receptor target gene. *Oncogene, 24,* 8167–8175.

Badve, S., Turbin, D., Thorat, M. A., Morimiya, A., Nielsen, T. O., Perou, C. M., et al. (2007). FOXA1 expression in breast cancer—Correlation with luminal subtype A and survival. *Clinical Cancer Research, 13,* 4415–4421.

Banham, A. H., Beasley, N., Campo, E., Fernandez, P. L., Fidler, C., Gatter, K., et al. (2001). The FOXP1 winged helix transcription factor is a novel candidate tumor suppressor gene on chromosome 3p. *Cancer Research, 61,* 8820–8829.

Banham, A. H., Boddy, J., Launchbury, R., Han, C., Turley, H., Malone, P. R., et al. (2007). Expression of the forkhead transcriptional factor FOXP1 is associated both with hypoxia inducible factors (HIFs) and the androgen receptor in prostate cancer but is not directly regulated by androgens or hypoxia. *Prostate, 67,* 1091–1098.

Banham, A. H., Connors, J. M., Brown, P. J., Cordell, J. L., Ott, G., Sreenivasan, G., et al. (2005). Expression of the FOXP1 transcription factor is strongly associated with inferior survival in patients with diffuse large B-cell lymphoma. *Clinical Cancer Research, 11,* 1065–1072.

Barrans, S. L., Fenton, J. A., Banham, A., Owen, R. G., & Jack, A. S. (2004). Strong expression of FOXP1 identifies a distinct subset of diffuse large B-cell lymphoma (DLBCL) patients with poor outcome. *Blood, 104,* 2933–2935.

Bates, G. J., Fox, S. B., Han, C., Launchbury, R., Leek, R. D., Harris, A. L., et al. (2008). Expression of the forkhead transcription factor FOXP1 is associated with that of estrogen receptorβ in primary invasive breast carcinomas. *Breast Cancer Research and Treatment, 111,* 453–459.

Carroll, J. S., & Brown, M. (2006). Estrogen receptor target gene: An evolving concept. *Molecular Endocrinology, 20,* 1707–1714.

Carroll, J. S., Liu, X. S., Brodsky, A. S., Li, W., Meyer, C. A., Szary, A. J., et al. (2005). Chromosome-wide mapping of estrogen receptor binding reveals long-range regulation requiring the forkhead protein FoxA1. *Cell, 122,* 33–43.

Carroll, J. S., Meyer, C. A., Song, J., Li, W., Geistlinger, T. R., Eeckhoute, J., et al. (2006). Genome-wide analysis of estrogen receptor binding sites. *Nature Genetics, 38,* 1289–1297.

Craig, V. J., Cogliatti, S. B., Imig, J., Renner, C., Neuenschwander, S., Rehrauer, H., et al. (2011). Myc-mediated repression of microRNA-34a promotes high grade transformation of B-cell lymphoma by dysregulation of FoxP1. *Blood, 117,* 6227–6236.

Fox, S. B., Brown, P., Han, C., Ashe, S., Leek, R. D., Harris, A. L., et al. (2004). Expression of the forkhead transcription factor FOXP1 is associated with estrogen receptor α and improved survival in primary human breast carcinomas. *Clinical Cancer Research, 10,* 3521–3527.

Ghosh, M. G., Thompson, D. A., & Weigel, R. J. (2000). PDZK1 and GREB1 are estrogen-regulated genes expressed in hormone-responsive breast cancer. *Cancer Research, 60,* 6367–6375.

Goatly, A., Bacon, C. M., Nakamura, S., Ye, H., Kim, I., Brown, P. J., et al. (2008). FOXP1 abnormalities in lymphoma: Translocation breakpoint mapping reveals insights into deregulated transcriptional control. *Modern Pathology, 21,* 902–911.

Grange, T., Roux, J., Rigaud, G., & Pictet, R. (1991). Cell-type specific activity of two glucocorticoid responsive units of rat tyrosine aminotransferase gene is associated with multiple binding sites for C/EBP and a novel liver-specific nuclear factor. *Nucleic Acids Research, 19,* 131–139.

Habashy, H. O., Powe, D. G., Rakha, E. A., Ball, G., Paish, C., Gee, J., et al. (2008). Forkhead-box A1 (FOXA1) expression in breast cancer and its prognostic significance. *European Journal of Cancer*, *44*, 1541–1551.

Hall, J. M., & McDonnell, D. P. (2005). Coregulators in nuclear estrogen receptor action: From concept to therapeutic targeting. *Molecular Interventions*, *5*, 343–357.

Hoeller, S., Schneider, A., Haralambieva, E., Dirnhofer, S., & Tzankov, A. (2010). FOXP1 protein overexpression is associated with inferior outcome in nodal diffuse large B-cell lymphomas with non-germinal centre phenotype, independent of gains and structural aberrations at 3p14.1. *Histopathology*, *57*, 73–80.

Holmes, K. A., Hurtado, A., Brown, G. D., Launchbury, R., Ross-Innes, C. S., Hadfield, J., et al. (2012). Transducin-like enhancer protein 1 mediates estrogen receptor binding and transcriptional activity in breast cancer cells. *Proceedings of the National Academy of Sciences of the United States of America*, *109*, 2748–2753.

Hurtado, A., Holmes, K. A., Ross-Innes, C. S., Schmidt, D., & Carroll, J. S. (2011). FOXA1 is a key determinant of estrogen receptor function and endocrine response. *Nature Genetics*, *43*, 27–33.

Ijichi, N., Shigekawa, T., Ikeda, K., Horie-Inoue, K., Shimizu, C., Saji, S., et al. (2012). Association of double-positive FOXA1 and FOXP1 immunoreactivities with favorable prognosis of tamoxifen-treated breast cancer patients. *Hormones & Cancer*, *3*, 147–159.

Kastner, P., Krust, A., Turcotte, B., Stropp, U., Tora, L., Gronemeyer, H., et al. (1990). Two distinct estrogen-regulated promoters generate transcripts encoding the two functionally different human progesterone receptor forms A and B. *EMBO Journal*, *9*, 1603–1614.

Laganière, J., Deblois, G., Lefebvre, C., Bataille, A. R., Robert, F., & Giguère, V. (2005). From the cover: Location analysis of estrogen receptor α target promoters reveals that FOXA1 defines a domain of the estrogen response. *Proceedings of the National Academy of Sciences of the United States of America*, *102*, 11651–11656.

Lai, K., Harnish, D. C., & Evans, M. J. (2003). Estrogen receptor α regulates expression of the orphan receptor small heterodimer partner. *Journal of Biological Chemistry*, *278*, 36418–36429.

Li, S., Weidenfeld, J., & Morrisey, E. E. (2004). Transcriptional and DNA binding activity of the Foxp1/2/4 family is modulated by heterotypic and homotypic protein interactions. *Molecular and Cellular Biology*, *24*, 809–822.

Lupien, M., Eeckhoute, J., Meyer, C. A., Wang, Q., Zhang, Y., Li, W., et al. (2008). FoxA1 translates epigenetic signatures into enhancer-driven lineage-specific transcription. *Cell*, *132*, 958–970.

Mehta, R. J., Jain, R. K., Leung, S., Choo, J., Nielsen, T., Huntsman, D., et al. (2012). FOXA1 is an independent prognostic marker for ER-positive breast cancer. *Breast Cancer Research and Treatment*, *131*, 881–890.

Perou, C. M., Sørlie, T., Eisen, M. B., van de Rijn, M., Jeffrey, S. S., Rees, C. A., et al. (2000). Molecular portraits of human breast tumours. *Nature*, *406*, 747–752.

Platet, N., Cathiard, A. M., Gleizes, M., & Garcia, M. (2004). Estrogens and their receptors in breast cancer progression: A dual role in cancer proliferation and invasion. *Critical Reviews in Oncology/Hematology*, *51*, 55–67.

Prown, P. J., Ashe, S. L., Leich, E., Burek, C., Barrans, S., Fenton, J. A., et al. (2008). Potentially oncogenic B-cell activation induced smaller isoforms of FOXP1 are highly expressed in the activated B cell-like subtype of DLBCL. *Blood*, *111*, 2816–2824.

Rayoo, M., Yan, M., Takano, E. A., Bates, G. J., Brown, P. J., Banham, A. H., et al. (2009). Expression of the forkhead box transcription factor FOXP1 is associated with oestrogen receptor alpha, oestrogen receptor beta and improved survival in familial breast cancers. *Journal of Clinical Pathology*, *62*, 896–902.

Ross-Innes, C. S., Stark, R., Teschendorff, A. E., Holmes, K. A., Ali, H. R., Dunning, M. J., et al. (2012). Differential oestrogen receptor binding is associated with clinical outcome in breast cancer. *Nature, 481*, 389–393.

Sagaert, X., De Paepe, P., Libbrecht, L., Vanhentenrijk, V., Verhoef, G., Thomas, J., et al. (2006). Forkhead box protein P1 expression in mucosa-associated lymphoid tissue lymphomas predicts poor prognosis and transformation to diffuse large B-cell lymphoma. *Journal of Clinical Oncology, 24*, 2490–2497.

Schuur, E. R., Loktev, A. V., Sharma, M., Sun, Z., Roth, R. A., & Weigel, R. J. (2001). Ligand-dependent interaction of estrogen receptor-α with members of the forkhead transcription factor family. *Journal of Biological Chemistry, 276*, 33554–33560.

Shigekawa, T., Ijichi, N., Ikeda, K., Horie-Inoue, K., Shimizu, C., Saji, S., et al. (2011). FOXP1, an estrogen-inducible transcription factor, modulates cell proliferation in breast cancer cells and 5-year recurrence-free survival of patients with tamoxifen-treated breast cancer. *Hormones & Cancer, 2*, 286–297.

Sørlie, T., Perou, C. M., Tibshirani, R., Aas, T., Geisler, S., Johnsen, H., et al. (2001). Gene expression patterns of breast carcinomas distinguish tumor subclasses with clinical implications. *Proceedings of the National Academy of Sciences of the United States of America, 98*, 10869–10874.

Takayama, K., Horie-Inoue, K., Ikeda, K., Urano, T., Murakami, K., Hayashizaki, Y., et al. (2008). FOXP1 is an androgen-responsive transcription factor that negatively regulates androgen receptor signaling in prostate cancer cells. *Biochemical and Biophysical Research Communications, 374*, 388–393.

Tan, S. K., Lin, Z. H., Chang, C. W., Varang, V., Chng, K. R., Pan, Y. F., et al. (2011). AP-2γ regulates oestrogen receptor-mediated long-range chromatin interaction and gene transcription. *EMBO Journal, 30*, 2569–2581.

Thorat, M. A., Marchio, C., Morimiya, A., Savage, K., Nakshatri, H., Reis-Filho, J. S., et al. (2008). Forkhead box A1 expression in breast cancer is associated with luminal subtype and good prognosis. *Journal of Clinical Pathology, 61*, 327–332.

Wang, B., Lin, D., Li, C., & Tucker, P. (2003). Multiple domains define the expression and regulatory properties of Foxp1 forkhead transcriptional repressors. *Journal of Biological Chemistry, 278*, 24259–24268.

Wang, B., Weidenfeld, J., Lu, M. M., Maika, S., Kuziel, W. A., Morrisey, E. E., et al. (2004). Foxp1 regulates cardiac outflow tract, endocardial cushion morphogenesis and myocyte proliferation and maturation. *Development (Cambridge, England), 131*, 4477–4487.

Wolf, I., Bose, S., Williamson, E. A., Miller, C. W., Karlan, B. Y., & Koeffler, H. P. (2007). FOXA1: Growth inhibitor and a favorable prognostic factor in human breast cancer. *International Journal of Cancer, 120*, 1013–1022.

Zhang, Y., Li, S., Yuan, L., Tian, Y., Weidenfeld, J., Yang, J., et al. (2010). Foxp1 coordinates cardiomyocyte proliferation through both cell-autonomous and nonautonomous mechanisms. *Genes & Development, 24*, 1746–1757.

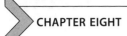

CHAPTER EIGHT

Role of KLF5 in Hormonal Signaling and Breast Cancer Development

Rong Liu*, Jin-Tang Dong[†,1], Ceshi Chen[*,1]

*Key Laboratory of Animal Models and Human Disease Mechanisms of Chinese Academy of Sciences & Yunnan Province, Kunming Institute of Zoology, Kunming, Yunnan, China
[†]Winship Cancer Institute, Emory University School of Medicine, Atlanta, Georgia, USA
[1]Corresponding authors: e-mail address: j.dong@emory.edu; chenc@mail.kiz.ac.cn

Contents

Abstract

Steroid hormones, including ovarian steroid hormones progesterone and estrogen and androgen, play vital roles in the development of normal mammary gland and breast cancer via their receptors. How these hormones regulate these physiological and pathological processes remains to be elucidated. Krüppel-like factor 5 (KLF5) is a transcription factor playing significant roles in breast carcinogenesis, whose expression has been shown to be regulated by hormones. In this review, the relationships among hormonal signaling, KLF5, and breast cancer are summarized and discussed.

1. INTRODUCTION

Ovarian steroid hormones, including estrogen and progesterone, play vital roles in the development and growth of normal breast. However, estrogen and progesterone, working through their cognate receptors, estrogen receptor (ER) and progesterone receptor (PR), respectively, have also been implicated in the pathogenesis of breast cancer due to their significant effects on breast cell proliferation, survival, and differentiation (Abdulkareem &

Vitamins and Hormones, Volume 93
ISSN 0083-6729
http://dx.doi.org/10.1016/B978-0-12-416673-8.00002-2
213

Zurmi, 2012). The incidence of breast cancer is increased by hormone factors, such as early menarche and delayed menopause (Chen, 2009), although the functional mechanisms of these hormones are not completely understood. Besides the ovarian steroid hormones, androgen also plays important roles in breast development beyond its essential roles in male traits and reproductive activity. Meanwhile, androgen, working through androgen receptor (AR), has also been implicated in breast cancer. However, the relationship between androgen and breast cancer is often contradictory and inconclusive from various studies (Kenemans & van der Mooren, 2012).

Human Krüppel-like factor 5 (KLF5/IKLF/BTEB2), a member of the Krüppel-like transcription factor family, was first identified as an intestinal-enriched member of the zinc-finger transcription factors of the Sp1 subfamily (Conkright, Wani, Anderson, & Lingrel, 1999). KLF5 has been reported to be regulated by several important developmental pathways, such as TGF-β (Guo, Dong, Zhang, et al., 2009; Guo, Dong, Zhao, et al., 2009; Guo, Zhao, Dong, Sun, & Dong, 2009), the Wnt (McConnell et al., 2011), retinoic acid (Chanchevalap, Nandan, Merlin, & Yang, 2004), Ras (Nandan et al., 2008), and Hippo (Zhao, Zhi, Zhou, & Chen, 2012; Zhi, Zhao, Zhou, Liu, & Chen, 2012), and regulates cell proliferation and differentiation in several organ systems. Specifically, KLF5 has been implicated in regulating cell proliferation, survival, differentiation, and embryonic stem cell (ESC) self-renewal.

It has been reported that KLF5 overexpression promotes the G1/S cell cycle progression (Chen et al., 2006) and breast cell proliferation, survival, and tumor growth (Liu, Zheng, Zhou, Dong, & Chen, 2009; Zheng et al., 2009). Furthermore, KLF5 has been reported to regulate smooth muscle cell and adipocyte differentiation (Fujiu et al., 2005; Oishi et al., 2005). On the other hand, KLF5 can also suppress cell proliferation upon acetylation induced by TGF-β (Guo, Dong, Zhang, et al., 2009; Guo, Dong, Zhao, et al., 2009; Guo, Zhao, Dong, Sun, & Dong, 2009). Most recently, KLF5 was shown to promote the self-renewal of ESC and to maintain ESC in an undifferentiated state (Jiang et al., 2008; Parisi et al., 2008). Interestingly, the gene expression signature of basal-like breast cancer cells is similar to that of ESC through analyzing the microarray data from 1211 breast tumors (Ben-Porath et al., 2008). KLF5 and eight other genes are highly expressed in basal-type breast tumors (Ben-Porath et al., 2008). Indeed, positive *KLF5* mRNA and protein expression is an unfavorable prognostic marker correlated with shorter survival for breast cancer patients (Takagi et al., 2012; Tong et al., 2006).

In this chapter, we focus on the regulation of KLF5 by steroid hormones and potential functions of KLF5 in hormone signaling pathways and breast tumorigenesis.

2. PROGESTERONE—PR SIGNALING, KLF5, AND BREAST CANCER

Progesterone is essential for normal postnatal mammary gland development during pregnancy and lactation by stimulating ductal side branching and development of lobuloalveolar structures (Conneely, Mulac-Jericevic, & Arnett-Mansfield, 2007). A recent study showed that progesterone promotes proliferation and activity of mammary stem cells (Joshi et al., 2010). In addition, PR knockout mice showed incomplete mammary gland ductal side branching due to insufficient cell proliferation (Ismail et al., 2003).

Accumulated evidence suggests that Pg and PR promote mammary tumorigenesis (Lanari et al., 2009; Lange, 2008). Administration of medroxyprogesterone acetate, a synthesized progesterone, induces mammary ductal carcinomas with a mean latency of 52 weeks and an incidence of about 80% in BALB/c female mice (Lanari et al., 2009). Moreover, Pg has been shown to increase breast cancer risk for menopausal women in several large-scale hormone-replacement therapy clinical studies (Beral, 2003; Kirsh & Kreiger, 2002; Schairer et al., 2000). In these studies, Pg plus estrogen significantly increased the risk of invasive breast cancer compared with estrogen alone. Additionally, Pg has been shown to have proliferative effects in the PR-positive breast cancer cell lines *in vitro* (Hissom & Moore, 1987; Liu, Zhou, Zhao, & Chen, 2011) and in nude mice (Liang, Besch-Williford, Brekken, & Hyder, 2007). Importantly, Pg was shown to reprogram a small subset of ER+/PR+/cytokeratin 5 (CK5)-differentiated luminal cells into ER−PR−CK5+ progenitor cancer cells (Horwitz, Dye, Harrell, Kabos, & Sartorius, 2008; Sartorius, Harvell, Shen, & Horwitz, 2005).

Our recent study showed that the KLF5 transcription factor is induced by Pg through PR and contributes to Pg-induced cell proliferation and dedifferentiation in PR-positive breast cancer cells (Liu et al., 2011; Fig. 8.1). First, KLF5 is an important Pg/PR downstream target gene promoting cell cycle progression. Pg increases the binding of PR and the KLF5 promoter. In the PR-positive breast cancer cell line T47D, Pg functions through KLF5 to promote the G1/S transition of the cell cycle by inducing the expression of a set of genes, including cyclin A, chromatin licensing and

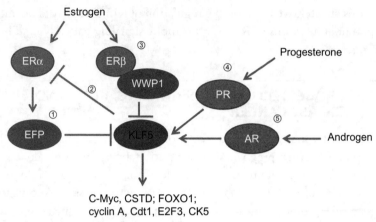

Figure 8.1 Relationships between steroid hormones and KLF5 in breast cells. ① Estrogen and ERα induce the expression of the EFP E3 ubiquitin ligase, which targets KLF5 for degradation in ERα-positive breast cancer cells. ② KLF5 interacts with ERα to suppress ERα-mediated transcription of c-Myc and CSTD in ERα-positive breast cancer cells. ③ KLF5 interacts with ERβ, which recruits the WWP1 E3 ubiquitin ligase to promote KLF5 proteolysis in the presence of estrogen, in prostate cancer cells. Because KLF5 induces the FOXO1 gene transcription, estrogen promotes prostate tumor growth in this scenario. Similar mechanism may exist in ERβ-positive breast cancer cells. ④ Progesterone and PR induce the expression of KLF5 in PR-positive breast cancer cells. KLF5 contributes to progesterone-induced cell proliferation and dedifferentiation by inducing the transcription of a subset of gene, including cyclin A, Cdt1, and E2F3. ⑤ Androgen and AR induce the expression of KLF5 in AR-positive breast cancer cells. KLF5 contributes to androgen-induced cell proliferation. (See Color Insert.)

DNA replication factor 1 (Cdt1), and E2F3 transcription factor (Graham et al., 2009; Liu et al., 2011). Second, progestins have been shown to reprogram a subset of ER + PR + CK5–differentiated cells into ER−PR−CK5 + basal-like progenitor cancer cells *in vitro* and *in vivo* (Horwitz et al., 2008; Kabos et al., 2011; Sartorius et al., 2005). The ER−PR−CK5 + cells have progenitor potential and are more resistant to drug-induced apoptosis during the endocrine therapy and chemotherapies (Kabos et al., 2011). Additionally, Pg increased the development of CK5 + basal-type breast cancer in rats (Haslam, 2010). Interestingly, KLF5 contributes to Pg-induced cell dedifferentiation as suggested by inducing the CK5 expression (Liu et al., 2011). These data imply that KLF5 mediates Pg's function in reprogramming ER+PR+CK5–differentiated luminal cells into ER−PR−CK5 + progenitor cancer cells. Given the significant role of KLF5 in maintaining ESC self-renewal and preventing their differentiation, it is very likely that KLF5 contributes to Pg-initiated cell reprogramming.

The induction of KLF5 by Pg is physiologically relevant because the expression of mouse Klf5 is upregulated after pregnancy in mice (Liu et al., 2011). It is well known that Pg begins to increase at early pregnancy so that the induction of Klf5 in mice is likely caused by Pg and PR. How the expression of KLF5 is maintained during the pregnancy and lactation is unknown at this time. Adult mice with the knockout of PR showed defects in normal mammary gland development (Lydon et al., 1995). Because the klf5 homozygous KO mice are lethal, a breast-specific klf5 KO mouse model will be essential to evaluate the physiological role of Klf5 in normal breast development (Wan et al., 2008). Given the essential role of KLF5 in the Pg/PR signaling pathway, klf5 may play a significant role in normal breast development.

Taken together, these findings suggest that KLF5 is an important downstream target gene of the Pg–PR signaling to regulate the development of normal breast and breast cancer.

3. ESTROGEN—ER SIGNALING AND KLF5 IN BREAST CANCER

Estrogen regulates normal breast cell growth and differentiation and maintains homeostasis of the normal mammary gland (Edwards, 2005). However, sustained exposure of ERα with endogenous or exogenous estrogen has been well known to cause breast cancer (Colditz, 1998; Hankinson, Colditz, & Willett, 2004). Sustained stimulation of ERα-positive breast epithelial cells by estrogen leads to the hyperactivation of cell proliferation and survival pathways, which induces breast cancers (Rana, Rangasamy, & Mishra, 2010). Approximately 70% of human breast cancers express ERα (Johnston & Dowsett, 2003). The growth of ERα-positive breast cancers usually depends on estrogen, and the cells undergo apoptosis in the absence of estrogen (Thiantanawat, Long, & Brodie, 2003).

Estrogen promotes breast cancer progression; therefore, drugs that inhibit estrogen function (either block estrogen synthesis, such as aromatase inhibitors, or antagonize estrogen's action, such as selective ERα modulators, SERMs) can inhibit the growth of ERα-positive breast cancer cells. Clinically, tamoxifen, a SERM, is the first-line therapy for ERα-positive breast cancer (Jensen & Jordan, 2003). More than 50% of patients with ERα-positive breast cancers achieve an objective response or tumor stabilization with tamoxifen treatment since 1978 (Campbell et al., 1981; Jaiyesimi, Buzdar, Decker, & Hortobagyi, 1995; Lippman & Allegra, 1980). However, long-term use of tamoxifen leads to drug resistance and other side effects (Rana et al., 2010); and around 40% of patients receiving adjuvant tamoxifen eventually relapse (Ring & Dowsett, 2004). Although the mechanisms have not been clearly illustrated, loss of ERα expression and/or function would confer to tamoxifen resistance (Ring & Dowsett, 2004). A few ERα−PR−CK5+ basal-like cells in ERα+PR+CK5-luminal breast cancers have been considered to be one of the important mechanisms for drug resistance and tumor relapse (Horwitz et al., 2008).

KLF5 is highly expressed in immortalized breast epithelial cells and a sub-set of ERα/PR/HER2 triple negative breast cancer cells lines, such as HCC1937 and HCC1806, but lowly expressed in ERα-positive breast cancer cell lines (Chen, Bhalala, Qiao, & Dong, 2002; Liu et al., 2011). We recently found that estrogen negatively regulates the KLF5 protein expression in ERα-positive breast cancer cells (Zhao et al., 2011). The proteasomal degradation of KLF5 protein in MCF7 and T47D appears to be mediated by the estrogen-inducible E3 ubiquitin ligase EFP (estrogen-responsive finger protein; Fig. 8.1). Although EFP interacts with KLF5, it could not promote KLF5 ubiquitination like other KLF5 E3 ligases, WWP1 (Chen et al., 2005), Fbw7 (Zhao, Zheng, Zhou, & Chen, 2010), and Smurf2 (Du et al., 2011). The detailed mechanism by which EFP promotes KLF5 ubiquitin-independent degradation (Chen, Zhou, Guo, &Dong, 2007) is unknown. Consistently, Nakajima et al. (2011) also found that estrogen causes KLF5 degradation in prostate cancer cells, although the degradation there is medi-ated by WWP1. In addition, ERα signaling inhibits the KLF5 expression at the RNA level at 72 h through an unknown mechanism (Zhao et al., 2011).

While estrogen signaling inhibits the KLF5 expression, KLF5 feedback inhibits estrogen-promoted cell proliferation and gene expression in ERα-positive breast cancer cells (Guo et al., 2010). Estrogen induces the interaction between KLF5 and ERα, which, in turn, suppresses the binding of ERα to the promoters of its target genes such as c-Myc and CSTD (Fig. 8.1). In this scenario, KLF5 may function as a transcription corepressor.

In addition to ERα, KLF5 also interacts with ERβ (Nakajima et al., 2011). In prostate cancer cells, the KLF5 and ERβ complex directly bind to the promoter of the FOXO1 tumor suppressor gene. Estrogen-loaded ERβ recruits the KLF5 E3 ubiquitin ligase WWP1 to promote the KLF5 degradation (Fig. 8.1), therefore inhibiting the FOXO1 transcription and promoting tumor growth. In contrast, the ERβ antagonist ICI 182,780 increases the FOXO1 expression and suppresses tumor growth. Whether the same mechanism sustains in breast cancer has not been investigated.

Taken together, the interplay between the estrogen–ER signaling and KLF5 might play important roles in breast carcinogenesis.

4. ANDROGEN/AR SIGNALING, KLF5, AND BREAST CANCER

Besides the ovarian steroid hormones discussed above, another important steroid hormone, androgen, also plays important roles in breast development. In contrast to the role of estrogen in breast development, androgens suppress breast epithelial cell proliferation and inhibit breast development independent of genetic sex (Dimitrakakis & Bondy, 2009; Forsbach, Guitron-Cantu, Vazquez-Lara, Mota-Morales, & Diaz-Mendoza, 2000).

Currently, the relationship between androgens and breast cancer is controversial. On one hand, epidemiological studies showed that the risk of breast cancer in postmenopausal women using testosterone supplementation, either testosterone alone or together with estrogen plus progestin, does not appear to have significant increase (Davis, Hirschberg, Wagner, Lodhi, & von Schoultz, 2009; van Staa & Sprafka, 2009); on the other hand, studies on androgen serum levels in postmenopausal women suggest a positive association between high levels of androgens and an increase risk of breast cancer. In postmenopausal women diagnosed with breast cancer, serum testosterone levels were significantly higher than those in controls, and postmenopausal women with high estrogen and testosterone have a higher risk of breast cancer (Eliassen & Hankinson, 2008; Secreto et al., 2009; Shimono et al., 2009). Meanwhile, AR, androgen's cognate receptor, was reported to be expressed in around 60–70% breast cancers (Ni et al., 2011), and clinical findings indicate that a significant number of poorly differentiated breast carcinomas are AR-positive while ERα-negative and PR-negative (Dimitrakakis & Bondy, 2009). Furthermore, specific targeting AR signaling could suppress androgen-stimulated breast tumor cell growth (Hu et al., 2011; Ni et al., 2011), suggesting that androgen promotes breast cancer growth.

Our earlier study suggests that *KLF5* mRNA can be induced by androgen R1881 in the 22Rv1 prostate cancer cells (Chen et al., 2004). Similar results were independently observed in LNCaP by another group (Lee et al., 2009). KLF5 was induced by androgen to increase the expression of the *fatty acid synthase* (*FASN*) gene in collaboration with SREBP-1 (Lee et al., 2009).

Recently, Takagi et al. showed that the KLF5 protein expression, as detected by immunohistochemical staining, is positively associated with the AR status in breast cancers (Takagi et al. 2012), and the KLF5 expression was suggested to be an independent prognostic factor for both disease-free and breast cancer-specific survival of the patients (Takagi et al., 2012). In this chapter, KLF5 was demonstrated to be induced by 5α-dihydrotestosterone in the MCF7 breast cancer cell line (Fig. 8.1), and the induction of KLF5 was blocked by AR antagonist bicalutamide (Takagi et al., 2012). When the expression of KLF5 was silenced by siRNA, cell proliferation was significantly decreased.

Taken together, current findings suggest that KLF5 is induced by androgen through AR, and KLF5 contributes to AR signaling by promoting cell proliferation and regulating the expression of AR downstream target genes such as *FASN*. Targeting AR-KLF5 signaling might provide new therapeutic approaches for AR-positive breast cancers.

5. SUMMARY AND PERSPECTIVES

Steroid hormones, including estrogen, progesterone, and androgen, play essential roles in the development of normal mammary gland and breast cancer. The link between hormone therapy for menopausal women and breast cancer risk has been extensively investigated. Not only estrogen plus progestin therapy but also estrogen therapy alone increases breast cancer risks in women if taken for more than 10 years (Brinton et al., 2008). Testosterone therapy in women has been utilized since 1938 to treat various endocrine and sexual disorders and benign and malignant tumors of the breast, uterus, and ovaries (Traish, Feeley, & Guay, 2009). Although the evidence so far is not so consistent, a host of clinical trials support a pro-breast carcinogenesis role of androgens. However, the mechanisms by which these steroid hormones affect breast cancer progression are largely unknown.

Accumulated studies have revealed that KLF5 promotes the proliferation and survival of breast cancer cells. Recently, KLF5 was found to be induced by progesterone and androgen to contribute to progesterone/androgen-induced breast cancer cell proliferation (Liu et al., 2011; Takagi et al., 2012). It is thus possible that KLF5 mediates these hormones' actions in breast carcinogenesis. Estrogen suppresses KLF5 expression in ERα-positive breast cancer cells and KLF5 also suppresses ERα-mediated gene transcription. Therefore, the relationship between estrogen and KLF5 is more complex. In addition, the ERα−PR−CK5+ breast cancer cells, which express higher levels of KLF5, have progenitor cell potential and are more resistant to drug-induced apoptosis during the endocrine therapy and chemotherapies (Kabos et al., 2011). Consistently, KLF5 has been reported to cause chemotherapeutic drug resistance via inducing the expression of anti-apoptotic proteins, such as survivin (Zhu et al., 2006) and Pim1 (Zhao et al., 2008). Given the role of KLF5 in progesterone-induced breast cancer cell dedifferentiation, it is likely that KLF5 also contributes to the drug resistance and breast cancer relapse.

Several key and fundamental questions remain to be answered. First, what are the physiological and pathological roles of KLF5 in the breast? Characterization of breast-specific Klf5 transgenic mouse models will provide with more precise answer. Accumulated evidence suggests that KLF5 may play a context-dependent role in different subtypes of breast tumors. Second, what are the coordinated regulatory mechanisms of KLF5 by steroid hormones in breast cells at different levels including cell, tissue, and whole body? Finally, how shall we translate this knowledge into the clinic? Endocrine therapies have been widely applied to treat metastatic breast cancer. Interference of KLF5 may become novel strategy for improving the efficacy of current treatments.

In summary, steroid hormones including estrogen, progesterone, and androgen play important roles in the development of normal breast tissue and breast cancer. As a common downstream target of these hormones in breast cells, KLF5 contributes to the signaling pathways of these hormones by regulating gene transcription, cell proliferation, survival, and dedifferentiation. Targeting these steroid hormone–nuclear receptors–KLF5 pathways may be effective approaches for breast cancer prevention and therapy.

ACKNOWLEDGMENTS

Our studies have been supported by the Strategic Priority Research Program of the Chinese Academy of Sciences, Stem Cell and Regenerative Medicine Research (XDA01040406) (C. C.), and the US National Institutes of Health (J.-T. D.).

REFERENCES

Abdulkareem, I. H., & Zurmi, I. B. (2012). Review of hormonal treatment of breast cancer. *Nigerian Journal of Clinical Practice*, *15*, 9–14.

Ben-Porath, I., Thomson, M. W., Carey, V. J., Ge, R., Bell, G. W., Regev, A., et al. (2008). An embryonic stem cell-like gene expression signature in poorly differentiated aggressive human tumors. *Nature Genetics*, *40*, 499–507.

Beral, V. (2003). Breast cancer and hormone-replacement therapy in the Million Women Study. *Lancet*, *362*, 419–427.

Brinton, L. A., Richesson, D., Leitzmann, M. F., Gierach, G. L., Schatzkin, A., Mouw, T., et al. (2008). Menopausal hormone therapy and breast cancer risk in the NIH-AARP Diet and Health Study Cohort. *Cancer Epidemiology, Biomarkers & Prevention, 17,* 3150–3160.

Campbell, F. C., Blamey, R. W., Elston, C. W., Morris, A. H., Nicholson, R. I., Griffiths, K., et al. (1981). Quantitative oestradiol receptor values in primary breast cancer and response of metastases to endocrine therapy. *Lancet, 2,* 1317–1319.

Chanchevalap, S., Nandan, M. O., Merlin, D., & Yang, V. W. (2004). All-trans retinoic acid inhibits proliferation of intestinal epithelial cells by inhibiting expression of the gene encoding Kruppel-like factor 5. *FEBS Letters, 578,* 99–105.

Chen, F. P. (2009). Postmenopausal hormone therapy and risk of breast cancer. *Chang Gung Medical Journal, 32,* 140–147.

Chen, C., Benjamin, M. S., Sun, X., Otto, K. B., Guo, P., Dong, X. Y., et al. (2006). KLF5 promotes cell proliferation and tumorigenesis through gene regulation and the TSU-Pr1 human bladder cancer cell line. *International Journal of Cancer, 118,* 1346–1355.

Chen, C., Bhalala, H. V., Qiao, H., & Dong, J. T. (2002). A possible tumor suppressor role of the KLF5 transcription factor in human breast cancer. *Oncogene, 21,* 6567–6572.

Chen, C., Sun, X., Guo, P., Dong, X. Y., Sethi, P., Cheng, X., et al. (2005). Human Kruppel-like factor 5 is a target of the E3 ubiquitin ligase WWP1 for proteolysis in epithelial cells. *The Journal of Biological Chemistry, 280,* 41553–41561.

Chen, C., Zhou, Z., Guo, P., & Dong, J. T. (2007). Proteasomal degradation of the KLF5 transcription factor through a ubiquitin-independent pathway. *FEBS Letters, 581,* 1124–1130.

Chen, C., Zhou, Y., Zhou, Z., Sun, X., Otto, K. B., Uht, R. M., et al. (2004). Regulation of KLF5 involves the Sp1 transcription factor in human epithelial cells. *Gene, 330,* 133–142.

Colditz, G. A. (1998). Relationship between estrogen levels, use of hormone replacement therapy, and breast cancer. *Journal of the National Cancer Institute, 90,* 814–823.

Conkright, M. D., Wani, M. A., Anderson, K. P., & Lingrel, J. B. (1999). A gene encoding an intestinal-enriched member of the Kruppel-like factor family expressed in intestinal epithelial cells. *Nucleic Acids Research, 27,* 1263–1270.

Conneely, O. M., Mulac-Jericevic, B., & Arnett-Mansfield, R. (2007). Progesterone signaling in mammary gland development. *Ernst Schering Foundation Symposium Proceedings,* 45–54.

Davis, S. R., Hirschberg, A. L., Wagner, L. K., Lodhi, I., & von Schoultz, B. (2009). The effect of transdermal testosterone on mammographic density in postmenopausal women not receiving systemic estrogen therapy. *The Journal of Clinical Endocrinology and Metabolism, 94,* 4907–4913.

Dimitrakakis, C., & Bondy, C. (2009). Androgens and the breast. *Breast Cancer Research, 11,* 212.

Du, J. X., Hagos, E. G., Nandan, M. O., Bialkowska, A. B., Yu, B., & Yang, V. W. (2011). The E3 ubiquitin ligase SMAD ubiquitination regulatory factor 2 negatively regulates Kruppel-like factor 5 protein. *The Journal of Biological Chemistry, 286,* 40354–40364.

Edwards, D. P. (2005). Regulation of signal transduction pathways by estrogen and progesterone. *Annual Review of Physiology, 67,* 335–376.

Eliassen, A. H., & Hankinson, S. E. (2008). Endogenous hormone levels and risk of breast, endometrial and ovarian cancers: Prospective studies. *Advances in Experimental Medicine and Biology, 630,* 148–165.

Forsbach, G., Guitron-Cantu, A., Vazquez-Lara, J., Mota-Morales, M., & Diaz-Mendoza, M. L. (2000). Virilizing adrenal adenoma and primary amenorrhea in a girl with adrenal hyperplasia. *Archives of Gynecology and Obstetrics, 263,* 134–136.

Fujiu, K., Manabe, I., Ishihara, A., Oishi, Y., Iwata, H., Nishimura, G., et al. (2005). Synthetic retinoid Am80 suppresses smooth muscle phenotypic modulation and in-stent neointima formation by inhibiting KLF5. *Circulation Research, 97,* 1132–1141.

Graham, J. D., Mote, P. A., Salagame, U., van Dijk, J. H., Balleine, R. L., Huschtscha, L. I., et al. (2009). DNA replication licensing and progenitor numbers are increased by progesterone in normal human breast. *Endocrinology*, *150*, 3318–3326.

Guo, P., Dong, X. Y., Zhang, X., Zhao, K. W., Sun, X., Li, Q., et al. (2009). Pro-proliferative factor KLF5 becomes anti-proliferative in epithelial homeostasis upon signaling-mediated modification. *The Journal of Biological Chemistry*, *284*, 6071–6078.

Guo, P., Dong, X. Y., Zhao, K. W., Sun, X., Li, Q., & Dong, J. T. (2009). Opposing effects of KLF5 on the transcription of Myc in epithelial proliferation in the context of TGFbeta. *The Journal of Biological Chemistry*, *284*, 28243–28252.

Guo, P., Dong, X. Y., Zhao, K. W., Sun, X., Li, Q., & Dong, J. T. (2010). Estrogen-induced interaction between KLF5 and estrogen receptor (ER) suppresses the function of ER in ER-positive breast cancer cells. *International Journal of Cancer*, *126*, 81–89.

Guo, P., Zhao, K. W., Dong, X. Y., Sun, X., & Dong, J. T. (2009). Acetylation of KLF5 alters the assembly of P15 transcription factors in TGFbeta-mediated induction in epithelial cells. *The Journal of Biological Chemistry*, *284*, 18184–18193.

Hankinson, S. E., Colditz, G. A., & Willett, W. C. (2004). Towards an integrated model for breast cancer etiology: The lifelong interplay of genes, lifestyle, and hormones. *Breast Cancer Research*, *6*, 213–218.

Haslam, S. (2010). Role of progesterone in the etiology of breast cancer in an animal model. In *BIT's 3rd world cancer congress: Breast cancer conference* (p. 146).

Hissom, J. R., & Moore, M. R. (1987). Progestin effects on growth in the human breast cancer cell line T-47D—Possible therapeutic implications. *Biochemical and Biophysical Research Communications*, *145*, 706–711.

Horwitz, K. B., Dye, W. W., Harrell, J. C., Kabos, P., & Sartorius, C. A. (2008). Rare steroid receptor-negative basal-like tumorigenic cells in luminal subtype human breast cancer xenografts. *Proceedings of the National Academy of Sciences of the United States of America*, *105*, 5774–5779.

Hu, R., Dawood, S., Holmes, M. D., Collins, L. C., Schnitt, S. J., Cole, K., et al. (2011). Androgen receptor expression and breast cancer survival in postmenopausal women. *Clinical Cancer Research*, *17*, 1867–1874.

Ismail, P. M., Amato, P., Soyal, S. M., DeMayo, F. J., Conneely, O. M., O'Malley, B. W., et al. (2003). Progesterone involvement in breast development and tumorigenesis—As revealed by progesterone receptor "knockout" and "knockin" mouse models. *Steroids*, *68*, 779–787.

Jaiyesimi, I. A., Buzdar, A. U., Decker, D. A., & Hortobagyi, G. N. (1995). Use of tamoxifen for breast cancer: Twenty-eight years later. *Journal of Clinical Oncology*, *13*, 513–529.

Jensen, E. V., & Jordan, V. C. (2003). The estrogen receptor: A model for molecular medicine. *Clinical Cancer Research*, *9*, 1980–1989.

Jiang, J., Chan, Y. S., Loh, Y. H., Cai, J., Tong, G. Q., Lim, C. A., et al. (2008). A core Klf circuitry regulates self-renewal of embryonic stem cells. *Nature Cell Biology*, *10*, 353–360.

Johnston, S. R., & Dowsett, M. (2003). Aromatase inhibitors for breast cancer: Lessons from the laboratory. *Nature Reviews. Cancer*, *3*, 821–831.

Joshi, P. A., Jackson, H. W., Beristain, A. G., Di Grappa, M. A., Mote, P. A., Clarke, C. L., et al. (2010). Progesterone induces adult mammary stem cell expansion. *Nature*, *465*, 803–807.

Kabos, P., Haughian, J. M., Wang, X., Dye, W. W., Finlayson, C., Elias, A., et al. (2011). Cytokeratin 5 positive cells represent a steroid receptor negative and therapy resistant subpopulation in luminal breast cancers. *Breast Cancer Research and Treatment*, *128*, 45–55.

Kenemans, P., & van der Mooren, M. J. (2012). Androgens and breast cancer risk. *Gynecological Endocrinology*, *28*(Suppl. 1), 46–49.

Kirsh, V., & Kreiger, N. (2002). Estrogen and estrogen-progestin replacement therapy and risk of postmenopausal breast cancer in Canada. *Cancer Causes & Control*, *13*, 583–590.

Lanari, C., Lamb, C. A., Fabris, V. T., Helguero, L. A., Soldati, R., Bottino, M. C., et al. (2009). The MPA mouse breast cancer model: Evidence for a role of progesterone receptors in breast cancer. *Endocrine-Related Cancer*, *16*, 333–350.

Lange, C. A. (2008). Challenges to defining a role for progesterone in breast cancer. *Steroids*, *73*, 914–921.

Lee, M. Y., Moon, J. S., Park, S. W., Koh, Y. K., Ahn, Y. H., & Kim, K. S. (2009). KLF5 enhances SREBP-1 action in androgen-dependent induction of fatty acid synthase in prostate cancer cells. *The Biochemical Journal*, *417*, 313–322.

Liang, Y., Besch-Williford, C., Brekken, R. A., & Hyder, S. M. (2007). Progestin-dependent progression of human breast tumor xenografts: A novel model for evaluating antitumor therapeutics. *Cancer Research*, *67*, 9929–9936.

Lippman, M. E., & Allegra, J. C. (1980). Quantitative estrogen receptor analyses: The response to endocrine and cytotoxic chemotherapy in human breast cancer and the disease-free interval. *Cancer*, *46*, 2829–2834.

Liu, R., Zheng, H. Q., Zhou, Z., Dong, J. T., & Chen, C. (2009). KLF5 promotes breast cell survival partially through fibroblast growth factor-binding protein 1-pERK-mediated dual specificity MKP-1 protein phosphorylation and stabilization. *The Journal of Biological Chemistry*, *284*, 16791–16798.

Liu, R., Zhou, Z., Zhao, D., & Chen, C. (2011). The induction of KLF5 transcription factor by progesterone contributes to progesterone-induced breast cancer cell proliferation and dedifferentiation. *Molecular Endocrinology*, *25*, 1137–1144.

Lydon, J. P., DeMayo, F. J., Funk, C. R., Mani, S. K., Hughes, A. R., Montgomery, C. A., Jr., et al. (1995). Mice lacking progesterone receptor exhibit pleiotropic reproductive abnormalities. *Genes & Development*, *9*, 2266–2278.

McConnell, B. B., Kim, S. S., Yu, K., Ghaleb, A. M., Takeda, N., Manabe, I., et al. (2011). Kruppel-like factor 5 is important for maintenance of crypt architecture and barrier function in mouse intestine. *Gastroenterology*, *141*(1302–1313), e1306.

Nakajima, Y., Akaogi, K., Suzuki, T., Osakabe, A., Yamaguchi, C., Sunahara, N., et al. (2011). Estrogen regulates tumor growth through a nonclassical pathway that includes the transcription factors ERbeta and KLF5. *Science Signaling*, *4*, ra22.

Nandan, M. O., McConnell, B. B., Ghaleb, A. M., Bialkowska, A. B., Sheng, H., Shao, J., et al. (2008). Kruppel-like factor 5 mediates cellular transformation during oncogenic KRAS-induced intestinal tumorigenesis. *Gastroenterology*, *134*, 120–130.

Ni, M., Chen, Y., Lim, E., Wimberly, H., Bailey, S. T., Imai, Y., et al. (2011). Targeting androgen receptor in estrogen receptor-negative breast cancer. *Cancer Cell*, *20*, 119–131.

Oishi, Y., Manabe, I., Tobe, K., Tsushima, K., Shindo, T., Fujiu, K., et al. (2005). Kruppel-like transcription factor KLF5 is a key regulator of adipocyte differentiation. *Cell Metabolism*, *1*, 27–39.

Parisi, S., Passaro, F., Aloia, L., Manabe, I., Nagai, R., Pastore, L., et al. (2008). Klf5 is involved in self-renewal of mouse embryonic stem cells. *Journal of Cell Science*, *121*, 2629–2634.

Rana, A., Rangasamy, V., & Mishra, R. (2010). How estrogen fuels breast cancer. *Future Oncology*, *6*, 1369–1371.

Ring, A., & Dowsett, M. (2004). Mechanisms of tamoxifen resistance. *Endocrine-Related Cancer*, *11*, 643–658.

Sartorius, C. A., Harvell, D. M., Shen, T., & Horwitz, K. B. (2005). Progestins initiate a luminal to myoepithelial switch in estrogen-dependent human breast tumors without altering growth. *Cancer Research*, *65*, 9779–9788.

Schairer, C., Lubin, J., Troisi, R., Sturgeon, S., Brinton, L., & Hoover, R. (2000). Estrogen-progestin replacement and risk of breast cancer. *JAMA: The Journal of the American Medical Association*, *284*, 691–694.

Secreto, G., Venturelli, E., Meneghini, E., Greco, M., Ferraris, C., Gion, M., et al. (2009). Testosterone and biological characteristics of breast cancers in postmenopausal women. *Cancer Epidemiology, Biomarkers & Prevention, 18*, 2942–2948.

Shimono, Y., Zabala, M., Cho, R. W., Lobo, N., Dalerba, P., Qian, D., et al. (2009). Down-regulation of miRNA-200c links breast cancer stem cells with normal stem cells. *Cell, 138*, 592–603.

Takagi, K., Miki, Y., Onodera, Y., Nakamura, Y., Ishida, T., Watanabe, M., et al. (2012). Kruppel-like factor 5 in human breast carcinoma: A potent prognostic factor induced by androgens. *Endocrine-Related Cancer, 19*, 741–750.

Thiantanawat, A., Long, B. J., & Brodie, A. M. (2003). Signaling pathways of apoptosis activated by aromatase inhibitors and antiestrogens. *Cancer Research, 63*, 8037–8050.

Tong, D., Czerwenka, K., Heinze, G., Ryffel, M., Schuster, E., Witt, A., et al. (2006). Expression of KLF5 is a prognostic factor for disease-free survival and overall survival in patients with breast cancer. *Clinical Cancer Research, 12*, 2442–2448.

Traish, A. M., Feeley, R. J., & Guay, A. T. (2009). Testosterone therapy in women with gynecological and sexual disorders: A triumph of clinical endocrinology from 1938 to 2008. *The Journal of Sexual Medicine, 6*, 334–351.

van Staa, T. P., & Sprafka, J. M. (2009). Study of adverse outcomes in women using testosterone therapy. *Maturitas, 62*, 76–80.

Wan, H., Luo, F., Wert, S. E., Zhang, L., Xu, Y., Ikegami, M., et al. (2008). Kruppel-like factor 5 is required for perinatal lung morphogenesis and function. *Development, 135*, 2563–2572.

Zhao, Y., Hamza, M. S., Leong, H. S., Lim, C. B., Pan, Y. F., Cheung, E., et al. (2008). Kruppel-like factor 5 modulates p53-independent apoptosis through Pim1 survival kinase in cancer cells. *Oncogene, 27*, 1–8.

Zhao, K. W., Sikriwal, D., Dong, X., Guo, P., Sun, X., & Dong, J. T. (2011). Oestrogen causes degradation of KLF5 by inducing the E3 ubiquitin ligase EFP in ER-positive breast cancer cells. *The Biochemical Journal, 437*, 323–333.

Zhao, D., Zheng, H. Q., Zhou, Z., & Chen, C. (2010). The Fbw7 tumor suppressor targets KLF5 for ubiquitin-mediated degradation and suppresses breast cell proliferation. *Cancer Research, 70*, 4728–4738.

Zhao, D., Zhi, X., Zhou, Z., & Chen, C. (2012). TAZ antagonizes the WWP1-mediated KLF5 degradation and promotes breast cell proliferation and tumorigenesis. *Carcinogenesis, 33*, 59–67.

Zheng, H. Q., Zhou, Z., Huang, J., Chaudhury, L., Dong, J. T., & Chen, C. (2009). Kruppel-like factor 5 promotes breast cell proliferation partially through upregulating the transcription of fibroblast growth factor binding protein 1. *Oncogene, 28*, 3702–3713.

Zhi, X., Zhao, D., Zhou, Z., Liu, R., & Chen, C. (2012). YAP promotes breast cell proliferation and survival partially through stabilizing the KLF5 transcription factor. *The American Journal of Pathology, 180*, 2452–2461.

Zhu, N., Gu, L., Findley, H. W., Chen, C., Dong, J. T., Yang, L., et al. (2006). KLF5 interacts with p53 in regulating survivin expression in acute lymphoblastic leukemia. *The Journal of Biological Chemistry, 281*, 14711–14718.

Dynamic Regulation of Steroid Hormone Receptor Transcriptional Activity by Reversible SUMOylation

Todd P. Knutson[*,†], Carol A. Lange[*,†,1]

[*]Department of Medicine (Division of Hematology, Oncology, and Transplantation), Masonic Cancer Center, University of Minnesota, Minneapolis, Minnesota, USA
[†]Department of Pharmacology (Division of Hematology, Oncology, and Transplantation), Masonic Cancer Center, University of Minnesota, Minneapolis, Minnesota, USA
[1]Corresponding author: e-mail address: lange047@umn.edu

Contents

Abstract

Transcription complexes containing steroid hormone receptors (SRs) have been well characterized at selected canonical target genes. More recently, the advent of whole genome technologies has allowed for complete SR transcriptome analyses in diverse cell types and in response to a variety of cellular stimuli. These types of studies have revealed little overlap between the tissue or cell type-specific transcriptomes of a given

Vitamins and Hormones, Volume 93
ISSN 0083-6729
http://dx.doi.org/10.1016/B978-0-12-416673-8.00008-3

SR, suggesting that all SRs are highly context-dependent transcription factors. However, the mechanisms controlling SR promoter selectivity have not been fully elucidated. Many factors may influence SR promoter selectivity, including chromatin structure, cofactor availability, and posttranslational modifications to SRs and/or their numerous coregulators; this review focuses on the impact that covalent attachment of small ubiquitin-like modifier (SUMO) moieties to SRs (i.e., SUMOylation) have on the transcriptional regulation of SR target genes.

1. INTRODUCTION

Multiple mechanisms modulate the functional activity of steroid hormone receptors (SRs) and posttranslational modifications have a major impact on cellular function, including protein–protein interactions, DNA repair, replication, transcription, chromosome segregation, genomic stability, and intracellular trafficking (for reviews, see Gareau & Lima, 2010; Gill, 2003; Hay, 2005; Johnson, 2004). Here, we discuss specific examples of how SUMOylation affects the major type I SRs, including progesterone receptor (PR), androgen receptor (AR), glucocorticoid receptor (GR), and estrogen receptor (ER).

Nuclear receptors are defined as ligand-activated transcription factors that become localized in the nucleus upon ligand binding where they regulate transcriptional programs necessary for development, metabolism, and homoeostasis. The nuclear receptor superfamily includes approximately 50 genes (Robinson-Rechavi, Carpentier, Duffraisse, & Laudet, 2001), many of which are conserved among vertebrates, and mediates multiple unique functions including almost all aspects of physiology. Steroid hormone receptors (SRs) are a subset of proteins within the nuclear receptor superfamily that include ER, PR, GR, AR, and mineralocorticoid receptor (MR). Each receptor binds unique steroid hormone ligands (agonists) that induce a conformational change in the receptor protein that initiates unique functional actions, including precise transcriptional transactivation at various gene loci (Danielian, White, Lees, & Parker, 1992; Shiau et al., 1998). These receptors are highly selective to their endogenous ligands, which are lipid molecules (derived from cholesterol) that can freely diffuse across plasma membranes (Strauss, Schuler, Rosenblum, & Tanaka, 1981). Endogenous SR ligands are synthesized primarily by the cyctochrome P450 family of enzymes in the adrenal glands, gonads (testis and ovary), placenta and, to a lesser extent, other glandular tissues (including breast adipose; Locke et al., 2008; Su, Wong, Hong, & Chen, 2011; Suzuki et al., 2005).

Additionally, SRs can also bind multiple closely related synthetic ligands, many of which contain antagonistic properties. Furthermore, recent studies have revealed that SRs participate in kinase signaling pathways, multiprotein complexes/scaffolds, and regulate transcription independent of ligand (Lange, 2008). These receptors exhibit diverse functions in tissue development and homoeostasis.

SRs contain multiple conserved functional protein domains, including a ligand-binding domain (LBD), hinge region (H), DNA-binding domain (DBD), transcriptional activation function (AF) domains, and variable length amino-terminal regions. SR tertiary structures resemble a molecule folded upon itself at the hinge region, resulting in N- and C-terminal interactions that regulate SR function (Takimoto et al., 2003). The AF domains contain residues important for transcriptional transactivation and often mediate protein–protein interactions (including coactivator and corepressor binding; Heery, Kalkhoven, Hoare, & Parker, 1997; Kamei et al., 1996; Onate, Tsai, Tsai, & O'Malley, 1995). The DBD is crucial for efficient DNA binding at conserved sequences, hormone response elements (HREs), within DNA, and the LBD is necessary for determining hormone-binding specificity (Hollenberg et al., 1985; Lieberman, Bona, Edwards, & Nordeen, 1993; Misrahi et al., 1987; Tang et al., 2011). Both of these domains are needed for effective SR dimerization on chromatin, a fundamental process required for transcriptional transactivation (Tetel, Giangrande, Leonhardt, McDonnell, & Edwards, 1999). The classical mechanism of SR action follows this general process: (i) steroid hormone ligands diffuse through the plasma membrane and bind cytoplasmic SRs causing their disassociation from heat shock chaperone proteins, (ii) SRs accumulate in the nucleus where they dimerize on HREs in enhancer/promoter sequences (or tether to other transcription factors), (iii) coregulatory molecules and basal transcriptional machinery are recruited and directly interact with SRs and the basal transcriptional machinery, (iv) coregulatory molecules remodel the chromatin structure (acetylation/deacetylation, methylation/demethylation, etc.), (v) resulting in transcriptional activation or repression. Recent studies have identified regulatory mechanisms that alter SR action at every step described earlier, indicating this process is very dynamic and highly sensitive to changes that mediate SR activity (for reviews, see Edwards, 2005; O'Malley & Kumar, 2009; Xu, Wu, & O'malley, 2009). Deregulation of these processes can have severe consequences for hormonally regulated tissues, including the facilitation of tumor development.

SUMOylation, like other posttranslational modifications including phosphorylation, acetylation, and methylation, is a mechanism cells use to dynamically alter generalized functions of substrate proteins. SRs are master regulators of many cellular functions, including development, proliferation, metabolism, and survival. Many SRs also participate in "nongenomic" actions involving cross talk signaling with multiple protein kinase pathways, including c-Src, IGF, and MAPK (for reviews, see Bjornstrom & Sjoberg, 2005; Edwards, 2005; Lange, 2008; Losel & Wehling, 2003). Because SR SUMOylation is a dynamic process, this modification can rapidly alter receptor function in response to various cellular stimuli. Transcriptional transactivation assays initially revealed that SR SUMOylation is primarily associated with transcriptional repression. More recently, it has become appreciated that small ubiquitin-like modifier (SUMO) modification of SRs significantly alters their protein–protein interactions that are critical for almost all SR tasks. New reports are detailing the diverse implications that SR SUMO modification has on transcriptional profiles and cell programs.

In this review, we focus on how SUMOylation impacts the major SRs activities with regard to their transcriptional action, interaction with coregulators, how SUMOylation controls promoter selectivity, and the implications of SR SUMOylation in cancer and other diseases.

2. MECHANISMS OF PROTEIN SUMOYLATION

2.1. The SUMO conjugation pathway

The SUMO conjugation pathway is similar to the ubiquitin conjugation pathway and has been extensively studied. Four SUMO proteins are expressed in mammalian cells, where SUMO2 and -3 are 97% identical, and SUMO1 is approximately 55% similar to SUMO2/3 (Saitoh & Hinchey, 2000). A fourth variant, SUMO4, was recently discovered because it resides in a locus containing multiple single nucleotide polymorphisms (SNPs) that are highly correlated with type 1 diabetes (Guo et al., 2004). However, subsequent studies have shown that SUMO4 cannot be conjugated to substrate proteins and likely functions through noncovalent interactions (Owerbach, McKay, Yeh, Gabbay, & Bohren, 2005). Each SUMO peptide is approximately 11.5 kDa and covalently attached to the ε-amino group of a Lys residue in substrate proteins through an isopeptide bond with the carboxy-terminal Gly of SUMO (Hay, 2005). Substrate proteins contain a conserved SUMO attachment consensus motif, ψKx(D/E), where

SUMO moieties are attached to the Lys residue, ψ is a large hydrophobic residue, and x is any residue (Iniguez-Lluhi & Pearce, 2000). Interestingly, SUMO2/3 itself contains a SUMO-conjugation motif and can form polySUMO chains, whereas SUMO1 does not contain a SUMO-conjugation motif and is not believed to form chains (Tatham et al., 2001). Mutating the conserved Lys residue to another basic residue (e.g., Arg) can abolish substrate protein SUMOylation. In fact, Holmstrom, Van Antwerp, and Iniguez-Lluhi (2003) showed that mutating the other conserved, non-Lys, residue within the motif (i.e., Asp/Glu) also substantially reduced GR SUMOylation; thus, efficient substrate SUMOylation depends on the complete motif sequence. For example, a naturally occurring germline mutation within a SUMO-conjugation motif was discovered in the microphthalmia-associated transcription factor (MITF), where the fourth position, Glu, was mutated to Lys (Bertolotto et al., 2011). This substitution substantially decreased the ability for MITF to be SUMOylated (Bertolotto et al., 2011). Thus far, UBC9 is the only known E2 SUMO-conjugation enzyme that is necessary and sufficient for SUMO attachment, unlike the ubiquitin conjugation cascade where hundreds of E2 and E3 enzymes are involved in ubiquitin attachment. However, in cooperation with UBC9, SUMO attachment can be catalyzed by a limited number of SUMO E3 ligases, including members of the PIAS, Pc2, and histone deacetylases (HDAC) protein families. With only a limited number of enzymes involved in substrate protein SUMOylation, specificity for SUMO attachment is unknown but under active investigation. A small number of SUMO (also called Sentrin) proteases (SENPs) reverse the reaction and remove SUMO molecules from protein substrates through cleavage of the isopeptide bond (Gong, Millas, Maul, & Yeh, 2000; Nishida, Kaneko, Kitagawa, & Yasuda, 2001). A number of studies have revealed that cells dynamically modulate the expression of SUMO-conjugation pathway proteins (including the upregulation of SENPs) to drive various cellular actions (Bawa-Khalfe, Cheng, Lin, Ittmann, & Yeh, 2010; Cheng, Bawa, Lee, Gong, & Yeh, 2006).

2.2. Protein phosphorylation affects substrate SUMOylation

Phosphorylation of substrate proteins can have positive or negative effects on the SUMO-conjugation machinery. A number of SUMOylated proteins have been discovered to contain expanded SUMO consensus motifs, ψKx(D/E)xxSP, where phosphorylation at the downstream Ser residue enhanced substrate SUMOylation (Hietakangas et al., 2006). Thus, these consensus motifs were named phosphorylation-dependent SUMO motifs (PDSM; Mohideen et al., 2009). Multiple transcriptional regulators contain PDSMs, including HSF1, MEF2, GATA1, PPARgamma, and NCoR (Hietakangas et al., 2006; Shalizi et al., 2006). The negative charge of the phospho-species facilitates interaction with the basic residues of the E2 (UBC9). In fact, many substrate proteins can be SUMOylated without requiring an E3 ligase; however, the kinetics are much faster when an E3 ligase is available. Through a similar mechanism, negatively charged amino acid-dependent SUMO motifs facilitate E2 binding and SUMO conjugation (Yang, Galanis, Witty, & Sharrocks, 2006). Thus, it is likely that phosphorylation at nearby residues affects substrate protein conformation or localization, allowing efficient E2 and/or E3 access to the consensus Lys attachment site. Indeed, a unique nonconsensus SUMO-conjugation motif was recently described, where the consensus D/E residue is substituted for a Ser residue, whose phosphorylation enhances nearby SUMOylation (Picard et al., 2012). This phosphorylated SUMOylation motif (pSuM; Picard et al., 2012) is another example highlighting the importance of negative charge within SUMO-conjugation motifs.

Conversely, substrate protein phosphorylation at residues outside the SUMO-conjugation motif can also regulate substrate SUMOylation. For example, phosphorylation of KAP1 by ataxia telangiectasia mutated results in decreased KAP1 SUMOylation (Li et al., 2007). Similar mechanisms have been described for c-Fos (Bossis et al., 2005), AIB1 (Wu et al., 2006), and PR (Daniel, Faivre, & Lange, 2007) (discussed below).

2.3. SUMOylated proteins interact through specialized motifs

The primary molecular consequence of substrate SUMOylation is altered protein–protein interactions. Thus, noncovalent binding occurs between SUMO moieties and specific surfaces in protein-binding partners called SUMO-interacting motifs (SIMs). The SIM, V/I-x-V/I-V/I, binds all SUMO isoforms and is found in almost all proteins that depend on SUMO regulation (Song, Durrin, Wilkinson, Krontiris, & Chen, 2004). Antibody variants, called monobodies, have been genetically developed to bind selective SUMO isoforms and inhibit SUMO/SIM interaction, allowing for new studies to unravel the differences between the diverse functions of SUMO isoforms (Gilbreth et al., 2011).

3. SR SUMOYLATION/DESUMOYLATION

3.1. SRs are SUMOylated

SRs are critical mediators of transcriptional programs necessary for organ development and tissue maintenance. Thus, the mechanisms controlling SR action are under intense investigation. Many critical cell regulators are mutated in various cancers (e.g., *PTEN, TP53, RB1, BRAF, BRCA1/2, PIK3CA*, etc.), but few mutations in SRs have been linked with malignant disease. Instead, it appears that SR transcriptional action is primarily modulated via posttranslational modifications, including SUMOylation. Some estimates suggest that one-third of all proteins are endogenously SUMOylated in dynamic fashion (Yang, Jaffray, Senthinathan, Hay, & Sharrocks, 2003), but for technical reasons, only a few have been observed *in vivo* (without overexpression of SUMO isoforms), including RanGAP1 (Mahajan, Delphin, Guan, Gerace, & Melchior, 1997) and Daxx (Lin et al., 2006). However, many SUMOylated proteins have been characterized *in vitro* through the overexpression of unconjugated "free" SUMO precursor proteins in cell culture assays. Cell signaling mechanisms are very sensitive to large changes in the concentration of available SUMO proteins, which may cause unexpected or nonphysiological results. Therefore, studying the molecular or cellular effects of substrate SUMOylation may be more informative using models exploiting the mutation of key SUMO-conjugation motifs.

Poukka, Karvonen, Janne, and Palvimo (2000) showed that AR is SUMOylated at two residues (Lys386 and Lys520) but primarily at Lys386 (Fig. 9.1). Engineered point mutations at these AR residues demonstrated total loss of AR SUMOylation. GR SUMOylation was characterized at three SUMO-conjugation motifs (Le Drean, Mincheneau, Le Goff, & Michel, 2002; Poukka et al., 2000; Tian, Poukka, Palvimo, & Janne, 2002) originally described as synergy control (SC) motifs (Iniguez-Lluhi & Pearce, 2000). GR Lys277 and Lys293 are the major GR SUMO-acceptor sites, as Lys-to-Arg (KR) mutation at these residues fully blocks GR SUMOylation; thus GR Lys703 does not appear to contribute to the overall GR SUMOylation status (Fig. 9.1; Tian et al., 2002). Individual GR SUMO-deficient mutants (K277R or K293R) are significantly deSUMOylated and drive greater transcriptional transactivation in luciferase reporter assays, compared to wild-type (SUMOylated) GR. The double mutant (K277R/K293R) has even greater transactivation activity over a wide range of GR expression levels (Tian et al., 2002).

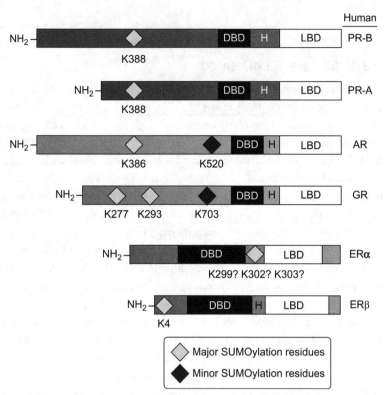

Figure 9.1 Steroid hormone receptor domain structures and key SUMOylation residues. All SRs depicted contain a DNA-binding domain (DBD) and a ligand-binding domain (LBD) separated by a hinge region (H). PR-A and PR-B are derived from the same gene, where PR-B is the full-length receptor containing an additional 164 amino acids that PR-A lacks. PR-B SUMOylation occurs at Lys388, and PR-A is SUMOylated at the analogous residue (technically PR-A Lys224). AR SUMOylation primarily occurs at Lys386. SUMOylation of AR at Lys520 is a very minor contribution of the overall AR SUMOylation. Similar to AR, SUMOylation of GR occurs primarily at two lysine residues, Lys277 and Lys293, where Lys703 is not an important SUMOylation site *in vivo*. The precise SUMOylation residues of ER-alpha have not been confidently mapped. The lysine rich hinge region of ER-alpha contains multiple possible SUMOylation conjugation sites, including Lys299, Lys302, and/or Lys303. Recent data have shown that ER-beta is SUMOylated at its N-terminal Lys4. (See Color Insert.)

Both PR–A and PR–B isoforms are primarily SUMOylated at Lys388 in the N-terminal region upstream from the activation function 1 (AF-1) domain (Fig. 9.1; Abdel–Hafiz, Takimoto, Tung, & Horwitz, 2002; Man et al., 2006). However, PR SUMOylation at Lys7 and Lys531 has also been suggested (Man et al., 2006). PR (and AR and GR) modification by

SUMO1 or SUMO2/3 is largely ligand dependent and occurs rapidly (i.e., within 15 min; Daniel et al., 2007) at consensus IKxE SUMO-conjugation motifs (Abdel-Hafiz et al., 2002; Han et al., 2011). PR-A is more heavily SUMOylated than PR-B and thus is more transcriptionally repressed in reporter assays (Daniel et al., 2007). Ligand-dependent PR SUMOylation contributes to PR autoinhibition and transrepression of PR and ER isoforms (Abdel-Hafiz et al., 2002). PR Ser294 phosphorylation facilitates PR ubiquitination and proteasome degradation, and also antagonizes PR SUMOylation at Lys388 (Daniel et al., 2007; Lange, Shen, & Horwitz, 2000). It has been demonstrated that kinase-directed phosphorylation at PR Ser294 (by CDK2, MAPK, etc.) blocks PR SUMOylation and thus dere-presses PR transcriptional action (Daniel et al., 2007; Daniel & Lange, 2009). Indeed, mutation of Ser294 causes increased PR SUMOylation, transcrip-tional repression, and receptor stabilization (thereby antagonizing receptor activity; Daniel et al., 2007).

ER-alpha is the primary ER isoform driving breast cancer progression and its regulation has been shown to be affected by SUMOylation among other posttranslational modifications, including phosphorylation, acetylation, meth-ylation, and ubiquitination (Kato et al., 1995; Le Romancer et al., 2008; Lonard, Nawaz, Smith, & O'Malley, 2000; Wang et al., 2001). Sentis, Le Romancer, Bianchin, Rostan, and Corbo (2005) provided convincing data that SUMO1 is conjugated to ER-alpha in a strictly estrogen-dependent man-ner. ER-alpha SUMOylation may be somewhat unique from other SRs because the receptor lacks a consensus SUMO-conjugation motif. However, domain deletion studies (combined with *in vivo* and *in vitro* SUMO-conjugation assays) have determined that ER-alpha SUMOylation is targeted to the hinge region, residues 251–305 (Sentis et al., 2005). Detailed mapping suggests possible ER-alpha SUMO-acceptor sites may include K266, K268, K299, K302, and K303, but the major SUMOylated lysines are K299, K302, and K303 (Fig. 9.1; Sentis et al., 2005). From simple transcriptional reporter assays, it appears that ER-alpha SUMOylation enhances transactivation, a mechanism contrary to other SRs (Sentis et al., 2005). However, these studies were conducted via reporter assays, and it is plausible that ER SUMOylation also impacts endogenous promoter selectivity. Despite these findings, one study found that ER-alpha and ER-beta SUMOylation was not observed fol-lowing *in vitro* translation and SUMO1 conjugation assays (Poukka et al., 2000). Perhaps a specific factor(s) is required for stable ER-alpha SUMOylation *in vivo*. Clearly, further studies are needed to expand our understanding of ER-alpha SUMOylation.

ER-beta undergoes dynamic SUMOylation at Lys4 after estrogen treatment and is deSUMOylated by catalytically active SENP1 (Fig. 9.1; Picard et al., 2012). Mutation of this SUMO-acceptor residue, K4R, completely abolishes ER-beta SUMOylation (Picard et al., 2012). ER-beta is SUMOylated at a unique phosphorylated SUMOylation motif (pSuM; Picard et al., 2012). The N-terminal motif, ψKxS, contains a Lys residue necessary for SUMO attachment, flanked by a large hydrophobic group (ψ) and nearby Ser residue (Picard et al., 2012). Phosphorylation at Ser6 is required for ER-beta SUMOylation, and phosphorylation mimics (substitutions with Asp or Glu at Ser6) also allow efficient ER-beta SUMOylation (Picard et al., 2012). Mutation of Ser6 to Ala completely abrogated ER-beta SUMOylation (Picard et al., 2012). Thus, phosphorylation at Ser6 provides the necessary negative charge required for substrate SUMOylation (usually provided by the presence of Asp or Glu in the consensus SUMO-conjugation motif) and is phosphorylated by MAPK pathway activation. Unlike ER-alpha SUMOylation, ER-beta SUMOylation repressed ER-beta-mediated transcriptional transactivation in reporter gene assays and at multiple endogenous ER-beta target genes (Picard et al., 2012). In addition, ChIP assays demonstrated that recruitment of deSUMOylated ER-beta (K4R) was substantially higher at ER-beta target gene promoters, compared to SUMO-competent receptors (i.e., WT, S6E, S6D; Picard et al., 2012). These data support the discovery that deSUMOylated ER-beta is transcriptionally hyperactive at these genes (Picard et al., 2012). It appears that multiple kinases mediate ER-beta phosphorylation, enhancing its SUMOylation. ERK1/2, p38 MAPK, JNK, Src, and PKA inhibition modestly reduced ER-beta SUMOylation, whereas GSK3-beta inhibition or knockdown significantly reduced ER-beta SUMOylation (Picard et al., 2012). However, it appears that GSK-beta phosphorylation of ER-beta occurs at two nearby residues (Ser8, Ser12) and their phosphorylation is required for efficient ER-beta SUMOylation (Picard et al., 2012). This demonstrates that dynamic regulation of ER-beta SUMOylation at the pSuM includes key downstream hormone-dependent GSK3-beta phosphorylation sites.

3.2. Interplay between SR ubiquitination and SUMOylation

There is an interesting interplay between PR SUMOylation and ubiquitination-mediated proteasome turnover. Highly SUMOylated receptors are greatly stabilized (Daniel et al., 2007), whereas Ser294-phosphorylated and deSUMOylated PR are transcriptionally hyperactive and undergo rapid turnover (Lange et al., 2000). Experiments have shown that a small ubiquitin-binding protein, CUEDC2, interacts with PR and promotes progesterone-dependent degradation via the ubiquitin-proteasome pathway (Zhang et al., 2007). CUEDC2 expression promoted ligand-dependent ubiquitination and reduced PR SUMOylation. CUEDC2 knockdown substantially reduced progestin-dependent WT PR degradation (Zhang et al., 2007). In experiments expressing SUMO-deficient mutant PR (K388R), CUEDC2 could not mediate progestin-dependent PR turnover, suggesting that Lys388 is a possible PR ubiquitination site. Indeed, K388R PR was less ubiquitinated (compared to WT PR), thus indicating that Lys388 may be involved (directly or indirectly) in PR ubiquitination (Zhang et al., 2007). These experiments suggest that Lys388 is modified by both SUMO and ubiquitin and that these modifications compete. However, other reports clearly indicate that K388R PR undergoes considerable ligand-dependent turnover (with similar kinetics or even faster relative to WT PR; Abdel-Hafiz, Dudevoir, & Horwitz, 2009; Daniel et al., 2007; Knutson et al., 2012), reflecting that PR must also be ubiquitinated at other residues besides Lys388. Further investigation into the relative levels of PR SUMOylation and ubiquitination at candidate residues is needed, and thus far, native PR ubiquitination residues have not been thoroughly investigated.

Hormone-dependent degradation of ER-beta was inhibited, compared to WT, when SUMOylation-facilitating mutants were expressed (i.e., S6D, S6E), suggesting that ER-beta SUMOylation inhibits receptor turnover (Picard et al., 2012). However, the K4R SUMO-deficient mutant was also greatly stabilized compared to WT. In time course experiments, K4R receptors did undergo hormone-dependent turnover, indicating Lys4 is not the sole ubiquitination site (Picard et al., 2012), although ubiquitination assays demonstrated that SUMO and ubiquitin compete for attachment at Lys4, thus implicating Lys4 as an important regulatory site.

3.3. Expression of SUMO-conjugation pathway factors impact SR function

3.3.1 PIAS

Early studies investigating the functional consequences of SR SUMOylation started by modulating the expression of SUMO-pathway proteins and measuring their transcriptional effects using luciferase reporter assays. SR SUMOylation is catalyzed primarily by the PIAS family of SUMO E3 ligases. When overexpressed in cells, PIAS1 and PIAS3 caused the appearance of multiple high-molecular-weight ER-alpha bands via SDS-PAGE, indicating that PIAS1 and PIAS3 facilitate ER-alpha SUMOylation at multiple sites or may facilitate ER-alpha polySUMOylation (Sentis et al., 2005). Because ER-alpha SUMOylation is enhanced upon 17-beta-estradiol treatment, but to a lesser extent in response to 4-OH-tamoxifen (Kobayashi et al., 2004; Sentis et al., 2005), there may be a ligand-specific mechanism controlling ER-alpha SUMOylation. Thus, modulating ER-alpha SUMOylation by various ligands may contribute to ER-alpha promoter selectivity. However, this does not appear to hold true for PR, where both progestin and antiprogestin treatment stimulate rapid PR SUMOylation equally (Daniel et al., 2007). PIAS3 expression has also been implicated in mediating PR SUMOylation (Daniel et al., 2007).

Similar to PR and ER, ligand (testosterone) binding greatly enhances AR SUMOylation. PIAS proteins (PIASxalpha/ARIP3 and PIAS1) facilitate AR SUMOylation, resulting in decreased transcriptional transactivation (Kotaja, Karvonen, Janne, & Palvimo, 2002; Nishida & Yasuda, 2002). However, PIAS1, but not ARIP3, was able to facilitate GRIP1 SUMOylation, suggesting that despite a single known E2 (UBC9), PIAS proteins provide specificity for substrate SUMOylation. PIASxalpha/ARIP3 interact with free SUMO1 through noncovalent interactions within a stretch of Ser-, Glu-, and Asp-rich amino acids, and when these residues were deleted from ARIP3, its interaction with SUMO1 was diminished and ARIP3 recruitment of other SUMOylated proteins was diminished. Thus, this suggests that PIAS proteins may tether to interaction partners through SUMO modifications. However, deletion of these residues did not affect ARIP3 SUMOylation (Kotaja, Karvonen, et al., 2002). The E3 activity of PIAS proteins appears to depend on the RING finger-like domain, because mutation of the conserved cysteine residue causes loss of ARIP3 and UBC9 interaction as well as loss of AR SUMOylation and SUMO-mediated AR transcriptional repression (Nishida & Yasuda, 2002). PIASy was also shown to inhibit AR transactivation. However, this occurred via SUMOylation-independent mechanisms (Gross, Yang, Top, Gasper, & Shuai, 2004). PIASy directly interacts with HDAC1 and HDAC3 through its repression domain 1, and mutations that destroy the PIASy E3 SUMO-ligase activity, or mutations in the AR SUMO-acceptor sites, do not affect the ability for PIASy to repress AR transcription. Therefore, PIASy appears to alter AR transcriptional action through a SUMOylation-independent mechanism that can be relieved through HDAC inhibitor treatment (Gross et al., 2004).

3.3.2 SENP

Like PIAS overexpression, SENP1 activity can also modulate SR SUMO-ylation. Despite the transcriptionally repressive effect of AR SUMOylation, transient overexpression of SENP1 augmented AR-mediated transactivation (Cheng, Wang, Wang, & Yeh, 2004). Paradoxically, transcriptional trans-activation of the SUMO-deficient AR mutant was also augmented. This sug-gests that the effects of SENP1 overexpression were likely independent of AR deSUMOylation (Cheng et al., 2004). Interestingly, SENP1 expression levels are induced by ligand-dependent AR action and can be inhibited by treatment with AR antagonist, bicalutamide (Bawa-Khalfe, Cheng, Wang, & Yeh, 2007). Further, the authors identified an ARE in the core promoter sequences of SENP1, and ChIP assays at the SENP1 promoter confirmed AR recruit-ment (Bawa-Khalfe et al., 2007). Thus, it appears that AR drives the expres-sion of SENP1, and SENP1 activity elevates AR transcriptional transactivation, however, not through direct AR deSUMOylation. Instead, other studies revealed that SENP1 deSUMOylates HDAC1, relieving its repressive effects on AR (further discussed below; Cheng et al., 2004).

Notably, SENP1 transiently overexpressed in breast cancer cells medi-ated PR deSUMOylation and increased PR transcriptional activity in both reporter transcription assays and at PR-target genes, as measured by increased *HBEGF* transcript levels (Abdel-Hafiz & Horwitz, 2012; Daniel et al., 2007). In reporter assays, SENP1 expression sensitizes WT PR to low concentrations of ligand, whereas SUMO-deficient PR tran-scriptional activity was not affected, indicating that SENP1 mediates PR hypersensitivity via deSUMOylation of the receptor (Abdel-Hafiz & Horwitz, 2012; Daniel et al., 2007). Catalytically inactive SENP1 expressed in breast cancer cells repressed PR-mediated gene expression through dominant negative action (Daniel et al., 2007). SENP2 did not affect PR-mediated transcriptional activity, possibly due to SENP2's more diffuse nuclear and cytoplasmic localization (Daniel et al., 2007).

Despite the variability of *in vitro* SENP overexpression studies, recent work has revealed that some prostate cancers express high levels of SENP1, which contributes to elevated AR-dependent gene expression (Bawa-Khalfe et al., 2010; Cheng et al., 2006). In the normal parental prostate epi-thelial cell line, RWPE1, endogenous levels of SENP1 mRNA expression levels are relatively low, whereas the transformed (RWPE2) and malignant (LNCaP) prostate cancer cells contain high levels of SENP1 mRNA expres-sion (Bawa-Khalfe et al., 2007). Indeed, high levels of SENP1 expression in patient tumors were correlated with high Gleason scores and increased risk of prostate cancer recurrence (Wang et al., 2013). SENP1 action also contributes to tumor aggressiveness through the stabilization of HIF-1alpha (via its deSUMOylation), allowing the transcription factor to upregulate matrix metalloproteinases (e.g., MMP2, MMP9) that are important drivers of metastasis (Wang et al., 2013). These experiments revealed that SENP1-mediated deSUMOylation of important transcriptional mediators (e.g., HDAC1, PR, AR, HIF-1alpha) contributes to SR-driven malignancies.

3.3.3 UBC9

UBC9 is the only known SUMO E2 conjugating enzyme and mediates the attachment of processed SUMO moieties to substrate proteins. UBC9 expression levels are precisely regulated, as fluctuations in expression can dramatically impact the regulation of many SUMO substrates including SR transactivation. The first SR shown to interact with UBC9 was GR, where researchers were searching for factors mediating GR (and/or c-Jun)-mediated transcriptional repression (Gottlicher et al., 1996). Subsequently, UBC9 was also shown to physically interact with AR through its nuclear localization signal sequence (Poukka, Aarnisalo, Karvonen, Palvimo, & Janne, 1999). These early studies characterizing interactions between SRs and UBC9 led to the hypothesis that SRs were covalently modified by SUMO and that SUMO governs transcriptional repression. However, UBC9 was shown to be a GR transcriptional adapter protein that increases GR transactivation when cells were treated with agonists or antagonists, independent of UBC9 SUMO-conjugation activity (as conjugation-deficient UBC9 mutant, C93S, expression also sensitizes GR to ligand as measured by transactivation dose–response curves; Kaul, Blackford, Cho, & Simons, 2002). Similarly, UBC9 overexpression greatly enhances AR-mediated transactivation, through a SUMO-conjugation-independent mechanism (Poukka et al., 1999).

Like GR and AR, UBC9 was discovered to interact with ER-alpha via yeast-two-hybrid assay and shown to enhance ER-alpha mediated transactivation in COS-1 cells, independent of UBC9 SUMO-conjugation activity (Kobayashi et al., 2004). Thus, it appears that UBC9 is present in the multiprotein transcriptional complex assembled by SRs and can function to enhance transcription, regardless of its SUMO-conjugation activities (i.e., as determined by expression of UBC9 mutant C93S). In addition, other studies have shown that SUMOylation of SR cofactors has significant impact on SR transactivation; thus overexpression of UBC9 in cell lines may not result in predictable transcriptional outcomes. However, a recent analysis showed that women carrying a dominant SNP in UBC9 had increased risk for grade 1 breast tumors, indicating UBC9 expression does impact disease outcomes (and further discussed below; Dünnebier et al., 2010). Thus, it appears that UBC9 is, first, a multifunctional protein that is required for SUMO conjugation to substrate proteins and, second, a SR transcriptional coactivator. Further studies are needed to characterize the role of UBC9 in transcriptional activator complexes.

3.3.4 SUMO

The critical amino acid residues of SUMO2 that make up its functionally repressive surface, and are required for its transcriptionally repressive effects, are located at the end of its second beta sheet following the alpha helix (Chupreta, Holmstrom, Subramanian, & Iniguez-Lluhi, 2005). Based on functional reporter assays, the repressive surface of SUMO2 is not found in other ubiquitin-like proteins (e.g., NEDD8 or ubiquitin), consistent with the lack of transcriptionally repressive effects of these molecules. Like SUMO2/3, these residues are also conserved in SUMO1 and are responsible for its repressive effects. Mutation of these residues restores GR transcriptional activity (derepression); moreover, these SUMO2 mutants are appropriately processed by the SUMO-conjugation machinery, thus retaining other basic functions. Based on the crystal structures, SUMO contains four basic (positively charged) residues (K33, K35, K42, and R50) that extend into the solvent to form a rectangular shape (Huang, Ko, Li, & Wang, 2004). These important residues are required for SUMO-mediated transcriptional repression, and the protein structure (Huang et al., 2004) is conserved between SUMO2, SUMO1, and SMT3 (the *Saccharomyces cerevisiae* SUMO homolog). Thus, these positively charged residues likely interact with acidic surfaces of corepressors to mediate transcriptional inhibition. However, it is unclear whether the inhibitory surface of SUMO can mediate transcriptional inhibition over long distances or is limited to the local chromatin structure (Chupreta et al., 2005).

A less studied consequence of AR SUMOylation involves polyglutamine tract repeats in the neurodegenerative disorder, spinal and bulbar muscular atrophy (also called Kennedy disease; Mukherjee, Thomas, Dadgar, Lieberman, & Iniguez-Lluhi, 2009). The CAG trinucleotide repeat expansion within the N-terminal domain of the AR gene causes this disease through AR misfolding (and is not dependent on transcriptional activity). Mukherjee et al. (2009) showed that cells expressing a polyglutamine-expanded form of AR caused its aggregation in the cytoplasm after ligand treatment. However, cells overexpressing SUMO3 block the ligand-dependent aggregation of polyglutamine-expanded-AR molecules, and the receptor is localized to the nucleus. Thus, SUMO-modified AR appears to be excluded from cytoplasmic aggregates, which cause neural toxicity. This effect is completely dependent on the direct SUMOylation of AR because SUMOylation-deficient AR mutants remain fully aggregated within the cytoplasm. This research reveals a novel functional role for AR SUMOylation (i.e., to prevent cytoplasmic aggregation), independent of SUMO-mediated transcriptional effects (Mukherjee et al., 2009).

4. SR SUMOYLATION MODULATES TRANSCRIPTIONAL ACTION AND PROMOTER SELECTIVITY

4.1. The impact of SR SUMOylation on promoter selectivity

Early studies reported that SUMO-modified SRs were transcriptionally repressed (Abdel-Hafiz et al., 2002; Iniguez-Lluhi & Pearce, 2000; Poukka et al., 2000); however, new information has revealed that SUMO modifications allow substrate proteins to function in altogether different ways than previously known. Early data were primarily collected using luciferase reporter assays that cannot recapitulate the topology or diversity of chromatin structure at endogenous enhancer and promoter loci that is essential for tissue-specific or disease-dependent transcriptional regulation (Lupien et al., 2008; Verzi et al., 2010). It is becoming clear that multiple factors are required for efficient SR transcriptional action and SUMO modification of SRs may significantly alter SR interactions with essential cofactors and/or chromatin.

Multiple studies have reported that only a small proportion of SRs in cells are SUMO modified (~5–10% of total protein) at any given time (when measured by Western blotting techniques); therefore, the significance of SR SUMOylation has been questioned. The low level of SUMO-modified proteins measured using *in vitro* assays may be artificially low due to rapid deSUMOylation upon cell lysis. Alternatively, SUMOylated SRs may need only to be transiently modified to initiate the recruitment of corepressors that will sustain transcriptional inhibition, thus relieving the need for sustained high-level SR SUMOylation. These mechanisms are not fully understood. Unfortunately, measuring cellular levels of SUMOylated proteins is difficult because antibodies targeting specific SUMO-conjugated proteins are not available (as phospho-specific antibodies are available). However, immunoprecipitation of substrate proteins followed by immunoblotting for SUMO isoforms is an effective technique to determine the level of substrate protein SUMOylation. Using this technique, Shao et al. (2004) demonstrated that in ovarian granulosa cells, PR is substantially SUMOylated in response to gonadotropin stimulation *in vivo*. Despite these detection limitations, engineered mutations of a substrate protein's SUMO-acceptor sites clearly demonstrate that SUMO modification has significant transcriptional impact in cell culture and mouse models. *In vivo* evidence that SUMO-modified receptors have substantially altered function comes from experiments with a SUMOylation-deficient knockin mouse model (expressing a Lys-to-Arg (KR) mutation at the endogenous locus) of nuclear receptor SF-1 (NR5A1). Analysis of this KR knockin mouse revealed a dramatically different phenotype compared to SF-1 knockout or overexpression (Lee et al., 2011). Mice expressing the SF-1 KR knockin displayed altered SF-1 promoter selectivity and had a distinct endocrine physiology (Lee et al., 2011). Thus, for the first time, *in vivo* mouse models demonstrate that SUMO conjugation to nuclear receptors (e.g., SF-1) can significantly affect normal development through altered transcriptional function.

Another example of the powerful effects that SUMOylation has on substrate proteins was discovered in melanoma and hepatacellular carcinoma (HCC) patients (Bertolotto et al., 2011). MITF is a member of the Myc family of transcription factors and drives cell proliferation and invasion through the regulation of important target genes (e.g., MET and CDKN2A/p16INK4A; Cheli, Ohanna, Ballotti, & Bertolotto, 2010). Patients with melanoma and/or HCC are 4–14 times more likely to carry a germline missense mutation in MITF (E318K) that dramatically reduces MITF SUMOylation (at nearby Lys316 within a SUMO-conjugation motif; Bertolotto et al., 2011). Subsequent gene expression profiling and ChIP-seq analyses demonstrated that deSUMOylated MITF transcriptionally regulates a distinct set of genes, compared to wild-type MITF. Thus, alterations in MITF SUMOylation contribute to its promoter selectivity, driving melanoma and HCC incidence and malignant progression (Bertolotto et al., 2011), suggesting that SUMOylation is a clinically relevant modification of proteins (e.g., transcription factors).

4.2. SR cross talk with growth factor signaling pathways modulate SR SUMOylation and promoter selectivity

Fuqua et al. (Giordano et al., 2010) discovered a naturally occurring somatic mutation in ER-alpha, converting Lys303 to Arg in approximately 30–50%

of malignant or invasive breast cancers (Fuqua et al., 2000; Herynk et al., 2007). Although unknown, it has been suggested that K303 may be a key SUMO-attachment residue in ER-alpha. Cells expressing this mutant receptor are hypersensitive to low levels of estrogen in anchorage-independent growth assays; mouse xenografts (Herynk et al., 2010) and these cells are resistant to tamoxifen treatment when HER2 signaling is active. The ER-alpha K303 mutant displays bidirectional cross talk with the HER2 signaling pathway, where cells expressing this mutant are constitutively phosphorylated at Ser305 and HER2 phosphorylation is also greatly increased. The elevated levels of growth factor signaling in these cells greatly contribute to their tamoxifen resistance phenotype. Indeed, the ER-alpha K303R mutation was associated with elevated HER2 levels (Herynk et al., 2007). These authors also suggest that cells expressing ER-alpha K303R drives tamoxifen resistance through altered coregulatory recruitment to transcriptional promoters/enhancers. For example, ER-alpha K303R displayed increased binding and altered promoter cycling of various coactivators, including SRC2 (Fuqua et al., 2000), AIB1 (Herynk et al., 2010), and TIF-2, and reduced interaction with corepressors NCOR1 and BRCA1 (Herynk et al., 2010). Transcription factor SUMOylation is known to alter cofactor binding; thus mutated (and deSUMOylated) ER-alpha may be driving tamoxifen resistance through altered cofactor recruitment and/or altered promoter selectivity. This hypothesis has yet to be investigated.

SUMO-dependent PR promoter selectivity at multiple endogenous genes in T47D breast cancer cells was recently described. Cells expressing either WT or SUMO-deficient PR were assayed for differentially regulated genes using whole genome gene expression microarrays and validated in multiple cell line models, including MCF-7 and BT-474 (Knutson et al., 2012). These data clearly demonstrated dramatic differences in PR transcriptional activity depending on its SUMOylation status; unique up- and down-regulated gene sets were defined under ligand-dependent and independent conditions. Gene sets upregulated specifically by SUMO-deficient PR (compared to WT) were discovered to be significantly associated with highly expressed genes (top 5–10%) in ERBB2-positive tumors and cell lines (Knutson et al., 2012). Additionally, in unmodified ERBB2-overexpressing BT-474 breast cancer cells, multiple genes upregulated by SUMO-deficient PR were transcriptionally hyperactive and MAPK pathway inhibition reduced mRNA levels and cellular proliferation (Knutson et al., 2012). Thus, in breast cancer cells, it appears that deSUMOylated PR (receptors likely to be phosphorylated at the MAPK consensus site, Ser294) drive a gene expression program to enforce ERBB/MAPK pathway activation necessary for tumor cell proliferation.

4.3. Mechanistic interaction between SRs and DNA substrates impact promoter selectivity

4.3.1 Receptor SUMOylation does not influence DNA-binding affinity

Data from the *in vivo* SF-1 and MITF experiments (described earlier) demonstrated that SUMOylated or deSUMOylated transcription factors have different transcriptional action that contributes to broad cellular and physiological consequences. The molecular mechanisms explaining how transcription factor SUMOylation modulates promoter selectivity are not fully understood. One hypothesis is that WT and SUMO-deficient SRs differ in DNA-binding affinities. However, this does not appear to be true. Wild-type and SUMO-deficient (mutant) PR or AR receptors had similar DNA-binding affinity for HREs (within DNA fragments) measured in electrophoretic mobility shift assays (Callewaert, Verrijdt, Haelens, & Claessens, 2004; Iniguez-Lluhi & Pearce, 2000). However, SR-interacting proteins may alter SR/DNA-binding complexes in a SUMO-dependent manner; *in vitro* gel shift assays show that PIAS3 overexpression reduces PR binding to PRE-containing DNA sequences (Man et al., 2006). However, it seems more likely that differences in SR DNA-binding sequence motifs contribute to the altered transcriptional activity of SUMO-modified and unmodified SRs. Experiments involving GR demonstrated that DNA itself serves as a sequence specific allosteric ligand, where single base pair changes in the DNA motif can alter GR structural conformation, revealing substantially different GR surfaces (Meijsing et al., 2009). These conformational changes altered cofactor recruitment and gene regulation (Meijsing et al., 2009). Thus, variation in SR DNA-binding sequence motifs may alter the structural presentation of SUMOylated SRs, likely influencing cofactor involvement and promoter selectivity.

4.3.2 HRE positioning and transcriptional synergy control

Iniguez-Lluhi and Pearce (2000) discovered that the composition of HREs within promoter DNA sequences influence the transcriptional action of SUMOylated GR. Initially, they screened a library of GR mutants to identify regulatory domains that affect GR transcriptional action (Iniguez-Lluhi & Pearce, 2000). They identified two particular GR mutants that contain substitutions in the AF-1 domain that resulted in nonadditive (synergistic) transcriptional activity in response to ligand, but only on promoters containing multiple HREs. Thus, the mutant regions conferring increased transcriptional activity were named SC motifs (Iniguez–Lluhi & Pearce, 2000), and it was subsequently shown that synergy control (SC) motifs are sites of receptor SUMOylation (i.e., a conserved SUMO-attachment consensus motif; Le Drean et al., 2002; Tian et al., 2002). The SC motifs in GR are conserved across multiple nuclear receptors, including AR, PR, and MR. These researchers showed that GR transcriptional synergy requires mutations in the SC motif (i.e., a deSUMOylated receptor) and depends on compound HREs (multiple HREs in tandem) for greatly increased GR transcriptional transactivation. Promoters with up to three tandem HREs were tested and synergy increased with HRE number. Notably, when the conserved Lys residue within the SC motif was mutated to Glu (switching from positive to negative charge), synergy was enhanced, although switching the residue charge was not necessary for transcriptional synergy. Mutating the conserved Lys to Arg (both positive) also disrupted the transcriptional repression mediated by SC motifs. These data suggested that a posttranslational modification occurred at this residue and that mutation to any other residue would relieve transcriptional repression (Iniguez–Lluhi & Pearce, 2000). Similar observations were realized for AR-dependent transcriptional transactivation (Callewaert et al., 2004). However, in GR transcriptional reporter assays using different promoters (i.e., the ARE4-tk promoter contains four HREs and the MMTV promoter contains one HRE), the SUMO-deficient GR mutants were not more transcriptionally active, compared to wild type (Tian et al., 2002). Thus, the authors concluded that GR SUMOylation affects its transcriptional activity in a promoter selective manner (Tian et al., 2002) that also depends on the number of nearby (tandem) HREs (Iniguez–Lluhi & Pearce, 2000).

Similar to GR and AR, PR also displays transcriptional synergy when its key SUMO-conjugation site is mutated (K388R). However, this transcriptional synergy is restricted in assays involving the PRE2-luc promoter that contains two palindromic PREs (Abdel-Hafiz & Horwitz, 2012). However, SUMO-deficient PR does not drive transcriptional synergy in MMTV-luc reporter assays; the MMTV promoter contains a single palindromic PRE and three PRE half-sites (Abdel-Hafiz & Horwitz, 2012). In intact cells, PR promoter selectivity on endogenous genes does indeed depend on PR SUMOylation status and may also depend on the number of nearby functional PREs (Daniel et al., 2007). Only SUMO-deficient PR greatly upregulated *HBEGF* expression (which contains 22 PRE half-sites) relative to WT PR, whereas modest upregulation of *MUC1* expression (which contains few PRE half-sites) remained similar between WT and SUMO-deficient (K388R) PRs (Daniel et al., 2007).

Using recent ChIP-chip data investigating genome-wide binding site of GR (So, Chaivorapol, Bolton, Li, & Yamamoto, 2007), Holmstrom, Chupreta, So, and Iñiguez-Lluhí (2008) characterized multiple GR-binding sites for transcriptional synergy. They investigated eight GR-binding sites that contained multiple GREs and found that three sites had some level of transcriptional synergy when GR SUMO-attachment sites were mutated. For one of those three genes, *FKBP5*, endogenous mRNA expression was higher in cells expressing SC mutants, compared to WT (Holmstrom et al., 2008). With the availability of many SR cistromes and transcriptomes (Tang et al., 2011), it will be interesting to investigate how the number of HREs within SR-binding regions affects nearby gene expression levels on a global scale.

4.3.3 SUMO localized to the promoter region causes transcriptional repression

The idea that the presence of SUMO moieties at transcriptional promoters is transcriptionally repressive has been extensively explored (Holmstrom et al., 2003). To demonstrate the *in trans* effects of SUMO presence on GR transcriptional activity, researchers used synthetic promoters containing two Gal and either one or three GRE sequences and forced the presence of SUMO proteins to nearby Gal4 DNA-binding sequences (through noncleavable SUMO-Gal4 fusion protein expression). In these studies, the presence of Gal4-SUMO near single or multiple GREs inhibited both WT and SUMO-deficient GR transcription (Holmstrom et al., 2003). To demonstrate that SUMO is sufficient to inhibit *in cis* transcriptional synergy, WT or SUMO-deficient GRs were fused to SUMO1 or SUMO2. SUMO attachment did not affect the activity of WT or SUMO-deficient GR mutants in reporter assays containing single GREs. However, in assays containing multiple GREs, SUMO attachment significantly reduced both WT and SUMO-deficient GR mutant transactivation. In fact, SUMO2 appears to inhibit GR transactivation more than SUMO1 (Holmstrom et al., 2003). Thus, the authors concluded that the inhibitory effect of receptor SC motifs (i.e., receptor SUMOylation) is a direct consequence of the presence of SUMO moieties located near the promoter, regardless of their attachment to SRs.

In reporter assays measuring the transcriptional transactivation of various GR deletion mutants, it appears that the inhibitory effects of SUMOylated

GR only require stable binding of its N-terminus (containing the SC motifs) for GR-dependent transcriptional repression (Holmstrom et al., 2008). Further, a functional DBD and LBD provide additional stability and thus contribute to the overall stability of GR at the promoter, allowing the inhibitory effects of GR SUMOylation to be observed Holmstrom et al. (2008). These data suggest that transcriptional synergy at multiple GREs is transcriptionally repressed primarily by the stable assembly of SUMOylated GR (and other corepressors) on promoter DNA.

4.3.4 The need for high-throughput transcriptional and chromatin-binding assays

The major findings related to the influence of SUMO on SR transcriptional action have been found using luciferase reporter assays, containing various promoter sequences: some from endogenous genes (e.g., rat tyrosine aminotransferase, TAT), others from viruses (e.g., MMTV), and others from highly manipulated promoter sequences. The field needs to further transition this work toward measuring endogenous gene activities within chromatin using less manipulated cells, where the effects of SR SUMOylation can be more fully understood. In fact, it has been shown that most SR-binding sites are not in the proximal promoters of regulated genes (Carroll et al., 2006; Tang et al., 2011); thus, the relevance of reporter assay data containing only proximal promoters is somewhat questionable. However, mechanistic findings related to multiple HREs in promoters may also be relatable in the context of endogenous DNA looping, thus combining multiple distant HREs to a single transcriptional enhancer hub (Grontved & Hager, 2012). New work is emerging to define functional SR enhancer regions via DNaseI hypersensitivity mapping, FAIRE (formaldehyde-assisted isolation of regulatory elements), paired nucleosome positioning, histone acetylation, methylation markers, etc. Combined data from these chromatin studies, along with global SR ChIP-seq mapping, and gene expression studies will provide greater insight into SR interaction with DNA/chromatin and the regulation of their target genes. Thus far, few global studies have directly investigated endogenous transcriptional differences between SUMOylated and SUMO-deficient SR action (Knutson et al., 2012).

4.4. The impact of SR coregulators on promoter selectivity

4.4.1 SR coactivators

Multiple transcriptional coregulators have been implicated in modulating the actions of SUMOylated SRs. The p160 family of SR coactivators

(SRC1, SRC2, SRC3) are proteins that directly interact with SRs via LXXLL motifs (nuclear receptor boxes) and facilitate SR-dependent transcriptional activation (for review, Xu et al., 2009). *STC1* (an endogenous ligand-independent PR-target gene) mRNA levels were specifically upregulated in cells expressing SUMO-deficient PR and reduced upon SRC1 knockdown (Daniel & Lange, 2009). In addition, both SUMO-deficient PR mutants and SRC1, but not WT PR, were preferentially recruited to *STC1* enhancer regions (Daniel & Lange, 2009). These experiments demonstrate that SR coactivators (e.g., SRC1) cooperate to regulate selected SR target genes through SUMO-dependent mechanisms.

In fact, SRC1 itself is SUMOylated at five potential Lys residues that enhance the PR/SRC1 interaction through LXXLL motifs in the PR N-terminus and the SRC1 C-terminus (Chauchereau, Amazit, Quesne, Guiochon-Mantel, & Milgrom, 2003). This was discovered because overexpression of SUMO1 augmented PR transactivation, even in cells expressing SUMO-deficient PR mutants. Instead, overexpression of SUMO1 was found to drive SRC1 SUMOylation, thus stabilizing the interaction between PR and SRC1. Expression of completely SUMO-deficient SRC1 reduced PR/SRC1 binding. Therefore, SUMOylation of a prominent PR transcriptional coactivator, SRC1, facilitates the PR/SRC1 interaction, resulting in greatly enhanced PR transactivation, regardless of PR SUMOylation status (Chauchereau et al., 2003). Similar assays testing multiple SR target genes are needed to determine the extent of SRC1 contribution to SR promoter selectivity.

4.4.2 Histone deacetylases

Like SRC1, other coregulatory proteins involved in SR-mediated transactivation are also SUMOylated, including HDAC1. Generally, chromatin regions with high levels of histone acetylation are associated with transcriptional activation and these regions are reset through the actions of HDACs, resulting in transcriptional repression. HDACs also deacetylate nonhistone proteins to modulate their function. SUMOylation of HDAC1 promotes its deacetylase activity, whereas SENP1 overexpression inhibits this activity, thus relieving the repressive effects of HDAC1 on AR-dependent transcription (Cheng et al., 2004). Indeed, expression of catalytically inactive SENP1 was unable to deSUMOylate HDAC1 and unable to block its deacetylase activity, indicating that the repressive effects of HDAC1 on AR transcription are mediated through HDAC1 SUMOylation (Cheng et al., 2004). This was further validated when siRNA knockdown of HDAC1 relived repression of AR-mediated transactivation. Hence, in addition to being described as general SR corepressors, HDACs can influence SUMO-dependent SR transcriptional transactivation.

For example, Daniel and Lange (2009) demonstrated that *STC1* and *HBEGF* gene expression was primarily driven by SUMO-deficient mutant PR, and only WT (SUMOylated) PR recruited HDAC3 to their enhancer regions via ChIP assay. In agreement with the ChIP studies, treating cells with an HDAC inhibitor (trichostatin A) reduced *STC1* gene expression (Daniel & Lange, 2009). Additionally, siRNA knockdown of HDAC3 allowed PR-dependent *STC1* gene expression, thus implicating HDAC3 as a PR transcriptional corepressor that is dependent on the SUMOylation status of PR for repression of selected PR-target genes (Daniel & Lange, 2009). The transcriptional impact of HDAC expression on the trans-activation potential of AR was also tested. AR is acetylated in the KLKK region near the DBD by acetyltransferases p300, PCAF (Fu et al., 2000), and Tip60 (Gaughan, Logan, Cook, Neal, & Robson, 2002), resulting in increased AR transcriptional activity. Overexpression of HDAC1, HDAC4, and HDAC7 were shown to deacetylate AR and all three reduced AR tran-scriptional activity (via ARE-luciferase reporter expression assays), but HDAC4 was most repressive (Gaughan et al., 2002; Yang et al., 2011). Indeed, HDAC4 knockdown via siRNA reduced HDAC4 protein levels and increased AR-mediated transcriptional activation, indicating that endogenous HDAC4 mediates AR transcriptional repression. Surprisingly, the HDAC4-mediated AR repression did not occur through AR deacetylation because the transcriptional activity of acetylation-mutant AR (K632A/K633A; Thomas et al., 2004) was equally repressed by HDAC4 expression (Yang et al., 2011). However, these authors noted that HDAC4-mediated repression of AR was relieved in cells expressing the SUMOylation-deficient AR mutant. Protein levels for WT and SUMO-deficient AR remained equal; therefore, the repressive effect of HDAC4 expression was mediated through changes in AR SUMOylation (Yang et al., 2011). Both *in vivo* and *in vitro* assays confirmed that HDAC4 expres-sion facilitates the SUMOylation of WT AR. Increasing amounts of HDAC4 transfection into AR-negative PC-3 prostate cancer cells resulted in a dose-dependent increase in AR SUMOylation and dose-dependent decrease in reporter assay transcriptional activity (Yang et al., 2011). Finally, knockdown of endogenous HDAC4 in LNCaP prostate cells resulted in decreased endogenous AR SUMOylation, and elevated the expression of endogenous androgen-dependent AR target genes, Probasin and prostate specific antigen (PSA; Yang et al., 2011). The finding that HDAC4 drives SR transcriptional repression not through deacetylation but through enhanced receptor SUMOylation is novel. However, AR is also transcriptionally repressed through receptor deacetylation via HDAC1 and others (Fu et al., 2000; Gaughan et al., 2002), and SUMO-deficient AR is modestly repressed by HDAC4. These data suggest that HDAC4 may also function as a SUMO E3 ligase for AR (Yang et al., 2011).

4.4.3 Other coactivators

These findings are interesting because mechanisms describing how SUMO-conjugation proteins alter SR transactivation are not completely understood. Early publications identified interactions between UBC9 and multiple SRs (Gottlicher et al., 1996; Kaul et al., 2002; Kobayashi et al., 2004; Poukka et al., 1999; Sentis et al., 2005; Tirard, Almeida, Hutzler, Melchior, & Michaelidis, 2007) driving SR SUMOylation. Yet, new data suggest that the interactions between SUMO-conjugation proteins (e.g., UBC9, PIAS) may also function to SUMOylate SR coactivators within the complex, thereby indirectly altering SR-dependent transcriptional activity. GRIP1 (also called SRC2) is involved with SR-mediated transactivation. ARIP3 (AR-interacting protein 3, also called PIASxalpha) and its C-terminal splice variant Miz1 are members of the PIAS protein family and directly interact with GRIP1 (Kotaja, Vihinen, Palvimo, & Janne, 2002). ARIP3 and GRIP1 interact synergistically to upregulate AR- and GR-dependent transcriptional transactivation. PIAS proteins require zinc finger domains for their efficient protein SUMOylation abilities and their interaction between ARIP3 and GRIP1 is dependent on zinc finder motifs in ARIP3. Miz1 also directly interacts with GRIP1 and all three PIAS proteins (ARIP3, Miz1, PIAS1, but not PIAS3) depend on GRIP1 interaction for synergistic upregulation of both AR- and GR-dependent transcriptional transactivation (Kotaja, Vihinen et al., 2002). Mutation of the ARIP3 LXXLL motifs did not inhibit ARIP3 interaction with GRIP1 or significantly block AR- or GR-dependent transactivation; however, this finding may be promoter selective (Kotaja, Vihinen et al., 2002). Thus, SR SUMO-conjugation molecules likely interact within the transcriptional complex, impacting both SR and coregulator SUMOylation (e.g., SRC1, HDAC1, and GRIP1).

Converging data indicate that SR-dependent transcriptional complexes include multiple proteins involved in mediating efficient gene activation or repression. For example, at enhancer loci of genes (e.g., *MSX2*) regulated specifically by SUMO-deficient PR (compared to WT), higher levels of the general transcriptional coactivator CREB-binding protein were preferentially recruited (Knutson et al., 2012). Chromatin regions associated with transcriptionally active genes displayed higher levels of histone H3 Lys4 di/trimethylation; these marks serve to recruit transcriptional coactivator complexes and/or chromatin remodeling enzymes (for reviews, Baker, Allis, & Wang, 2008; Ruthenburg, Allis, & Wysocka, 2007; Taverna, Li, Ruthenburg, Allis, & Patel, 2007). In cells expressing deSUMOylated PR, higher levels of histone H3 Lys4 dimethylation were observed at the *MSX2* enhancer region (Knutson et al., 2012). Indeed, increased recruitment of the SR coactivator and histone methyltransferase, MLL2, was also observed at genes regulated by SUMO-deficient PR (Knutson et al., 2012). These studies indicated that PR SUMO-dependent promoter selectivity involves the differential recruitment of coactivator molecules that impact the chromatin structure, thereby facilitating the dynamic formation of complexes involved in transcriptional activation.

4.4.4 Other corepressors
Mutation of SR SUMO-conjugation motifs often results in transcriptional activation, indicating that SUMOylation is transcriptionally repressive and the SUMO moiety may be directly responsible for interaction with transcriptional corepressors. Daxx was identified as a SUMO1-interacting protein (Ryu, Chae, & Kim, 2000) and subsequently was identified as a coregulator primarily associated with transcriptional repression for multiple proteins, including SRs (Kim, Park, & Um, 2003; Li, Pei, Watson, & Papas, 2000; Lin et al., 2004; Lin, Lai, Ann, & Shih, 2003). Using coimmunoprecipitation, yeast-two-hybrid, and GST-pulldown assays, Lin et al. (2004) showed that AR and Daxx physically interact independent of ligand. Reporter assays demonstrated that overexpression of Daxx resulted in dose-dependent decrease in AR-dependent transactivation. In addition, LNCaP cells stably overexpressing Daxx reduced AR-induced (ligand-dependent) endogenous PSA mRNA levels, whereas Daxx knockdown in LNCaP cells caused elevated AR-mediated transcriptional transactivation (Lin et al., 2004). Daxx expression did not alter AR nuclear/cytoplasmic localization (Lin et al., 2004). Instead, it appeared that Daxx inhibited AR-mediated transcription through direct interaction with the AR N-terminal and DBD, causing interference of AR binding to its target DNA elements (Lin et al., 2004). SUMO-deficient AR mutants have reduced binding with Daxx, and SUMO-deficient AR mutants also lacking

the DBD almost completely lose AR/Daxx interaction. Daxx possesses an SIM that promotes noncovalent binding with SUMOylated proteins, and the Daxx SIM is necessary for its subnuclear localization and transcriptional repression (Lin et al., 2006).

It appears that Daxx-mediated transcriptional repression is relieved by its sequestration from SUMOylated factors (e.g., AR) in chromatin to subnuclear foci containing concentrated levels of SUMO-modified PML proteins, called promyelocytic leukemia (PML) oncogenic domains (PODs; Li, Leo, et al., 2000). The Daxx SIM is required for its interaction with AR or GR, and mutation of the Daxx SIM allowed for enhanced AR or GR-dependent reporter transactivation (Lin et al., 2006).

In Daxx$^{+/+}$ embryonic mouse cells, SUMO-deficient GR reporter activity was higher than wild-type (SUMOylated) GR at promoters containing two or four GREs, in agreement with the SC data (Holmstrom et al., 2003; Iniguez-Lluhi & Pearce, 2000). However, in Daxx$^{-/-}$ embryonic mouse cells, wild-type GR transactivation was derepressed and approached the activity of SUMO-deficient GR, suggesting that Daxx likely mediates SUMO-dependent GR transcriptional repression. However, other data refute this idea, showing that the inhibitory effects of Daxx are independent of GR SUMOylation (Holmstrom et al., 2008). Further studies will be needed to delineate the mechanisms of Daxx-mediated SR repression, preferably at an expanded number of endogenous gene loci.

5. CONCLUSIONS

There appears to be a complex balance between SR transcriptional activation and repression that is dependent in part on SR posttranslational modifications, including SUMOylation (Fig. 9.2). SR SUMOylation is a rapid and dynamic modification that is tightly regulated by the expression and activity of a limited number of conjugation and deconjugation enzymes and heavily influenced phosphorylation events. SRs control many cellular and physiological processes, and their deregulation can contribute to various disease states, including cancer. Thus, a better understanding of the precise signaling inputs and corresponding regulatory mechanisms of these master transcriptional factors is paramount.

SUMOylation of substrate proteins has been shown to alter protein interaction partners, compete for substrate ubiquitination, alter substrate localization, and influence transcription factor activity. Here, we have reviewed how SUMOylation mediates SR transcriptional action in a promoter/gene selective manner, through differential recruitment of coregulatory molecules within the context of specific DNA-binding sequences. Thus far, only a few studies have directly measured the impact of SR SUMOylation at endogenous target genes, yet the evidence suggests that these modifications are critical mediators of SR promoter selectivity. Endogenous gene activation is highly susceptible to a multitude to transcriptional regulatory factors, and SR

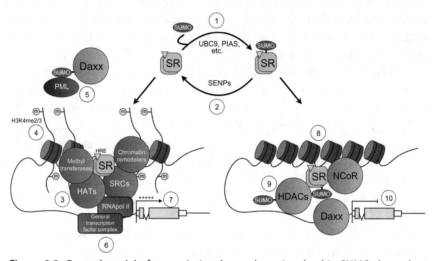

Figure 9.2 General model of transcriptional complexes involved in SUMO-dependent SR promoter selectivity. Dynamic transcriptional complexes are involved in SUMO-dependent SR promoter selectivity at unique genes. Herein, we stress that SUMO-dependent SR transcriptional complexes have diverse interaction partners, unique DNA sequence contexts, and cellular localization that may contribute to their promoter selectivity. In this example, a subset of ligand-bound receptors are rapidly SUMOylated via UBC9 and PIAS enzymes (1), and this modification can be cleaved by a family of SENP isopeptidases (2). In many cases, deSUMOylated receptors bind hormone response elements (HRE) and recruit or interact with coactivators, including histone methyltransferases, histone deacetylases (HATs), steroid receptor coactivators (SRCs), and chromatin remodeling enzyme complexes (3). These enhancer regions are characterized by nucleosome spreading (i.e., DNaseI hypersensitive sites) and histone H3 di/trimethylation (H3K4me2/3) (4). The transcriptionally repressive effects mediated by SUMOylated Daxx are blocked via Daxx sequestration by PML proteins (5). The combination of these factors allows for the recruitment of the general transcription factor machinery (6) and transcriptional initiation and elongation (7). Alternatively, many SUMOylated SRs can mediate promoter selective transcriptional repression through chromatin condensation (8) and recruitment of multiple transcriptional corepressors, including histone deacetylases (HDACs), Nuclear Receptor Corepressor (NCoR), and/ or Daxx (9). These molecules can be recruited by SUMOylated receptors at enhancers and promoters to mediate transcriptional repression (10). (See Color Insert.)

SUMOylation appears to fine-tune SR action in relation to unique chromatin environments. The past decade has made great strides to understand SR SUMOylation and its role on receptor actions, where future studies will need to delineate the impact of SR SUMOylation on disease initiation and progression, especially with regard to cancer, where novel therapeutics may target SUMOylating or deSUMOylating enzymes.

REFERENCES

Abdel-Hafiz, H. A., Dudevoir, M. L., & Horwitz, K. B. (2009). Mechanisms underlying the control of progesterone receptor transcriptional activity by sumoylation. *Journal of Biological Chemistry*, *284*, 9099–9108.

Abdel-Hafiz, H. A., & Horwitz, K. B. (2012). Control of progesterone receptor transcriptional synergy by SUMOylation and deSUMOylation. *BMC Molecular Biology*, *13*, 10.

Abdel-Hafiz, H., Takimoto, G. S., Tung, L., & Horwitz, K. B. (2002). The inhibitory function in human progesterone receptor N termini binds SUMO-1 protein to regulate autoinhibition and transrepression. *Journal of Biological Chemistry*, *277*, 33950–33956.

Baker, L. A., Allis, C. D., & Wang, G. G. (2008). PHD fingers in human diseases: Disorders arising from misinterpreting epigenetic marks. *Mutation Research*, *647*, 3–12.

Bawa-Khalfe, T., Cheng, J., Lin, S. H., Ittmann, M. M., & Yeh, E. T. (2010). SENP1 induces prostatic intraepithelial neoplasia through multiple mechanisms. *Journal of Biological Chemistry*, *285*, 25859–25866.

Bawa-Khalfe, T., Cheng, J., Wang, Z., & Yeh, E. T. (2007). Induction of the SUMO-specific protease 1 transcription by the androgen receptor in prostate cancer cells. *Journal of Biological Chemistry*, *282*, 37341–37349.

Bertolotto, C., Lesueur, F., Giuliano, S., Strub, T., de Lichy, M., Bille, K., et al. (2011). A SUMOylation-defective MITF germline mutation predisposes to melanoma and renal carcinoma. *Nature*, *480*, 94–98.

Bjornstrom, L., & Sjoberg, M. (2005). Mechanisms of estrogen receptor signaling: Convergence of genomic and nongenomic actions on target genes. *Molecular Endocrinology*, *19*, 833–842.

Bossis, G., Malnou, C. E., Farras, R., Andermarcher, E., Hipskind, R., Rodriguez, M., et al. (2005). Down-regulation of c-Fos/c-Jun AP-1 dimer activity by sumoylation. *Molecular and Cellular Biology*, *25*, 6964–6979.

Callewaert, L., Verrijdt, G., Haelens, A., & Claessens, F. (2004). Differential effect of small ubiquitin-like modifier (SUMO)-ylation of the androgen receptor in the control of cooperativity on selective versus canonical response elements. *Molecular Endocrinology*, *18*, 1438–1449.

Carroll, J., Meyer, C., Song, J., Li, W., Geistlinger, T., Eeckhoute, J., et al. (2006). Genome-wide analysis of estrogen receptor binding sites. *Nature Genetics*, *38*, 1289–1297.

Chauchereau, A., Amazit, L., Quesne, M., Guiochon-Mantel, A., & Milgrom, E. (2003). Sumoylation of the progesterone receptor and of the steroid receptor coactivator SRC-1. *Journal of Biological Chemistry*, *278*, 12335–12343.

Cheli, Y., Ohanna, M., Ballotti, R., & Bertolotto, C. (2010). Fifteen-year quest for microphthalmia-associated transcription factor target genes. *Pigment Cell & Melanoma Research*, *23*, 27–40.

Cheng, J., Bawa, T., Lee, P., Gong, L., & Yeh, E. T. (2006). Role of desumoylation in the development of prostate cancer. *Neoplasia*, *8*, 667–676.

Cheng, J., Wang, D., Wang, Z., & Yeh, E. T. (2004). SENP1 enhances androgen receptor-dependent transcription through desumoylation of histone deacetylase 1. *Molecular and Cellular Biology*, *24*, 6021–6028.

Chupreta, S., Holmstrom, S., Subramanian, L., & Iniguez-Lluhi, J. A. (2005). A small conserved surface in SUMO is the critical structural determinant of its transcriptional inhibitory properties. *Molecular and Cellular Biology*, *25*, 4272–4282.

Daniel, A. R., Faivre, E. J., & Lange, C. A. (2007). Phosphorylation-dependent antagonism of sumoylation derepresses progesterone receptor action in breast cancer cells. *Molecular Endocrinology*, *21*, 2890–2906.

Daniel, A. R., & Lange, C. A. (2009). Protein kinases mediate ligand-independent derepression of sumoylated progesterone receptors in breast cancer cells. *Proceedings of the National Academy of Sciences of the United States of America*, *106*, 14287–14292.

Danielian, P. S., White, R., Lees, J. A., & Parker, M. G. (1992). Identification of a conserved region required for hormone dependent transcriptional activation by steroid hormone receptors. *The EMBO Journal*, *11*, 1025–1033.

Dünnebier, T., Bermejo, J., Haas, S., Fischer, H., Pierl, C., Justenhoven, C., et al. (2010). Polymorphisms in the UBC9 and PIAS3 genes of the SUMO-conjugating system and breast cancer risk. *Breast Cancer Research and Treatment*, *121*, 185–194.

Edwards, D. P. (2005). Regulation of signal transduction pathways by estrogen and progesterone. *Annual Review of Physiology*, *67*, 335–376.

Fu, M., Wang, C., Reutens, A. T., Wang, J., Angeletti, R. H., Siconolfi-Baez, L., et al. (2000). p300 and p300/cAMP-response element-binding protein-associated factor acetylate the androgen receptor at sites governing hormone-dependent transactivation. *Journal of Biological Chemistry*, *275*, 20853–20860.

Fuqua, S. A., Wiltschke, C., Zhang, Q. X., Borg, A., Castles, C. G., Friedrichs, W. E., et al. (2000). A hypersensitive estrogen receptor-alpha mutation in premalignant breast lesions. *Cancer Research*, *60*, 4026–4029.

Gareau, J. R., & Lima, C. D. (2010). The SUMO pathway: Emerging mechanisms that shape specificity, conjugation and recognition. *Nature Reviews. Molecular Cell Biology*, *11*, 861–871.

Gaughan, L., Logan, I. R., Cook, S., Neal, D. E., & Robson, C. N. (2002). Tip60 and histone deacetylase 1 regulate androgen receptor activity through changes to the acetylation status of the receptor. *Journal of Biological Chemistry*, *277*, 25904–25913.

Gilbreth, R. N., Truong, K., Madu, I., Koide, A., Wojcik, J. B., Li, N. S., et al. (2011). Isoform-specific monobody inhibitors of small ubiquitin-related modifiers engineered using structure-guided library design. *Proceedings of the National Academy of Sciences of the United States of America*, *108*, 7751–7756.

Gill, G. (2003). Post-translational modification by the small ubiquitin-related modifier SUMO has big effects on transcription factor activity. *Current Opinion in Genetics & Development*, *13*, 108–113.

Giordano, C., Cui, Y., Barone, I., Ando, S., Mancini, M. A., Berno, V., et al. (2010). Growth factor-induced resistance to tamoxifen is associated with a mutation of estrogen receptor alpha and its phosphorylation at serine 305. *Breast Cancer Research and Treatment*, *119*, 71–85.

Gong, L., Millas, S., Maul, G. G., & Yeh, E. T. (2000). Differential regulation of sentrinized proteins by a novel sentrin-specific protease. *Journal of Biological Chemistry*, *275*, 3355–3359.

Gottlicher, M., Heck, S., Doucas, V., Wade, E., Kullmann, M., Cato, A. C., et al. (1996). Interaction of the Ubc9 human homologue with c-Jun and with the glucocorticoid receptor. *Steroids*, *61*, 257–262.

Grontved, L., & Hager, G. L. (2012). Impact of chromatin structure on PR signaling: Transition from local to global analysis. *Molecular and Cellular Endocrinology*, *357*, 30–36.

Gross, M., Yang, R., Top, I., Gasper, C., & Shuai, K. (2004). PIASy-mediated repression of the androgen receptor is independent of sumoylation. *Oncogene*, *23*, 3059–3066.

Guo, D., Li, M., Zhang, Y., Yang, P., Eckenrode, S., Hopkins, D., et al. (2004). A functional variant of SUMO4, a new I kappa B alpha modifier, is associated with type 1 diabetes. *Nature Genetics*, *36*, 837–841.

Han, B. Y., Li, F. C., Cheng, L., Xu, X. J., Jiang, K., Fu, J., et al. (2011). SUMO-2/3 can covalently bind to progesterone receptor B to regulate its transcriptional activity]. *Nan fang yi ke da xue xue bao = Journal of Southern Medical University*, *31*, 1493–1497.

Hay, R. T. (2005). SUMO: A history of modification. *Molecular Cell*, *18*, 1–12.

Heery, D. M., Kalkhoven, E., Hoare, S., & Parker, M. G. (1997). A signature motif in transcriptional co-activators mediates binding to nuclear receptors. *Nature*, *387*, 733–736.

Herynk, M. H., Hopp, T., Cui, Y., Niu, A., Corona-Rodriguez, A., & Fuqua, S. A. (2010). A hypersensitive estrogen receptor alpha mutation that alters dynamic protein interactions. *Breast Cancer Research and Treatment*, *122*, 381–393.

Herynk, M. H., Parra, I., Cui, Y., Beyer, A., Wu, M. F., Hilsenbeck, S. G., et al. (2007). Association between the estrogen receptor alpha A908G mutation and outcomes in invasive breast cancer. *Clinical Cancer Research: An Official Journal of the American Association for Cancer Research*, *13*, 3235–3243.

Hietakangas, V., Anckar, J., Blomster, H. A., Fujimoto, M., Palvimo, J. J., Nakai, A., et al. (2006). PDSM, a motif for phosphorylation-dependent SUMO modification. *Proceedings of the National Academy of Sciences of the United States of America*, *103*, 45–50.

Hollenberg, S. M., Weinberger, C., Ong, E. S., Cerelli, G., Oro, A., Lebo, R., et al. (1985). Primary structure and expression of a functional human glucocorticoid receptor cDNA. *Nature*, *318*, 635–641.

Holmstrom, S., Chupreta, S., So, A., & Iñiguez-Lluhí, J. (2008). SUMO-mediated inhibition of glucocorticoid receptor synergistic activity depends on stable assembly at the promoter but not on Daxx. *Molecular Endocrinology*, *22*, 2061–2075.

Holmstrom, S., Van Antwerp, M. E., & Iniguez-Lluhi, J. A. (2003). Direct and distinguishable inhibitory roles for SUMO isoforms in the control of transcriptional synergy. *Proceedings of the National Academy of Sciences of the United States of America*, *100*, 15758–15763.

Huang, W. C., Ko, T. P., Li, S. S., & Wang, A. H. (2004). Crystal structures of the human SUMO-2 protein at 1.6 A and 1.2 A resolution: Implication on the functional differences of SUMO proteins. *European Journal of Biochemistry/FEBS*, *271*, 4114–4122.

Iniguez-Lluhi, J. A., & Pearce, D. (2000). A common motif within the negative regulatory regions of multiple factors inhibits their transcriptional synergy. *Molecular and Cellular Biology*, *20*, 6040–6050.

Johnson, E. S. (2004). Protein modification by SUMO. *Annual Review of Biochemistry*, *73*, 355–382.

Kamei, Y., Xu, L., Heinzel, T., Torchia, J., Kurokawa, R., Gloss, B., et al. (1996). A CBP integrator complex mediates transcriptional activation and AP-1 inhibition by nuclear receptors. *Cell*, *85*, 403–414.

Kato, S., Endoh, H., Masuhiro, Y., Kitamoto, T., Uchiyama, S., Sasaki, H., et al. (1995). Activation of the estrogen receptor through phosphorylation by mitogen-activated protein kinase. *Science*, *270*, 1491–1494.

Kaul, S., Blackford, J. A., Jr., Cho, S., & Simons, S. S., Jr. (2002). Ubc9 is a novel modulator of the induction properties of glucocorticoid receptors. *Journal of Biological Chemistry*, *277*, 12541–12549.

Kim, E. J., Park, J. S., & Um, S. J. (2003). Identification of Daxx interacting with p73, one of the p53 family, and its regulation of p53 activity by competitive interaction with PML. *Nucleic Acids Research*, *31*, 5356–5367.

Knutson, T. P., Daniel, A. R., Fan, D., Silverstein, K. A., Covington, K. R., Fuqua, S. A., et al. (2012). Phosphorylated and sumoylation-deficient progesterone receptors drive proliferative gene signatures during breast cancer progression. *Breast Cancer Research*, *14*, R95.

Kobayashi, S., Shibata, H., Yokota, K., Suda, N., Murai, A., Kurihara, I., et al. (2004). FHL2, UBC9, and PIAS1 are novel estrogen receptor alpha-interacting proteins. *Endocrine Research*, *30*, 617–621.

Kotaja, N., Karvonen, U., Janne, O. A., & Palvimo, J. J. (2002). PIAS proteins modulate transcription factors by functioning as SUMO-1 ligases. *Molecular and Cellular Biology*, *22*, 5222–5234.

Kotaja, N., Vihinen, M., Palvimo, J. J., & Janne, O. A. (2002). Androgen receptor-interacting protein 3 and other PIAS proteins cooperate with glucocorticoid receptor-interacting protein 1 in steroid receptor-dependent signaling. *Journal of Biological Chemistry*, *277*, 17781–17788.

Lange, C. A. (2008). Integration of progesterone receptor action with rapid signaling events in breast cancer models. *The Journal of Steroid Biochemistry and Molecular Biology*, *108*, 203–212.

Lange, C. A., Shen, T., & Horwitz, K. B. (2000). Phosphorylation of human progesterone receptors at serine-294 by mitogen-activated protein kinase signals their degradation by the 26S proteasome. *Proceedings of the National Academy of Sciences of the United States of America*, *97*, 1032–1037.

Le Drean, Y., Mincheneau, N., Le Goff, P., & Michel, D. (2002). Potentiation of glucocorticoid receptor transcriptional activity by sumoylation. *Endocrinology*, *143*, 3482–3489.

Le Romancer, M., Treilleux, I., Leconte, N., Robin-Lespinasse, Y., Sentis, S., Bouchekioua-Bouzaghou, K., et al. (2008). Regulation of estrogen rapid signaling through arginine methylation by PRMT1. *Molecular Cell*, *31*, 212–221.

Lee, F. Y., Faivre, E. J., Suzawa, M., Lontok, E., Ebert, D., Cai, F., et al. (2011). Eliminating SF-1 (NR5A1) sumoylation in vivo results in ectopic hedgehog signaling and disruption of endocrine development. *Developmental Cell*, *21*, 315–327.

Li, X., Lee, Y. K., Jeng, J. C., Yen, Y., Schultz, D. C., Shih, H. M., et al. (2007). Role for KAP1 serine 824 phosphorylation and sumoylation/desumoylation switch in regulating KAP1-mediated transcriptional repression. *Journal of Biological Chemistry*, *282*, 36177–36189.

Li, H., Leo, C., Zhu, J., Wu, X., O'Neil, J., Park, E. J., et al. (2000). Sequestration and inhibition of Daxx-mediated transcriptional repression by PML. *Molecular and Cellular Biology*, *20*, 1784–1796.

Li, R., Pei, H., Watson, D. K., & Papas, T. S. (2000). EAP1/Daxx interacts with ETS1 and represses transcriptional activation of ETS1 target genes. *Oncogene*, *19*, 745–753.

Lieberman, B. A., Bona, B. J., Edwards, D. P., & Nordeen, S. K. (1993). The constitution of a progesterone response element. *Molecular Endocrinology*, *7*, 515–527.

Lin, D. Y., Fang, H. I., Ma, A. H., Huang, Y. S., Pu, Y. S., Jenster, G., et al. (2004). Negative modulation of androgen receptor transcriptional activity by Daxx. *Molecular and Cellular Biology*, *24*, 10529–10541.

Lin, D. Y., Huang, Y. S., Jeng, J. C., Kuo, H. Y., Chang, C. C., Chao, T. T., et al. (2006). Role of SUMO-interacting motif in Daxx SUMO modification, subnuclear localization, and repression of sumoylated transcription factors. *Molecular Cell*, *24*, 341–354.

Lin, D. Y., Lai, M. Z., Ann, D. K., & Shih, H. M. (2003). Promyelocytic leukemia protein (PML) functions as a glucocorticoid receptor co-activator by sequestering Daxx to the PML oncogenic domains (PODs) to enhance its transactivation potential. *Journal of Biological Chemistry*, *278*, 15958–15965.

Locke, J. A., Guns, E. S., Lubik, A. A., Adomat, H. H., Hendy, S. C., Wood, C. A., et al. (2008). Androgen levels increase by intratumoral de novo steroidogenesis during progression of castration-resistant prostate cancer. *Cancer Research*, *68*, 6407–6415.

Lonard, D. M., Nawaz, Z., Smith, C. L., & O'Malley, B. W. (2000). The 26S proteasome is required for estrogen receptor-alpha and coactivator turnover and for efficient estrogen receptor-alpha transactivation. *Molecular Cell, 5*, 939–948.

Losel, R., & Wehling, M. (2003). Nongenomic actions of steroid hormones. *Nature Reviews. Molecular Cell Biology, 4*, 46–56.

Lupien, M., Eeckhoute, J., Meyer, C. A., Wang, Q., Zhang, Y., Li, W., et al. (2008). FoxA1 translates epigenetic signatures into enhancer-driven lineage-specific transcription. *Cell, 132*, 958–970.

Mahajan, R., Delphin, C., Guan, T., Gerace, L., & Melchior, F. (1997). A small ubiquitin-related polypeptide involved in targeting RanGAP1 to nuclear pore complex protein RanBP2. *Cell, 88*, 97–107.

Man, J.-H., Li, H.-Y., Zhang, P.-J., Zhou, T., He, K., Pan, X., et al. (2006). PIAS3 induction of PRB sumoylation represses PRB transactivation by destabilizing its retention in the nucleus. *Nucleic Acids Research, 34*, 5552–5566.

Meijsing, S. H., Pufall, M. A., So, A. Y., Bates, D. L., Chen, L., & Yamamoto, K. R. (2009). DNA binding site sequence directs glucocorticoid receptor structure and activity. *Science, 324*, 407–410.

Misrahi, M., Atger, M., d'Auriol, L., Loosfelt, H., Meriel, C., Fridlansky, F., et al. (1987). Complete amino acid sequence of the human progesterone receptor deduced from cloned cDNA. *Biochemical and Biophysical Research Communications, 143*, 740–748.

Mohideen, F., Capili, A. D., Bilimoria, P. M., Yamada, T., Bonni, A., & Lima, C. D. (2009). A molecular basis for phosphorylation-dependent SUMO conjugation by the E2 UBC9. *Nature Structural & Molecular Biology, 16*, 945–952.

Mukherjee, S., Thomas, M., Dadgar, N., Lieberman, A. P., & Iniguez-Lluhi, J. A. (2009). Small ubiquitin-like modifier (SUMO) modification of the androgen receptor attenuates polyglutamine-mediated aggregation. *Journal of Biological Chemistry, 284*, 21296–21306.

Nishida, T., Kaneko, F., Kitagawa, M., & Yasuda, H. (2001). Characterization of a novel mammalian SUMO-1/Smt3-specific isopeptidase, a homologue of rat axam, which is an axin-binding protein promoting beta-catenin degradation. *Journal of Biological Chemistry, 276*, 39060–39066.

Nishida, T., & Yasuda, H. (2002). PIAS1 and PIASxalpha function as SUMO-E3 ligases toward androgen receptor and repress androgen receptor-dependent transcription. *Journal of Biological Chemistry, 277*, 41311–41317.

O'Malley, B. W., & Kumar, R. (2009). Nuclear receptor coregulators in cancer biology. *Cancer Research, 69*, 8217–8222.

Onate, S. A., Tsai, S. Y., Tsai, M. J., & O'Malley, B. W. (1995). Sequence and characterization of a coactivator for the steroid hormone receptor superfamily. *Science, 270*, 1354–1357.

Owerbach, D., McKay, E. M., Yeh, E. T., Gabbay, K. H., & Bohren, K. M. (2005). A proline-90 residue unique to SUMO-4 prevents maturation and sumoylation. *Biochemical and Biophysical Research Communications, 337*, 517–520.

Picard, N., Caron, V., Bilodeau, S., Sanchez, M., Mascle, X., Aubry, M., et al. (2012). Identification of estrogen receptor beta as a SUMO-1 target reveals a novel phosphorylated sumoylation motif and regulation by glycogen synthase kinase 3beta. *Molecular and Cellular Biology, 32*, 2709–2721.

Poukka, H., Aarnisalo, P., Karvonen, U., Palvimo, J. J., & Janne, O. A. (1999). Ubc9 interacts with the androgen receptor and activates receptor-dependent transcription. *Journal of Biological Chemistry, 274*, 19441–19446.

Poukka, H., Karvonen, U., Janne, O. A., & Palvimo, J. J. (2000). Covalent modification of the androgen receptor by small ubiquitin-like modifier 1 (SUMO-1). *Proceedings of the National Academy of Sciences of the United States of America, 97*, 14145–14150.

Robinson-Rechavi, M., Carpentier, A. S., Duffraisse, M., & Laudet, V. (2001). How many nuclear hormone receptors are there in the human genome? *Trends in genetics: TIG, 17,* 554–556.

Ruthenburg, A. J., Allis, C. D., & Wysocka, J. (2007). Methylation of lysine 4 on histone H3: Intricacy of writing and reading a single epigenetic mark. *Molecular Cell, 25,* 15–30.

Ryu, S. W., Chae, S. K., & Kim, E. (2000). Interaction of Daxx, a Fas binding protein, with sentrin and Ubc9. *Biochemical and Biophysical Research Communications, 279,* 6–10.

Saitoh, H., & Hinchey, J. (2000). Functional heterogeneity of small ubiquitin-related protein modifiers SUMO-1 versus SUMO-2/3. *Journal of Biological Chemistry, 275,* 6252–6258.

Sentis, S., Le Romancer, M., Bianchin, C., Rostan, M.-C., & Corbo, L. (2005). Sumoylation of the estrogen receptor alpha hinge region regulates its transcriptional activity. *Molecular Endocrinology, 19,* 2671–2684.

Shalizi, A., Gaudilliere, B., Yuan, Z., Stegmuller, J., Shirogane, T., Ge, Q., et al. (2006). A calcium-regulated MEF2 sumoylation switch controls postsynaptic differentiation. *Science, 311,* 1012–1017.

Shao, R., Zhang, F.-P., Rung, E., Palvimo, J. J., Huhtaniemi, I., & Billig, H. (2004). Inhibition of small ubiquitin-related modifier-1 expression by luteinizing hormone receptor stimulation is linked to induction of progesterone receptor during ovulation in mouse granulosa cells. *Endocrinology, 145,* 384–392.

Shiau, A. K., Barstad, D., Loria, P. M., Cheng, L., Kushner, P. J., Agard, D. A., et al. (1998). The structural basis of estrogen receptor/coactivator recognition and the antagonism of this interaction by tamoxifen. *Cell, 95,* 927–937.

So, A. Y., Chaivorapol, C., Bolton, E. C., Li, H., & Yamamoto, K. R. (2007). Determinants of cell- and gene-specific transcriptional regulation by the glucocorticoid receptor. *PLoS Genetics, 3,* e94.

Song, J., Durrin, L. K., Wilkinson, T. A., Krontiris, T. G., & Chen, Y. (2004). Identification of a SUMO-binding motif that recognizes SUMO-modified proteins. *Proceedings of the National Academy of Sciences of the United States of America, 101,* 14373–14378.

Strauss, J. F., 3rd., Schuler, L. A., Rosenblum, M. F., & Tanaka, T. (1981). Cholesterol metabolism by ovarian tissue. *Advances in Lipid Research, 18,* 99–157.

Su, B., Wong, C., Hong, Y., & Chen, S. (2011). Growth factor signaling enhances aromatase activity of breast cancer cells via post-transcriptional mechanisms. *The Journal of Steroid Biochemistry and Molecular Biology, 123,* 101–108.

Suzuki, T., Miki, Y., Nakamura, Y., Moriya, T., Ito, K., Ohuchi, N., et al. (2005). Sex steroid-producing enzymes in human breast cancer. *Endocrine-Related Cancer, 12,* 701–720.

Takimoto, G. S., Tung, L., Abdel-Hafiz, H., Abel, M. G., Sartorius, C. A., Richer, J. K., et al. (2003). Functional properties of the N-terminal region of progesterone receptors and their mechanistic relationship to structure. *The Journal of Steroid Biochemistry and Molecular Biology, 85,* 209–219.

Tang, Q., Chen, Y., Meyer, C., Geistlinger, T., Lupien, M., Wang, Q., et al. (2011). A comprehensive view of nuclear receptor cancer cistromes. *Cancer Research, 71,* 6940–6947.

Tatham, M. H., Jaffray, E., Vaughan, O. A., Desterro, J. M., Botting, C. H., Naismith, J. H., et al. (2001). Polymeric chains of SUMO-2 and SUMO-3 are conjugated to protein substrates by SAE1/SAE2 and Ubc9. *Journal of Biological Chemistry, 276,* 35368–35374.

Taverna, S. D., Li, H., Ruthenburg, A. J., Allis, C. D., & Patel, D. J. (2007). How chromatin-binding modules interpret histone modifications: Lessons from professional pocket pickers. *Nature Structural & Molecular Biology, 14,* 1025–1040.

Tetel, M. J., Giangrande, P. H., Leonhardt, S. A., McDonnell, D. P., & Edwards, D. P. (1999). Hormone-dependent interaction between the amino- and carboxyl-terminal domains of progesterone receptor in vitro and in vivo. *Molecular Endocrinology, 13,* 910–924.

Thomas, M., Dadgar, N., Aphale, A., Harrell, J. M., Kunkel, R., Pratt, W. B., et al. (2004). Androgen receptor acetylation site mutations cause trafficking defects, misfolding, and aggregation similar to expanded glutamine tracts. *Journal of Biological Chemistry, 279,* 8389–8395.

Tian, S., Poukka, H., Palvimo, J. J., & Janne, O. A. (2002). Small ubiquitin-related modifier-1 (SUMO-1) modification of the glucocorticoid receptor. *Biochemical Journal, 367,* 907–911.

Tirard, M., Almeida, O. F., Hutzler, P., Melchior, F., & Michaelidis, T. M. (2007). Sumoylation and proteasomal activity determine the transactivation properties of the mineralocorticoid receptor. *Molecular and Cellular Endocrinology, 268,* 20–29.

Verzi, M. P., Shin, H., He, H. H., Sulahian, R., Meyer, C. A., Montgomery, R. K., et al. (2010). Differentiation-specific histone modifications reveal dynamic chromatin interactions and partners for the intestinal transcription factor CDX2. *Developmental Cell, 19,* 713–726.

Wang, C., Fu, M., Angeletti, R. H., Siconolfi-Baez, L., Reutens, A. T., Albanese, C., et al. (2001). Direct acetylation of the estrogen receptor alpha hinge region by p300 regulates transactivation and hormone sensitivity. *Journal of Biological Chemistry, 276,* 18375–18383.

Wang, Q., Xia, N., Li, T., Xu, Y., Zou, Y., Zuo, Y., et al. (2013). SUMO-specific protease 1 promotes prostate cancer progression and metastasis. *Oncogene, 32*(19), 2493–2498. http://dx.doi.org/10.1038/onc.2012.250.

Wu, H., Sun, L., Zhang, Y., Chen, Y., Shi, B., Li, R., et al. (2006). Coordinated regulation of AIB1 transcriptional activity by sumoylation and phosphorylation. *Journal of Biological Chemistry, 281,* 21848–21856.

Xu, J., Wu, R.-C., & O'malley, B. W. (2009). Normal and cancer-related functions of the p160 steroid receptor co-activator (SRC) family. *Nature Reviews. Cancer, 9,* 615–630.

Yang, S. H., Galanis, A., Witty, J., & Sharrocks, A. D. (2006). An extended consensus motif enhances the specificity of substrate modification by SUMO. *The EMBO Journal, 25,* 5083–5093.

Yang, S. H., Jaffray, E., Senthinathan, B., Hay, R. T., & Sharrocks, A. D. (2003). SUMO and transcriptional repression: Dynamic interactions between the MAP kinase and SUMO pathways. *Cell Cycle, 2,* 528–530.

Yang, Y., Tse, A. K., Li, P., Ma, Q., Xiang, S., Nicosia, S. V., et al. (2011). Inhibition of androgen receptor activity by histone deacetylase 4 through receptor SUMOylation. *Oncogene, 30,* 2207–2218.

Zhang, P. J., Zhao, J., Li, H. Y., Man, J. H., He, K., Zhou, T., et al. (2007). CUE domain containing 2 regulates degradation of progesterone receptor by ubiquitin-proteasome. *The EMBO Journal, 26,* 1831–1842.

CHAPTER TEN

Beta-Endorphin Neuron Regulates Stress Response and Innate Immunity to Prevent Breast Cancer Growth and Progression

Dipak K. Sarkar[1], Changqing Zhang

Endocrinology Program and Department of Animal Sciences, Rutgers, The State University of New Jersey, New Brunswick, New Jersey, USA

[1]Corresponding author: e-mail address: sarkar@aesop.rutgers.edu

Contents

Abstract

Body and mind interact extensively with each other to control health. Emerging evidence suggests that chronic neurobehavioral stress can promote various tumor growth and progression. The biological reaction to stress involves a chemical cascade initiated within the central nervous system and extends to the periphery, encompassing the immune, endocrine, and autonomic systems. Activation of sympathetic nervous system, such as what happens in the "fight or flight" response, downregulates tumor-suppressive genes, inhibits immune function, and promotes tumor growth. On the other hand, an optimistic attitude or psychological intervention helps cancer patients to survive longer via increase in β-endorphin neuronal suppression of stress hormone levels and sympathetic outflows and activation of parasympathetic control of tumor suppressor gene and innate immune cells to destroy and clear tumor cells.

Vitamins and Hormones, Volume 93
ISSN 0083-6729
http://dx.doi.org/10.1016/B978-0-12-416673-8.00011-3

1. INTRODUCTION

Breast cancer is the most frequent malignant disease among women. The National Cancer Institute estimated that there would be 39,920 deaths due to breast cancer and 229,960 new cases of invasive breast cancer among American women in the year 2012 (Siegel, Naishadham, & Jemal, 2012). Stress has been shown to be a tumor-promoting factor (Marchetti, Spinola, Pelletier, & Labrie, 1991; Montgomery & McCrone, 2010; Reiche, Nunes, & Morimoto, 2004; Thaker & Sood, 2008; Thaker et al., 2006). Emerging evidence suggests that chronic neurobehavioral stress can promote various tumor growth and progression secondary to sustained activation of sympathetic nervous system (SNS) and inhibition of parasympathetic nervous system (Abo & Kawamura, 2002; Smyth, Cretney, Kershaw, & Hayakawa, 2004; Webster Marketon & Glaser, 2002). Stress can significantly affect many aspects of the body's immune systems. For example, higher levels of stress were shown to be associated with decrease in natural killer (NK) cell lysis activity, macrophage migration activity, decrease in T-cell population, decreased lymphocyte proliferation following infection, and decrease in interferon-γ (IFN-γ) levels (Webster, Tonelli, & Sternberg, 2002). These factors are reported to be important components of immunity against cancer (Herberman, 1984; Smyth et al., 2004). Therefore, controlling the body's stress response may be beneficial to increase immunity and fight against cancer. Hence, the purpose of this review is to briefly describe the process of how stress may affect immunity and cancer growth and how reducing body stress via β-endorphin (BEP) cell transplantation may prevent cancer growth and progression.

2. NEUROENDOCRINE RESPONSE TO STRESS

Stress is a state of threatened or perceived as threatened homeostasis. In response to a stressful condition, body initiate a cascade of physiological changes in the central nervous system (CNS) and periphery, which subsequently trigger the autonomic nervous system (ANS) and the hypothalamic–pituitary–adrenal axis (HPA) (Antoni et al., 2006; Tsigos & Chrousos, 2002). Stressful experiences activate components of the limbic system including the hippocampus and the amygdala that modulate the activity of hypothalamic and brainstem structures that control HPA axis and ANS activities. The hypothalamus secretes corticotrophin-releasing factor

(CRF) and vasopressin (VP) from the paraventricular nucleus (PVN) of the hypothalamus, both of which activate the pituitary to release hormones of the proopiomelanocortin (POMC) peptides such as adrenocorticotrophic hormone (ACTH) that stimulates the secretion of glucocorticoids from the adrenal cortex to the peripheral circulation. Stress response also involves the secretion of adrenaline (epinephrine) from the chromaffin cells of the adrenal medulla.

In addition to the activation of the HPA axis, stressful stimuli also activate the SNS, what is often termed the "fight or flight" response. Similar to other parts of the nervous system, the SNS operates through a series of inter-connected neurons, many of which have direct connections with the neurons of the PVN, run through the brainstem and the preganglionic neurons, and terminate in the ganglia near the spinal column. From these ganglia, post-ganglionic fibers run to the effector organs including spleen and many other lymphoid tissues (Murugan et al., 2013). The main neurotransmitter of the preganglionic sympathetic fibers is acetylcholine, a chemical messenger that binds and activates nicotinic acetylcholine receptors on postganglionic neu-rons. The principal neurotransmitter released by the postganglionic neurons is noradrenaline (norepinephrine, NE). The other division of the ANS is the parasympathetic nervous system, which is responsible for stimulation of "rest-and–digest" activities that occur when the body is at rest and is normally func-tioning in opposition to the sympathetic neurons. The main neurotransmitter of the parasympathetic fibers is acetylcholine. Acetylcholine acts on two types of receptors, the nicotinic cholinergic (at postganglionic neurons) and musca-rinic (at the target organ).

3. CHRONIC STRESS AND ITS EFFECT ON IMMUNE FUNCTIONS

Human body and mind responses to stress are tightly regulated. If reac-tion to stress is inadequate or excessive and/or prolonged, it may affect many physiological functions such as the inflammatory/immune response (Charmandari, Tsigos, & Chrousos, 2005). Chronic stress can significantly affect the body's immune system. For example, higher levels of stress were associated with increased prevalence of tuberculosis and vulnerability to common cold virus (Webster Marketon & Glaser, 2002).

Hormones produced in reaction to chronic stress have detrimental effect on immune functions, including reduced NK cell activity, lymphocyte pop-ulation, lymphocyte proliferation, antibody production, and reactivation of latent viral infections (Webster Marketon & Glaser, 2002). It is known that glucocorticoids can modulate the transcription of many cytokines. They suppress the proinflammatory cytokines such as IL-12, TNF-α, IFN-γ, and GM-CSF while upregulating the anti-inflammatory cytokines IL-4 and IL-10 (Webster et al., 2002). They also suppress maturation, differentiation, and proliferation of immune cells, including innate immune cells, T cells, and B cells. NE released by SNS activation also disturbs inflammatory cytokine network by inhibiting the production of immune-enhancing cytokines such as IL-12 and TNF-α, and by upregulating the production of inhibitory cytokines such as IL-10 and TGF-β (Webster et al., 2002). NK cells are a subset of lymphocytes, providing first-line defense against viral infection, tumor growth, and metastasis by their unique cytolytic action (Herberman & Ortaldo, 1981). Cytolytic activity of NK cells involves the synergistic action of pore-forming protein perforin and the serine protease granzyme B to cause apoptosis of target cells (Graubert, Russell, & Ley, 1996). Among the HPA hormones, glucocorticoid and CRH have been shown to be potent inhibitors of NK cell activity *in vitro* and *in vivo*. β-Adrenergic receptors were found on NK cells (Madden, Sanders, & Felten, 1995). Hypothalamic CRH inhibits NK activity and IFN-γ production through the activation of SNS, which causes release of catecholamines in spleen and activation of β-adrenergic receptor on NK cells (Irwin, Hauger, Jones, Provencio, & Britton, 1990). Thus, it appears that hormones secreted during stress from HPA axis and SNS have inhibitory effects on immune functions against infection and cancer. Therefore, ways to reduce the detrimental effect caused by hyperactive stress axis may form a novel method in recovering immunity in a variety of cases.

4. NEUROENDOCRINE-IMMUNE PATHWAY OF CANCER

Recently, the results of various studies on animals and humans all point that the body's psychophysiological reactions during stress are associated with a greater likelihood of incidence or relapse of cancer (Moreno-Smith, Lutgendorf, & Sood, 2010). At the cellular and molecular level, psychological stress associated increase in production of epinephrine, NE, and cortisol causing upregulation of DNA damage sensors Chk1 and Chk2 and the proto-oncogene CDC25A, which is involved in cell cycle delay following DNA damage, resulting in increased cell transformation and/or tumorigenicity (Flint, Baum, Chambers, & Jenkins, 2007). Transgenic, knockout, and *in vitro* models point that dysregulated stress response downregulates tumor suppressor genes such as phosphatase and tensin homolog (PTEN) or DNA repair genes such as BRCA1 (Hermes et al., 2009). Animal studies have shown that the activation of the SNS (that happens during various stresses) increases lung tumor metastases in liver carcinogen-given animals, whereas pretreatment of animals with β-adrenergic antagonists (to block the activity of SNS activation) and indomethacin (to block inflammation) synergistically blocked the effects of behavioral stress on lung tumor metastasis. Consistent with these are the recent data showing that β-adrenergic antagonists promote ovarian cancer cell spreading and adhesion to laminin-5 and promote adhesion to a fibronectin matrix (Bos, 2006). Thus, catecholamines may promote cancer cell–matrix attachments. NE and epinephrine can also promote migration and invasive potential of ovarian cancer cells, by increasing MMP-2 and MMP-9 by tumor cells and matrix metalloproteinases that are important for tumor cell penetration (Yang et al., 2006). In addition, it has been found that stress hormones may promote angiogenic mechanisms in human tumors by increasing the production of vascular endothelial growth factor. Interleukin 6, another key cytokine that plays a key role in tumor progression and angiogenesis, is also elevated by NE in various cancer animal models (Nilsson et al., 2007). Thus, chronic stress not only activates the HPA axis but also activates production of catecholamines, and several cytokines, which may promote cancer growth and progression at biochemical and molecular levels (Henry, 1992).

Studies from human and animal models also have shown that acute and chronic stressful events have adverse effects on a variety of immunological mechanisms, such as trafficking of neutrophils, macrophages, antigen-presenting cells, NK cells, and T- and B-lymphocytes (Capuron & Miller, 2011). Exposure to stress modulates cell-mediated immunity by suppressing lymphocyte proliferation and NK activation, lowering the number of CD4+ cells in the peripheral blood and altering CD4/CD8 T-cell ratios (Witek-Janusek, Gabram, & Mathews, 2007). Studies have also shown that depression and stress might have effects on carcinogenesis indirectly, through the poorer destruction or elimination of abnormal cells by reduced NK cell activity. Decreased NK cells activity is also associated with growth and progression of a variety of cancers in animals and humans, because NK cells appear to represent a first-line defense against the metastatic spread of tumor cells (Padgett & Glaser, 2003). Stress is associated with altered inflammatory and anti-inflammatory cytokine ratio in systemic circulation. It increases the expression of interleukin-1 beta and tumor necrosis factor-alpha (TNF-a) and reduced expression of IL-2 and interferon-gamma (IFN-g). Sustained elevation of TNF-a is known to inhibit the activity of protein tyrosine phosphatase, causing reduced production of MHC class

I antigen of the cell surface and leading to malignant cells escaping immune surveillance. Although there are many specific details yet to be delineated, it is becoming increasingly clear that stressful life events can impact cancer growth, progression, and metastasis by modulating nervous, endocrine, and immune system of body.

5. BETA-ENDORPHIN NEUROTRANSMISSION REDUCES THE BODY'S STRESS RESPONSE

BEP, an endogenous opioid polypeptide primarily produced by the hypothalamus and pituitary gland, is known to have the ability to inhibit stress hormone production and produce analgesia and a feeling of well-being (Akil, Watson, Young, & Lewis, 1984; Yermal, Witek-Janusek, Peterson, & Mathews, 2010). BEP is a cleavage product of POMC, which is also the precursor hormone for ACTH and a–melanocyte-stimulating hormone. BEP neuronal cell bodies are primarily localized in the arcuate nuclei of the hypothalamus, and its terminals are distributed throughout the CNS, including the PVN of the hypothalamus (Kawano & Masuko, 2000). In the PVN, these neurons innervate corticotropin-releasing hormone (CRH) neurons and inhibit CRH release (Plotsky, Thrivikraman, & Meaney, 1993), while a μ–opioid receptor antagonist increases it (Boyadjieva, Advis, & Sarkar, 2006). During stress, secretion of CRH and catecholamine stimulate the secretion of hypothalamic BEP and other POMC–derived peptides, which in turn inhibit the activity of the stress system (Plotsky et al., 1993). BEP is known to bind to δ– and μ–opioid receptors and modulate the neurotransmission in sympathetic and parasympathetic neurons via neuronal circuitry within the PVN to activate NK cell cytolytic functions in the spleen (Boyadjieva, Ortigüela, Arjona, Cheng, & Sarkar, 2009; Boyadjieva et al., 2006; Sarkar et al., 2011). Abnormalities in BEP neuronal function are correlated with a higher incidence of cancers and infections in patients with schizophrenia, depression, and fetal alcohol syndrome, and in obese patients (Bernstein et al., 2002; Giovannucci & Michaud, 2000; Grinshpoon et al., 2005; Lissoni et al., 1983; Pankov et al., 2002; Polanco et al., 2010; Zangen et al., 2002).

6. BETA-ENDORPHIN NEUROTRANSMISSION ENHANCES INNATE IMMUNITY

The BEP perikarya are located mainly in the ventromedial arcuate nucleus region that projects to widespread brain structures, including many areas of the hypothalamus and limbic system, where these peptides have been proposed to function as neurotransmitters or neuromodulators regulating a variety of brain functions. CNS opioid systems are implicated in many of the effects of stress and depression on immune system functions. Acute stress activates the HPA axis leading to elevated release of hypothalamic BEP and CRH, pituitary ACTH and BEP, and adrenal glucocorticoids (Rivier, 1995). Until recently, corticoids were the only hormones considered to have significant effects on the immune system. The detection of receptors for opioid peptides, CRH, and ACTH on lymphocytes (Plaut, 1987) and the demonstration that lymphocytes themselves express opioid peptides suggest a more complex connection between the HPA axis and immunity. Among the HPA hormones, glucocorticoid and CRH have been shown to be potent *in vitro* and *in vivo* inhibitors of NK cell activity (Gatti et al., 1987; Holbrook, Cox, & Horner, 1983; Masera et al., 1989; Parrillo & Fauci, 1978). In contrast, hypothalamic opioid peptides have a stimulatory action on NK cells.

How do two neuropeptides of the HPA axis, BEP and CRH, produce opposite actions on immune cells? Hypothalamic BEP is known to inhibit CRH release (Buckingham, 1986; Plotsky et al., 1993). It is interesting that the cytokine IL-1β, which is released during immune surveillance and stimulates CRH release (Rivier, 1995), has an inhibitory action on BEP neurons (Boyadjieva, Reddy, & Sarkar, 1997). Hence, it appears that hypothalamic BEP inhibits CRH secretion, and by doing so, it regulates sympathetic outflow to the spleen and other lymphoid glands and positively regulates NK cell cytolytic activity (Boyadjieva et al., 2006). Recent evidence also suggests the possibility that hypothalamic BEP may regulate NK cell and other immune cells by directly communicating with both sympathetic and parasympathetic outflows to lymphoid tissues (Sarkar et al., 2011; see also Fig. 10.1).

7. BETA-ENDORPHIN CELL TRANSPLANTATION EFFECTS ON THE NEUROENDOCRINE-IMMUNE PATHWAY OF CANCER

Previously, it has been shown that perfusion of BEP or an opioid receptor agonist stimulates NK cell cytolytic activity and lymphocyte proliferation, and these effects are blocked by intracranial administration of opiate antagonist (Boyadjieva et al., 2006). We have recently shown that the neural stem cell-derived BEP neurons, when transplanted in the PVN,

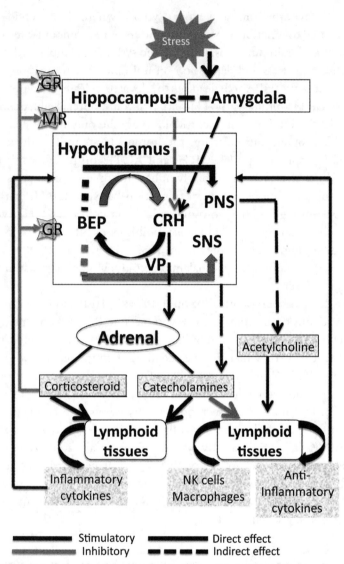

Figure 10.1 Bidirectional communication between the brain and the immune system, highlighting the influence of beta-endorphin (BEP). Stress signals reach the hypothalamus, causing secretion of corticotrophin-releasing hormone (CRH) and vasopressin (VP) from the neurons of the hypothalamus and resulting increased glucocorticoid secretion from the adrenal gland. Glucocorticoid crosses the blood–brain barrier and activates specific receptors in the hippocampus and other regions leading to regulation by negative inhibition. Stress signals also result in the activation of sympathetic nervous system (SNS) and inhibition of parasympathetic nervous system (PNS) neurons, and the neurotransmitters release from these neurons regulates cytokine production and

remained at the site of transplantation and increases NK cell cytolytic function and anti-inflammatory cytokines productions in response to immune challenges (Boyadjieva et al., 2009). Within the context of immune-related function, *in situ* BEP neurons in the hypothalamus are known to increase NK cell function. Interestingly, BEP transplant in the hypothalamus suppresses carcinogen-induced prostate cancer development in rats (Sarkar et al., 2008). Also, we recently showed that the supplementation of BEP neurons through transplants prevents mammary tumorigenesis (Sarkar et al., 2011). Importantly, when the BEP transplants were given at the early stage of tumor development, many tumors were destroyed possibly due to increased innate immune activity and the surviving tumors lost their ability to progress to high-grade cancer due to BEP cells' suppressive effects on EMT regulators. To address the question whether BEP alone and/or other peptide products from the transplanted neurons are responsible for the observed actions on the immune system and cancer, we tested the ability of a general opiate antagonist naloxone to block the effects of BEP neuron transplants on immune activation and metastasis prevention. Additionally, we tested the effects of NE agonist metaproterenol (MET) and a α7 nicotine acetylcholine receptor (α7 nAChR), antagonist methyllycaconitine (MLA). We found that naloxone, MET, and MLA all had moderate or strong inhibitory effect on basal and BEP-stimulated NK cell activity and macrophage migration activity. Consistent with these findings, we observed that naloxone, MET, and MLA prevented, at various degrees, the beneficial effect of BEP on eliminating tumor cell lung retention. These data suggest that BEP neurons activate innate immunity for cancer cell clearance via altering the function of the ANS.

Since NK cells and macrophages are critical components of the innate immune system and play a vital role in host defense against tumor cells (Mantovani and Sica, 2010; Wu & Van Kaer, 2011), the BEP cell transplants may have increased level of innate immunity which caused unfavorable conditions for cancer cell survival. In the BEP cell-treated animals, the lower inflammatory milieu that was achieved by the higher level of

---

the activity of innate immune cells including natural killer (NK) cells and macrophages. In the hypothalamus, the interaction of CRH and BEP involves negative inhibition; CRH increases the secretion of BEP, while BEP inhibits the secretion of CRH. Specific to immunity, BEP suppresses SNS control but activates the PNS control of lymphoid organs, activating innate immune cells (macrophages and NK cells) and increasing anti-inflammatory cytokine levels in circulation.

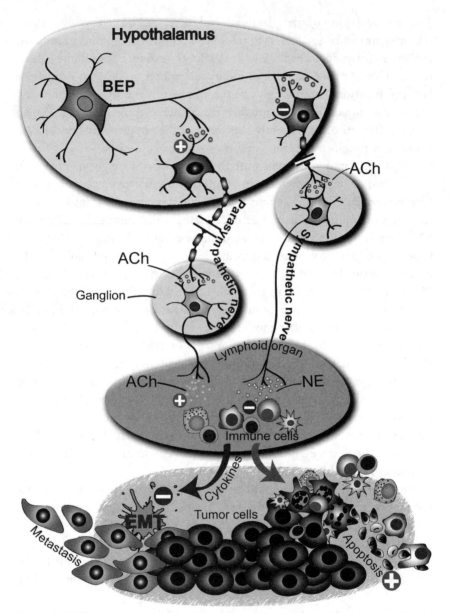

Figure 10.2 BEP neuron in the hypothalamus controls the growth and progression of tumor cells by modulating the neurotransmission in the autonomic nervous system and activating the innate immune system. Effects include the stimulation of parasympathetic nervous system and release of acetyl choline (Ach) and suppression of the sympathetic nervous system and release of norepinephrine, leading to activation of innate immune cells (including macrophages and natural killer cells) of the lymphoid organ

anti-inflammatory cytokines and the lower level of inflammatory cytokines may have also been involved in inhibiting cancer growth and transformation. Several studies have identified the involvement and roles of inflammatory cytokines in breast malignancy (Goldberg & Schwertfeger, 2010). The data obtained from these studies identified the importance of stress maintenance in regulating immune function in cancer patients and provided support for a potential therapeutic use of BEP cell transplantation for controlling breast cancer and possibly other cancers (see also Fig. 10.2).

8. CONCLUSIONS

Neurobehavioral stress has been shown to promote tumor growth and progression possibly by altering the production of hormones, catecholamine, and inflammatory cytokines. Reduction of body stress via BEP neural transplants in the brain reduces cancer growth and progression in animal models of breast cancers by altering the ANS functioning, leading to activation of innate immunity and reduction in systemic levels of inflammatory and anti-inflammatory cytokines ratios. Thus, it is apparent that stress prevention by BEP cell therapy might be beneficial in controlling breast and possibly other cancers. Current treatments of cancer focus on the physical removal of tumors and the destruction of dividing cells, such as chemotherapy and radiation therapy. These treatments are not specific, in that they also destroy normal cells that are programmed to be proliferating. This causes many side effects such as hair loss and nausea and, at the same time, weakens the body's defense against pathogens as well as tumors. These methods may also fail to kill cancer stem cells, which are in hibernation. Indeed, the body could recognize and kill cancerous cells by itself through immune surveillance. Thus, the BEP cell transplantation procedure to treat cancer could potentially be valuable because it utilizes and optimizes the body's own defense system to control abnormal cell proliferation, which is more specific, and bypasses the problem of current treatments.

and an increase in cytotoxic immune cells and anti-inflammatory cytokines levels in the circulation. In a tumor microenvironment, these immune cell and cytokine changes increase apoptotic death of tumor cells and reduce inflammation-mediated epithelial–mesenchymal transition, and thereby suppress cancer growth and metastasis. Collectively, these effects create an unfavorable environment for tumor initiation, growth, and progression. *From Zhang and Sarkar (2012)*. (See Color Insert.)

ACKNOWLEDGMENT

This work was partly supported by a National Institute of Health Grant R37AA08757.

REFERENCES

Abo, T., & Kawamura, T. (2002). Immunomodulation by the autonomic nervous system: Therapeutic approach for cancer, collagen diseases, and inflammatory bowel diseases. *Therapeutic Apheresis, 6,* 348–357.

Akil, H., Watson, S. J., Young, E., & Lewis, M. E. (1984). Endogenous opioids: Biology and function. *Annual Review of Neuroscience, 7,* 223–255.

Antoni, M. H., Lutgendorf, S. K., Cole, S. W., Dhabhar, F. S., Sephton, S. E., McDonald, P. G., et al. (2006). The influence of bio-behavioural factors on tumour biology: Pathways and mechanisms. *Nature Reviews. Cancer, 6,* 240–248.

Bernstein, H. G., Krell, D., Emrich, H. M., Baumann, B., Danos, P., Diekmann, S., et al. (2002). Fewer β-endorphin expressing arcuate nucleus neurons and reduced β-endorphinergic innervation of paraventricular neurons in schizophrenics and patients with depression. *Cellular & Molecular Biology, 48,* Online Pub:OL259-265.

Bos, J. L. (2006). Epac proteins: Multi-purpose cAMP targets. *Trends in Biochemical Sciences, 31,* 680–686.

Boyadjieva, N., Advis, J. P., & Sarkar, D. K. (2006). Role of BEP, corticotropin-releasing hormone and autonomic nervous system in mediation of the effect of chronic ethanol on natural killer cell cytolytic activity. *Alcoholism, Clinical and Experimental Research, 30,* 1761–1767.

Boyadjieva, N. I., Ortigüela, M., Arjona, A., Cheng, X., & Sarkar, D. K. (2009). β-Endorphin neuronal cell transplant reduces corticotropin releasing hormone hyperresponse to lipopolysaccharide and eliminates natural killer cell functional deficiencies in fetal alcohol exposed rats. *Alcoholism, Clinical and Experimental Research, 33,* 931–937.

Boyadjieva, N. Iv., Reddy, R. H., & Sarkar, D. K. (1997). Forskolin delays the ethanol-induced desensitization of hypothalamic beta-endorphin neurons in primary cultures. *Alcoholism, Clinical and Experimental Research, 21,* 477–482.

Buckingham, J. C. (1986). Stimulation and inhibition of corticotrophin releasing factor secretion by beta-endorphin. *Neuroendocrinology, 42,* 148–152.

Capuron, L., & Miller, A. H. (2011). Immune system to brain signaling: Neuropsychopharmacological implications. *Pharmacology & Therapeutics, 130,* 226–238.

Charmandari, E., Tsigos, C., & Chrousos, G. (2005). Endocrinology of the stress response. *Annual Review of Physiology, 67,* 259–284. ·

Flint, M. S., Baum, A., Chambers, W. H., & Jenkins, F. J. (2007). Induction of DNA damage, alteration of DNA repair and transcriptional activation by stress hormones. *Psychoneuroendocrinology, 32,* 470–479.

Gatti, G., Cavallo, R., Sartori, M. L., del Ponte, D., Masera, R., Salvadori, A., et al. (1987). Inhibition by cortisol of human natural killer (NK) cell activity. *Journal of Steroid Biochemistry, 26,* 49–58.

Giovannucci, E., & Michaud, D. (2000). The role of obesity and related metabolic disturbances in cancers of the colon, prostate, and pancreas. *Gastroenterology, 132,* 2208–2225.

Goldberg, J. E., & Schwertfeger, K. L. (2010). Proinflammatory cytokines in breast cancer: Mechanisms of action and potential targets for therapeutics. *Current Drug Targets, 11,* 1133–1146.

Graubert, T. A., Russell, J. H., & Ley, T. J. (1996). The role of granzyme B in murine models of acute graft-versus-host disease and graft rejection. *Blood, 87,* 1232–1237.

Grinshpoon, A., Barchana, M., Ponizovsky, A., Lipshitz, I., Nahon, D., Tal, O., et al. (2005). Cancer in schizophrenia: Is the risk higher or lower?. *Schizophr Research, 73,* 333–341.

Henry, J. P. (1992). Biological basis of the stress response. *Integrative Physiological and Behavioral Science, 27,* 66–83.

Herberman, R. B. (1984). Possible role of natural killer cells and other effector cells in immune surveillance against cancer. *The Journal of Investigative Dermatology, 83*, 137s–140s.

Herberman, R. B., & Ortaldo, J. R. (1981). Natural killer cells: Their roles in defenses against disease. *Science, 214*, 24–30.

Hermes, G. L., Delgado, B., Tretiakova, M., Cavigelli, S. A., Krausz, T., Conzen, S. D., et al. (2009). Social isolation dysregulates endocrine and behavioral stress while increasing malignant burden of spontaneous mammary tumors. *Proceedings of the National Academy of Sciences of the United States of America, 106*, 22393–22398.

Holbrook, N. J., Cox, W. I., & Horner, H. C. (1983). Direct suppression of natural killer activity in human peripheral blood leukocyte cultures by glucocorticoids and its modulation by interferon. *Cancer Research, 43*, 4019–4025.

Irwin, M., Hauger, R. L., Jones, L., Provencio, M., & Britton, K. T. (1990). Sympathetic nervous system mediates central corticotropin-releasing factor induced suppression of natural killer cytotoxicity. *The Journal of Pharmacology and Experimental Therapeutics, 255*, 101–107.

Lissoni, P., Barni, S., Paolorossi, F., Crispino, S., Rovelli, F., Ferri, L., et al. (1983). Evidence for altered opioid activity in patients with cancer. *British Journal of Cancer, 56*, 834–837.

Kawano, H., & Masuko, S. (2000). Beta-endorphin-, adrenocorticotrophic hormone- and neuropeptide y-containing projection fibers from the arcuate hypothalamic nucleus make synaptic contacts on to nucleus preopticus medianus neurons projecting to the paraventricular hypothalamic nucleus in the rat. *Neuroscience, 98*, 555–565.

Madden, K. S., Sanders, V. M., & Felten, D. L. (1995). Catecholamine influences and sympathetic neural modulation of immune responsiveness. *Annual Review of Pharmacology and Toxicology, 35*, 417–448.

Marchetti, B., Spinola, P. G., Pelletier, G., & Labrie, F. (1991). A potential role for catecholamines in the development and progression of carcinogen-induced mammary tumors: Hormonal control of beta-adrenergic receptors and correlation with tumor growth. *The Journal of Steroid Biochemistry and Molecular Biology, 38*, 307–320.

Masera, R., Gatti, G., Sartori, M. L., Carignola, R., Salvadori, A., Magro, E., et al. (1989). Involvement of Ca^{2+}-dependent pathways in the inhibition of human natural killer (NK) cell activity by cortisol. *Immunopharmacology, 18*, 11–22.

Mantovani, A., & Sica, A. (2010). Macrophages, innate immunity and cancer: Balance, tolerance, and diversity. *Current Opinion Immunology, 22*, 231–237.

Montgomery, M., & McCrone, S. H. (2010). Psychological distress associated with the diagnostic phase for suspected breast cancer: Systematic review. *Journal of Advanced Nursing, 66*, 2372–2390.

Moreno-Smith, M., Lutgendorf, S. K., & Sood, A. K. (2010). Impact of stress on cancer metastasis. *Future Oncology, 6*, 1863–1881.

Murugan, S., Zhang, C., Mojtehedzadeh, S. & Sarkar, D. K. (2013). Alcohol exposure *in utero* increases susceptibility to prostate tumorigenesis in rat offspring. *Alcoholism: Clinical and Experimental Research*, (in press).

Nilsson, M. B., Armaiz-Pena, G., Takahashi, R., Lin, Y. G., Trevino, J., Li, Y., et al. (2007). Stress hormones regulate interleukin-6 expression by human ovarian carcinoma cells through a Src-dependent mechanism. *The Journal of Biological Chemistry, 282*, 29919–29926.

Padgett, D. A., & Glaser, R. (2003). How stress influences the immune response. *Trends in Immunology, 24*, 444–448.

Pankov, IuA., Iatsyshina, S. B., Karpova, S. K., Chekhranova, M. K., Popova, IuP., Grigorian, O. N., et al. (2002). Screening of mutations in genes of pro-opiomelanocortin in patients with constitutional exogenous obesity. *Vopr Med Khim, 48*, 121–130.

Parrillo, J. E., & Fauci, A. S. (1978). Comparison of the effector cells in human spontaneous cellular cytotoxicity and antibody-dependent cellular cytotoxicity: Differential sensitivity of effector cells to in vivo and in vitro corticosteroids. *Scandinavian Journal of Immunology, 8*, 99–107.

Plaut, S. M. (1987). Lymphocyte hormone receptors. *Annual Review of Immunology*, *5*, 621–669.

Plotsky, P. M., Thrivikraman, K. V., & Meaney, M. J. (1993). Central and feedback regulation of hypothalamic corticotropin-releasing factor secretion. *Ciba Foundation Symposium*, *172*, 59–75.

Polanco, T. A., Crismale-Gann, C., Reuhl, K. R., Sarkar, D. K., & Cohick, W. S. (2010). Fetal alcohol exposure increases mammary tumor susceptibility and alters tumor phenotype in rats. *Alcoholism: Clinical and Experimental Research*, *34*, 1879–1887.

Reiche, E. M., Nunes, S. O., & Morimoto, H. K. (2004). Stress, depression, the immune system, and cancer. *The Lancet Oncology*, *5*, 617–625.

Rivier, C. (1995). Interaction between stress and immune signals on the hypothalamic-pituitary-adrenal axis of the rat: Influence of drugs. In D. K. Sarkar & C. D. Barnes (Eds.), *The reproductive neuroendocrinology of aging and drug abuse* (pp. 169–187). Boca Raton, Florida: CRC Press.

Sarkar, D. K., Boyadjieva, N. I., Chen, C. P., Ortigüela, M., Reuhl, K., Clement, E. M., et al. (2008). Cyclic adenosine monophosphate differentiated beta-endorphin neurons promote immune function and prevent prostate cancer growth. *Proceedings of the National Academy of Sciences of the United States of America*, *105*, 9105–9110.

Sarkar, D. K., Zhang, C., Murugan, S., Dokur, M., Boyadjieva, N. I., Ortigüela, M., et al. (2011). Transplantation of beta-endorphin neurons into the hypothalamus promotes immune function and restricts the growth and metastasis of mammary carcinoma. *Cancer Research*, *71*, 6282–6291.

Siegel, R., Naishadham, D., & Jemal, A. (2012). Cancer statistics, 2012. *CA: a Cancer Journal for Clinicians*, *62*, 10–29.

Smyth, M. J., Cretney, E., Kershaw, M. H., & Hayakawa, Y. (2004). Cytokines in cancer immunity and immunotherapy. *Immunological Reviews*, *202*, 275–293.

Thaker, P. H., Han, L. Y., Kamat, A. A., Arevalo, J. M., Takahashi, R., Lu, C., et al. (2006). Chronic stress promotes tumor growth and angiogenesis in a mouse model of ovarian carcinoma. *Nature Medicine*, *12*, 939–944.

Thaker, P. H., & Sood, A. K. (2008). Neuroendocrine influences on cancer biology. *Seminars in Cancer Biology*, *18*, 164–170.

Tsigos, C., & Chrousos, G. P. (2002). Hypothalamic-pituitary-adrenal axis, neuroendocrine factors and stress. *Journal of Psychosomatic Research*, *53*, 865–871.

Webster Marketon, J. I., & Glaser, R. (2002). Stress hormones and immune function. *Cellular Immunology*, *252*, 16–26.

Webster, J. I., Tonelli, L., & Sternberg, E. M. (2002). Neuroendocrine regulation of immunity. *Annual Review of Immunology*, *20*, 125–163.

Witek-Janusek, L., Gabram, S., & Mathews, H. L. (2007). Psychologic stress, reduced NK cell activity, and cytokine dysregulation in women experiencing diagnostic breast biopsy. *Psychoneuroendocrinology*, *32*, 22–35.

Wu, L., & Van Kaer, L. (2011). Natural killer T cells in health and disease. *Frontiers in Bioscience (Scholar Edition)*, *3*, 236–251.

Yang, E. V., Sood, A. K., Chen, M., Li, Y., Eubank, T. D., Marsh, C. B., et al. (2006). Norepinephrine up-regulates the expression of vascular endothelial growth factor, matrix metalloproteinase (MMP)-2, and MMP-9 in nasopharyngeal carcinoma tumor cells. *Cancer Research*, *66*, 10357–10364.

Yermal, S. J., Witek-Janusek, L., Peterson, J., & Mathews, H. L. (2010). Perioperative pain, psychological distress, and immune function in men undergoing prostatectomy for cancer of the prostate. *Biological Research for Nursing*, *11*, 351–362.

Zangen, A., Nakash, R., Roth-Deri, I., Overstreet, D. H., & Yadid, G. (2002). Impaired release of beta-endorphin in response to serotonin in a rat model of depression. *Neuroscience*, *110*, 389–393.

Zhang, C., & Sarkar, D. K. (2012). β-Endorphin neuron transplantation: A possible novel therapy for cancer prevention. *Oncoimmunology*, *1*(4), 552–554.

CHAPTER ELEVEN

The Functional Role of Notch Signaling in Triple-Negative Breast Cancer

Jodi J. Speiser[*], Çağatay Erşahin[*], Clodia Osipo[*,†,‡,1]

[*]Department of Pathology, Loyola University Chicago Division of Health Sciences, Maywood, Illinois, USA
[†]Oncology Institute, Loyola University Chicago Division of Health Sciences, Maywood, Illinois, USA
[‡]Department of Microbiology and Immunology, Loyola University Chicago Division of Health Sciences, Maywood, Illinois, USA
[1]Corresponding author: e-mail address: cosipo@lumc.edu

Contents

Abstract

The term "*triple-negative* breast cancer" (TNBC) is a heterogeneous subtype of breast cancer. Unfortunately, due to the lack of expression of hormone receptors and human epidermal growth factor receptor-2, therefore the lack of US Food and Drug Administration-approved targeted therapies, TNBC has the worst prognosis of all subtypes of breast cancer. Notch signaling has emerged as a pro-oncogene in several human malignancies and has particularly been associated with the triple-negative subtype of breast cancer. This chapter explores the role of Notch signaling in triple negative

Vitamins and Hormones, Volume 93
ISSN 0083-6729
http://dx.doi.org/10.1016/B978-0-12-416673-8.00013-7

277

and other subtypes of breast cancer, the relationship of Notch with other breast cancer biomarkers, prognostic indicators associated with Notch, and potential therapeutic strategies targeting Notch inhibition. Hopefully, better understanding of this signaling pathway in the future will lead to optimal molecular therapeutic treatments for TNBC patients, improving their quality of life and outcome.

1. BACKGROUND—TRIPLE-NEGATIVE BREAST CANCER AND NOTCH

1.1. Triple-negative breast cancer

Breast cancer is a heterologous disease that includes several molecular subtypes with different biochemical characteristics and clinical behaviors. These subtypes include estrogen receptor α-positive $(ER\alpha^+)$/progesterone receptor-positive (PR^+)/human epidermal growth factor receptor-2 $(HER-2^-)$ luminal A subtype, $ER\alpha^+/PR^+/HER-2^+$ luminal B subtype, $ER^-/PR^-/HER-2^+$ subtype, and basal-like subtype. Within the basal-like subtype, there is a group of cancers that are $ER^-/PR^-/HER-2^-$, or triple-negative breast cancers (TNBC), on which this chapter focuses.

The term TNBC is a heterogeneous disease, which represents 15% of breast cancers (Reis-Filho & Tutt, 2008). It encompasses several histological subgroups of breast cancer, including medullary tumors, small cell tumors metaplastic tumors and adenoid-cystic tumors, and others (Khalifeh et al., 2008). Additionally, recent research suggests that TNBCs may have a variety of molecular subtypes, including two basal-like (BL1 and BL2), an immuno-modulatory, a mesenchymal (M), a mesenchymal stem-like, and a luminal androgen receptor subtype (Lehmann et al., 2011). The biology of these subtypes is not identical to the "standard" high-grade invasive ductal TNBC; therefore, the topic of TNBC classification remains controversial. However, these subgroups do share a number of clinical, molecular, and morphological characteristics. TNBC most frequently affects young (<50 years) African-American, Hispanic (Bauer, Brown, Cress, Parise, & Caggiano, 2007), and obese (Vona-Davis et al., 2008) women. Due to the lack of expression of hormone receptors and HER-2, therefore the lack of US Food and Drug Administration-approved targeted therapies, TNBC has the worst prognosis of all subtypes of breast cancer. TNBC demonstrates with a high rate of local and systemic relapse (Weigelt, Baehner, & Reis-Filho, 2010) and shorter survival following metastases (Dent et al., 2007). Additionally, TNBC patients share several features with breast cancer susceptibility gene

(BRCA-1 and BRCA-2) outcome-associated breast cancer. Tumors arising in a BRCA-1 background most often display a basal-like genotype (Fasano & Muggia, 2009) and more than 80% of BRCA-1 mutation carriers have a triple-negative receptor expression profile (Yong et al., 2009).

1.2. Notch signaling pathway

Notch signaling has emerged as a pro-oncogene in several human malignancies (Miele, 2008; Miele, Miao, & Nickoloff, 2006) and may be a potential target for the treatment of breast cancer (Miele, 2008). In the mammalian system, there are four Notch receptors (Notch-1, Notch-2, Notch-3, and Notch-4; Blaumueller & Artiavanis-Tsakonas, 1997) and five known ligands (Delta-like 1, Delta-like 3, Delta-like 4, Jagged-1, and Jagged-2; Dunwoodie, Henrique, Harrison, & Beddington, 1997; Lindsell, Shawber, Boulter, & Weinmaster, 1995; Shawber, Boulter, Lindsell, & Weinmaster, 1996). Cell-to-cell contact is critical for the activation of Notch signaling, which subsequently enables the pathway to modulate genes involved in cell fate such as proliferation or differentiation (Callahan & Raafat, 2001). Notch is processed in the trans-Golgi apparatus, where it undergoes the first of three proteolytic cleavages. The single polypeptide is cleaved (S1) by furin-like convertase forming the mature Notch receptor, which is a heterodimer consisting of Notch extracellular (NEC) and Notch transmembrane (NTM) noncovalently bound with a Ca^{2+} cation. The receptor is trafficked to the plasma membrane, where it awaits engagement with its membrane-associated ligand. Upon ligand–receptor engagement, the second cleavage (S2) by a disintegrin and metalloproteases 10 and 17 (ADAM10 and ADAM17, respectively) (Brou et al., 2000) releases NEC to be trans-endocytosed into the ligand-expressing cell. Subsequently, NTM is cleaved (S3) by the γ-secretase complex, liberating the intracellular portion of Notch (NIC) (Saxena, Schroeter, Mumm, & Kopan, 2001). NIC translocates to the nucleus and binds to CBF-1, a constitutive transcriptional repressor, displacing corepressors and recruiting coactivators such as Mastermind (Hsieh, Zhou, Chen, Young, & Hayward, 1999; Wu et al., 2000). Notch activates many genes associated with differentiation and/or survival, including, but not limited to, the HES and HEY family of basic helix–loop–helix transcription factors (Maier & Gessler, 2000), cyclin D1 (Ronchini & Capobianco, 2001), and c-Myc (Weng et al., 2006). The third and final cleavage step is critical for active Notch signaling (Diagram 11.1).

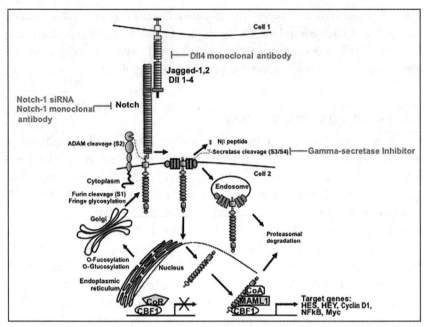

Diagram 11.1 The Notch signaling pathway (black) and potential therapeutic targets (red). (See Color Insert.)

2. NOTCH—BREAST ONCOGENES

The first evidence that Notch receptors are breast oncogenes was provided by mouse studies. Overexpression of constitutive, active forms of Notch-1 (N1IC) or Notch-4 (N4IC) forms spontaneous murine mammary tumors *in vivo* (Brou et al., 2000). Furthermore, elevated expression of Notch-1 and/or its ligand Jagged-1 in human breast tumors correlated with the poorest overall patient survival (Dickson et al., 2007; Reedijk et al., 2005, 2008) and was associated with increased expression of survivin, a tumor-associated cell death and mitotic regulator implicated in stem cell viability (Lee, Raskett, Prudovsky, & Altieri, 2008; Lee, Simin, et al., 2008; van Es et al., 2005). Mounting evidence suggests that Notch deregulation may engender critical tumor hallmarks, including oncogene expression (Sharma et al., 2006; Weng et al., 2006), angiogenesis (Keith & Simon, 2007), stem cell maintenance (van Es et al., 2005), deregulated cell cycle progression (Ronchini & Capobianco, 2001), and antiapoptotic mechanisms (Beverly, Felsher, & Capobianco, 2005). Notch-4, which is thought to be induced by Notch-1 (Weijzen et al., 2002), has been shown to be critical for the survival of tumor-initiating cells (TICs). Studies have demonstrated that Notch-4 mRNA levels (Raouf et al., 2008) and Notch-4 nuclear staining (Harrison et al., 2010) were increased in basal/stem cells compared with luminal progenitor cells. Similar to studies performed using Notch-1, mouse mammary tumor virus (MMTV)-driven Notch-3 receptor intracellular domain expression in transgenic mice showed enhanced mammary tumorigenesis (Hu et al., 2006). In HER-2$^-$ breast cancers, downregulation of Notch-3 resulted in suppressed proliferation and increased apoptosis (Yamaguchi et al., 2008). In contrast, overexpression of Notch-2 in MDA-MB-231 cells significantly decreased tumor growth and increased apoptosis *in vivo* (O'Neill et al., 2007), suggesting that Notch-2 is a breast tumor suppressor.

Additionally, there is evidence that the Notch pathway is involved in estrogen-induced angiogenesis in breast cancer cells (Soares et al., 2004; Soares, Guo, Gartner, Schmitt, & Russo, 2003). Estradiol (E2) has been shown to promote expression of Jagged-1 and Notch-1 in MCF-7 cells, which demonstrated an increased number of tumor microvessels and hypoxia-inducible factor α one gene, a well-known angiogenic factor (Soares et al., 2004). Increased expression of Jagged-1 and Notch-1 was also observed in endothelial cells, which demonstrated the formation of cord-like structures on Matrigel (Soares et al., 2004).

The factors that regulate Notch receptor expression in breast cancer cells are still widely unknown. It has been shown that p53 binds to the Notch-1 promoter and activates Notch-1 receptor transcription in human keratinocytes (Alimirah, Panchanathan, Davis, Chen, & Choubey, 2007). Activator protein 1 (AP-1) has been demonstrated to be a transcriptional activator of Notch-4 in human vascular endothelial cells (Wu et al., 2005).

3. NOTCH IN TNBC

Notch expression has particularly been associated with the triple-negative subtype of breast cancer. First, a study by Dickson et al. (2007) demonstrated that the high expression of JAG-1 and Notch-1 mRNA is associated with poor prognosis in breast cancers, including TNBC. Subsequently, Rizzo et al. (2008) demonstrated that estrogen receptor (ER)-negative breast cancer cell lines are highly sensitive to Notch inhibition *in vitro* and *in vivo*. The cells arrest in G2 and subsequently die when exposed to Notch-1 and Notch-4 small-interfering RNA (siRNA) or a γ-secretase inhibitor (GSI). Additionally, they found that estrogen causes accumulation of uncleaved Notch-1 at the cell membrane and prevents Notch activation in the nucleus. A study by Yao et al. (2011) confirmed these findings by demonstrating that ER-positive tumors express significantly more membranous staining of Notch-1 than ER-negative tumors, suggesting that tumors where the estrogen pathway is active tend to accumulate Notch-1 at the cell surface. In 2012, a study by Speiser et al. (2012) further confirmed these results by demonstrating Notch-1 and Notch-4 overexpression in TNBC with subcellular localization different from that of hormone receptor-positive breast cancer.

Determining subcellular localization of Notch in TNBC is important for understanding Notch signaling in this setting, as it may be a morphological illustration of function (Schroeter, Kisslinger, & Kopan, 1998). Notch receptors are activated at the membrane by at least two proteolytic cleavages, matured in the endoplasmic reticulum (perinuclear), and transferred to the nucleus, where they regulate transcription (Brennan & Brown, 2003). Therefore, the localization of the immunohistochemical staining for Notch may illustrate the functional activity of the Notch receptor. For example, membranous Notch staining may represent a mature receptor that is not yet active; cytoplasmic (perinuclear) staining may represent a newly synthesized receptor; and nuclear staining may represent an activated receptor. Speiser et al. (2012) demonstrated nuclear and cytoplasmic staining for Notch-1 and Notch-4 in TNBCs, which suggests an increased level of Notch transcription, with newly synthesized and activated receptors. In contrast, ER-positive tumors have shown an increased level of membranous staining, which suggests a decreased level of Notch transcription, with primarily mature, inactivated receptors. The aforementioned studies have demonstrated an overlap between ER-positive and ER-negative tumors, with both displaying cytoplasmic staining. However, the cytoplasmic staining may be occurring secondary to different mechanisms in each subtype. The cytoplasmic staining in ER-positive tumors may be due to Notch receptor maturation arrest and accumulation in the Golgi apparatus. In contrast, the cytoplasmic staining in ER-negative tumors may be due to increased receptor maturation secondary to induction of the Notch signaling pathway in the absence of estrogen. The expression rate and subcellular localization of Notch-1 and Notch-4 may represent a potentially promising therapeutic target for patients with TNBC.

4. NOTCH IN LUMINAL VERSUS BASAL-LIKE BREAST CANCER

Notch plays a significant role in both luminal breast cancers and basal-like breast cancer (BLBC). Luminal subtypes of breast cancer account for 70% of tumors and are classically characterized by the presence of ER and progesterone receptor (PR; Sotiriou et al., 2003), the expression of cytokeratin (CK) 8/18, and the absence of CK5 (Perou et al., 2000). Luminal breast cancer is further divided into two subtypes: luminal A, comprising those that are negative for the overexpression or gene amplification of ErbB-2/HER-2 and have low levels of genes responsible for proliferation, and luminal B, comprising those that are positive for HER-2 and have high expression of proliferation-associated genes (Sotiriou & Pusztai, 2009). Luminal breast cancers generally have a favorable prognosis and respond to antiestrogen or aromatase inhibitor therapy; however, development of hormone resistance associated with tumor recurrence is common (Dunnwald, Rossing, & Li, 2007).

In contrast, BLBC is characterized by an expression signature similar to that of the basal myoepithelial cells that express CK5/6, CK17, CK14, epidermal growth factor receptor (EGFR), and myoepithelial markers (Cheang et al., 2008; Diaz, Cryns, Symmans, & Sneige, 2007; Rakha et al., 2009). Currently, the triple-negative phenotype encompasses BLBC. However, although TNBC and BLBC share a number of molecular and morphological features, they are not identical. BLBC are classified as "triple-negative" phenotype if they lack ER, PR, HER2 but retain EFGR and/or CK5/6, and "5 negative" phenotype if they lack all five markers. It has been shown that BLBC defined by five biomarkers (ER$^-$, PR$^-$, HER-2$^-$, EGFR$^+$, and CK5/6) has more prognostic value than the triple-negative phenotype (Speirs et al., 1999). There is also a recently identified "claudin-low" phenotype associated with mesenchymal and stem cell markers (Prat et al., 2010). Clinically, BLBC is hormone independent, characterized by brief disease-free survival, a high proliferative index, and poor histologic grade, and requires aggressive chemotherapy (Iwao, Miyoshi, Egawa, Ikeda, & Noguchi, 2000; Iwao, Miyoshi, Egawa, Ikeda, Tsukamoto, et al., 2000; Rakha, Reis-Filho, & Ellis, 2008).

Although these two subtypes of breast cancer, luminal and basal, are currently considered completely different histological and clinical entities, new research has shown that there may be overlap between them. Molecular profiling of whole-tumor extracts demonstrated that molecular subtypes of breast cancer reflect the cellular hierarchy of the normal breast: the claudin-low signature matches a mammary stem cell profile, the basal-like signature is consistent with that of committed luminal progenitor cells, and the luminal signature resembles those of differentiated luminal epithelial cells (Haughian et al., 2012). However, these signatures are named based on the *majority* of cells within the tumor. It was demonstrated that there are heterogeneous cell types within the same tumor and that minor populations within a tumor can have tumor-initiating potential (Al-Hajj, Wicha, Benito-Hernandez, Morrison, & Clarke, 2003; Bonnet & Dick, 1997; Park, Gonen, Kim, Michor, & Polyak, 2010). Applying this theory to ER^+PR^+ luminal tumors, investigators identified an $ER^-PR^-CK5^+$ cell population, called "luminobasal" cells, that have tumor-initiating potential, express a TN basal-like and claudin-low phenotype and gene signature and demonstrate aggressive, estrogen-independent growth *in vivo* (Horwitz, Dye, Harrell, Kabos, & Sartorius, 2008). It is these "luminobasal" cells that have been shown to be increased in tumors that are resistant to chemo- and hormonal therapies (Kabos et al., 2011).

Luminal breast cancers are currently defined as positive for ER or PR if $\geq 1\%$ of tumor cell nuclei are immunoreactive (Hammond et al., 2010). However, the remaining minor cell subpopulations are largely ignored by these recommendations. In fact, Haughian et al. (2012) demonstrated that more than half of 72 ER^+PR^+ tumors contain a luminobasal subpopulation exceeding 1% of cells that expand when estrogen signaling is prevented. Therefore, the distinction between luminal and basal subtypes of breast cancer, especially status posttreatment with hormonal therapy, may not be as clear as originally thought. In fact, Haughian et al. (2012) demonstrated that despite the luminal derivation, luminobasal-rich cells after estrogen withdrawal cluster with TNBC cell lines and TNBC basal-like and claudin-low breast cancers when injected into the mammary glands of immune-compromised, ovariectomized mice with placebo or estrogen-releasing pellets.

When examining the role of Notch in luminal versus basal subtypes of cancer, Haughian et al. reported that (1) many Notch pathway genes were noted in the luminobasal gene signature, (2) Notch-1 transcripts were elevated in basal-like/claudin-low, ERα-negative tumors, and (3) strong constitutive Notch-dependent transcriptional activity was detected in the Notch-1-expressing luminobasal cells in ER^+PR^+ luminal breast cancers after estrogen withdrawal (Iwao, Miyoshi, Egawa, Ikeda, & Noguchi, 2000).

Therefore, the Notch signaling pathway plays a role in both subtypes of breast cancer and may do so through a similar mechanism—through possible selection and expansion of luminobasal cells. The relative dependence of these breast cancer subtypes on the Notch signaling pathway may be a result of the amount of estrogen present.

5. ER AND NOTCH

The steroid hormone 17β-E2 is a key regulator of growth, differentiation, and function in both reproductive and nonreproductive target tissues, including breast epithelial cells (Chang, Frasor, Komm, & Katzenellenbogen, 2006). Two subtypes of intracellular ERs, ERα and ERβ, mediate the actions of E2, via nuclear steroid hormone transcription factors with a broad range of physiological functions (Miele, 2008). Each receptor is encoded by unique genes, but has the hallmark modular structure of functional domains characteristic of the steroid/thyroid hormone super-family of nuclear receptors (Hall, Couse, & Korach, 2001).

Prolonged exposure to estrogens is associated with an increase in breast cancer risk with evidence of a dose–response relationship (Key, Appleby, Barnes, & Reeves, 2002). The tumorigenic effects of E2 are caused by increased cell proliferation through nuclear or extranuclear estrogen signaling pathways or from oxidative damage by estrogen metabolites (Bolton & Thatcher, 2008). There is a wide range of ER expression in normal and breast cancer tissues, with a large fraction expressing both ERα and ERβ (heterodimers), some expressing either ERα or ERβ (homodimers), and some that express neither ERα nor ERβ (Mann et al., 2001). A series of reports strongly indicated that estrogens, via ERα, stimulate proliferation and inhibit apoptosis (Fujita et al., 2003; Helguero, Faulds, Gustafsson, & Haldosen, 2005), whereas ERβ opposes the proliferative effect of ERα *in vitro* (Paruthiyil et al., 2004; Strom et al., 2004). However, data have indicated that ERβ functions differently when it is coexpressed with ERα than when it is expressed alone. TNBCs are defined as ERα negative, but may or may not be negative for ERβ (Skliris, Leygue, Watson, & Murphy, 2008). The relationship between Notch and estrogen in breast cancer must be examined separately for ERα$^+$ (luminal) and ERα$^-$ (TN) breast cancers.

A study by Lee, Raskett, et al. (2008) explored the role of Notch in ERα$^+$ and ERα$^-$ breast cancers. They found that the activation of Notch developmental signaling in ERα$^-$ breast cancer cells results in direct transcriptional upregulation of the apoptosis inhibitor and cell cycle regulator survivin, which is associated with increased expression of survivin at mitosis, enhanced cell proliferation, and heightened viability at cell division. In contrast, they found that untreated ERα^+ breast cancer cells, or various normal cell types, were insensitive to Notch stimulation. Therefore, they determined that ERα^- breast cancer cells become dependent on Notch-survivin signaling for their maintenance, *in vivo*.

A study by Rizzo et al. (2008) also explored this topic and found that estrogen inhibits Notch-1 (and downstream Notch-4) transcriptional activity in ERα^+ breast cancer cell lines by reducing levels of nuclear-cleaved Notch and increasing levels of cell membrane bound, uncleaved Notch-1. They also found that there is an increase in Notch activity when ERα^+ breast cancer cells become estrogen deprived or when estrogen is antagonized by selective ER modulators, which may indicate that these tumors become more dependent on Notch signaling when estrogen action is antagonized.

The potential role of ERβ in breast cancer progression is highly controversial. Herynk and Fuqua (2004) provided the following literature review of this topic.

Many studies have suggested that ERβ expression is a favorable prognostic indicator, whereas additional studies have suggested that ERβ expression is associated with known factors of poor clinical outcome. Basically, two types of prognostic studies have been performed to date: those evaluating RNA levels and those evaluating protein expression. It is interesting to note that many of the studies indicating that ERβ is a poor prognostic indicator have evaluated only the RNA levels by quantitative or semiquantitative PCR techniques. Many of these RNA-based studies have correlated ERβ expression with markers of a poor prognosis, such as EGF receptor expression and high tumor grade, and an inverse correlation between ERβ expression and PR status (Dotzlaw, Leygue, Watson, & Murphy, 1999; Iwao, Miyoshi, Egawa, Ikeda, Tsukamoto, et al., 2000; Knowlden, Gee, Robertson, Ellis, & Nicholson, 2000; Speirs et al., 1999). However, a few studies evaluating RNA have demonstrated that ERβ expression is reduced in breast cancer compared with normal epithelium and that it is inversely correlated with proliferation (evaluated by measuring Ki67 levels) (Iwao, Miyoshi, Egawa, Ikeda, & Noguchi, 2000; Roger et al., 2001), thereby suggesting that ERβ expression is a favorable prognostic indicator. However, PCR analysis of RNA levels from tumor samples will also measure ERβ mRNA in the "normal" surrounding cells, stroma, and contaminating immune cells present in homogenized tissues. Additionally, many

PCR primers may also amplify alternatively spliced RNA variants, thereby increasing the false-positive rate or perhaps skewing results toward higher expression levels. Thus, protein analyses would more precisely measure ERβ expression levels in clinical samples.

Studies evaluating ERβ protein expression appear to be much less contradictory. Direct protein analyses generally suggest that ERβ protein expression is a favorable prognostic indicator, correlating with known biomarkers such as low histological grade, ERα and PR expression, longer disease-free survival, and response to tamoxifen (Fuqua et al., 2003; Jarvinen, Pelto-Huikko, Holli, & Isola, 2000; Mann et al., 2001; Omoto et al., 2001, 2002; Skliris, Carder, Lansdown, & Speirs, 2001; Skliris et al., 2003). Although these studies do not always agree on the specific associations with known prognostic indicators, they do generally agree that similar to ERα, ERβ expression is a favorable prognostic indicator. A few protein-based studies have suggested that ERβ expression is associated with high proliferation (Ki67 expression) and high tumor grade (Jensen et al., 2001; Miyoshi, Taguchi, Gustafsson, & Noguchi, 2001). However, these studies have varying cutoff points for being classified as ERβ-positive, requiring 20–25% of the cells staining positive for ERβ. Furthermore, these later studies examined small tumor subsets. Mann et al. (2001) have demonstrated that tumors with as little as 10% of the cells expressing ERβ have a more favorable response to tamoxifen, thus suggesting that only 10% positive cells may be a reasonable cutoff point for the classification of ERβ status in tumors, as has been adopted for ERα and tamoxifen responses (Harvey, Clark, Osborne, & Allred, 1999). However, these methods give an estimate of the percentage of positive cells, but they do not account for expression levels in individual cells. The Allred score, used in several studies, measures both the percentage positive and the relative intensity, thus providing a semiquantitative method of ER protein expression (Allred, Harvey, Berardo, & Clark, 1998). It is clear that the role of ERβ in breast carcinogenesis has not been fully elucidated; however, direct protein analysis strongly suggests that ERβ is an indicator of a more favorable clinical outcome. A uniformly adopted classification of ERβ expression will be required to reconcile these issues and may help to clarify the potential role of ERβ in breast cancer progression. Furthermore, the major limitation for accurate ERβ protein expression has been reliable antibodies that can differentiate between ERα and ERβ.

It has also been suggested that it is not necessarily the individual level of ERα or ERβ that is clinically relevant, but the ratio of ERα:ERβ that may change and impact tumorigenesis. In support of this hypothesis, it has been shown that ER-positive breast cancer has a mean higher ERα:ERβ ratio when compared with the normal tissue; in contrast, estrogen independent, ER-negative cancer exhibits a low ERα:ERβ ratio (Farnie & Clarke, 2007; Leygue, Dotzlaw, Watson, & Murphy, 1998). Further complicating this hypothesis, however, is the existence of ERα and ERβ splice variants that may contribute to measurements and result in an overestimation of mRNA or protein expression. It is evident that the interplay between ERα and ERβ could be complicated; data exist that both may have roles within normal breast epithelial cells and that the upregulation or downregulation of one receptor could potentially upset a physiological balance. Thus, although a definitive role for ERβ in breast carcinogenesis has not yet been demonstrated, it can be concluded that ERα appears to play the dominant role in the breast.

There is virtually no literature addressing the interaction between ERβ and the Notch signaling pathway. Future studies will be needed to explore this area of TNBC.

6. PR AND NOTCH

Progesterone is an ovarian steroid hormone that is essential for normal breast development during puberty and in preparation for lactation and breastfeeding (Lange & Yee, 2008). In normal mammary glands, progesterone promotes epithelial cell proliferation and is essential for lobuloalveolar outgrowth (Lydon et al., 1995). This hormone mediates its effects through PRs, which belong to a large superfamily of ligand-activated nuclear receptor (Hopp et al., 2004). There are two distinct forms of the PR transcribed from a single gene by alternate initiation of transcription from two distinct promoters, giving rise to transcripts encoding two protein isoforms, PRA and PRB (Scarpin, Graham, Mote, & Clarke, 2009).

The role of progesterone in breast cancer was poorly understood until the publication of two studies demonstrating a statistically significant increase in breast cancer risk for women using combination estrogen and progesterone hormone replacement therapy versus estrogen replacement therapy alone (Colditz & Rosner, 2000; Ross, Paganini-Hill, Wan, & Pike, 2000). The tumorigenic potential of progesterone is thought to be mediated through progressive changes in PR isoform expression. A study by Mote, Bartow, Tran, and Clarke (2002) demonstrated that PRA and PRB are coexpressed in comparable amounts in normal breast and proliferative disease without atypia, while there is a predominant expression of one of the isoforms (either PRA or PRB) in atypical breast lesions. It is important to note that PRA and PRB proteins are expressed in a species-, tissue-, and cell type-specific manner; therefore, comparing results between species must be done with caution (Trimble, Xin, Guy, Muller, & Hassell, 1993). Mote et al. further established that PRs contribute to carcinogenesis in breast cancer specifically by (1) unbalanced expression of PRA and PRB results in altered hormonal response and aberrant targeting of genes that are not normally progestin-regulated, principally those involved in morphological changes and disruptions of the actin cytoskeleton, and in migration; (2) movement of PR into discrete nuclear domains, or foci, is a critical step in normal PR transcriptional activity that appears to be aberrant in cancers and likely related to alterations in nuclear morphology, gene expression, and cell function associated with tumor cells (Mote, Graham, & Clarke, 2007).

A study by Graham et al. (2009) demonstrated that progesterone increased the expression of genes in the Notch pathway in normal breast. Specifically, progesterone increased the human homologues of the Notch-Delta ligand (Delta-like 1 and 3) and the Notch receptor regulator presenilin 2. Delta- and presenilin-mediated cleavage of the receptor is required for release and nuclear translocation of the Notch intracellular signaling domain, which results in transcriptional effects on Notch target genes (Fortini, 2001). The finding that critical mediators of Notch signal transduction are positively regulated by progesterone suggests that the progesterone-mediated increase in breast progenitor cells may be mediated via Notch as a paracrine mediator. In other words, Notch may project the proliferative effects of progesterone from PR-positive cells to subsets of PR-negative cells that exhibit bipotent progenitor properties (Lydon & Edwards, 2009). Additionally, preliminary study results in mouse mammary epithelial cell lines have demonstrated that Notch expression causes a repression of PR activity (Osborne, 2000). Therefore, Notch appears to affect breast progenitor cells via paracrine activity with progesterone and perhaps via interaction with the PRs. Unfortunately, there is virtually no data addressing Notch and progesterone or PRs in breast cancer models.

7. HER-2 AND NOTCH

The HER-2 gene is amplified in approximately 25–30% of primary human breast cancers in which it is associated with aggressive disease and early development of metastasis (Slamon et al., 1989). The characteristic aggressive nature of HER-2-positive cancers may be due to a subpopulation of cells within a breast tumor that maintain or acquire stem cell character-istics (Korkaya & Wicha, 2007). A study by Korkaya, Paulson, Iovino, and Wicha (2008) demonstrated that HER-2 overexpression has effects on nor-mal and malignant mammary stem cells. In normal mammary epithelial cells, HER-2 overexpression is associated with increased proportion of stem/pro-genitor cells. In breast cancer cell populations, HER-2 overexpression is associated with increased expression of stem cell regulatory genes, increased invasion *in vitro,* and increased tumorigenesis.

As discussed earlier in this chapter, the Notch pathway also is associated with the function of normal and malignant breast cancer stem cells (Farnie & Clarke, 2007). A study by Osipo et al. (2008) demonstrated that ErbB-2-positive (HER-2) cells have low Notch transcriptional activity compared to nonoverexpressing cells and that Trastuzumab or a dual EGFR/ErbB-2 tyrosine kinase inhibitor (TKI) increased Notch activity. Additionally, they found that the increase in Notch activity was abrogated by a Notch inhib-itor, GSI, or Notch-1 siRNA. In a subsequent study, Korkaya and Wicha (2009) summarized findings that demonstrated the relationship between HER-2 overexpression and Notch, namely: (1) the HER-2 promoter con-tains Notch-binding sequences (Chen, Fischer, & Gill, 1997), (2) HER-2 overexpressing cells display activated Notch signaling (Magnifico et al., 2009), and (3) inhibition of Notch signaling using an siRNA or a GSI results in downregulation of HER2 expression resulting in decreased sphere forma-tion. It is hypothesized that this subpopulation of stem cells may be respon-sible for therapy-resistant breast cancer tumors. Therefore, understanding the relationship between HER-2 (both in the setting of overamplification and without overamplification), Notch, and stem cells will be important for guiding future treatment (Diagram 11.2).

8. PROGNOSTIC MAKERS FOR SURVIVAL ASSOCIATED WITH NOTCH IN TNBC

There are several Notch receptors, ligands, and effectors of Notch sig-naling that have demonstrated prognostic significance. These include Notch-1, Notch-4, Jagged-1, and survivin. This section provides a brief summary of each marker.

8.1. Notch-1, Notch-4, and Jagged-1

Notch-1 and Notch-4 are receptors within the Notch signaling pathway and human Jagged-1 (*JAG-1*) is the ligand for the Notch receptor. As stated

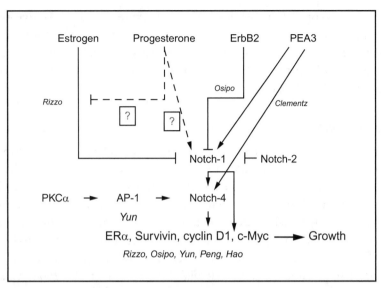

Diagram 11.2 Cross talk between Notch signaling pathway and key breast cancer-relevant pathways (⊢, inhibitory pathway; →, transcriptional activation pathway, *italic writing*—authors examining pathway). (See Color Insert.)

earlier in this chapter, elevated expression of Notch-1 and/or its ligand Jagged-1 in human breast tumors correlated with the poorest overall patient survival in several studies (Beverly et al., 2005; Ronchini & Capobianco, 2001; Weijzen et al., 2002). One study, which examined mRNA expression via *in situ* hybridization, showed that patients with high levels of Notch-1 and Jagged-1 demonstrated a 5-year survival rate of 42% compared with patients with low levels of Notch-1 and Jagged-1 with a 5-year survival rate of 65% (Beverly et al., 2005). A subsequent study, using immunohistochemical staining, demonstrated that tumors expressing high levels of Jagged-1 had a worse outcome than tumors expressing low levels (10-year survival rate of 26% versus 48%; Ronchini & Capobianco, 2001). Another study showed that moderate to high Jagged-1 mRNA expression was associated with reduced disease-free survival in univariate analysis and correlated with larger tumor size, ER and PR negativity, high tumor grade, and p53 antibody activity (Weijzen et al., 2002). Yao et al. (2011) further examined this topic and added Notch-4 to find a correlation between expression of Notch-1, Notch-4, and Jagged-1 via immunohistochemistry and poor prognostic markers in breast cancer, such as Ki67 (univariate analysis). They also found a correlation between Notch-1 expression and positive-node status (multivariate analysis), the most important prognostic factor in breast cancer. All of these studies show that Notch-1, Notch-4, and Jagged-1 may have a role in the biology of metastases and serve as poor prognostic indicators in breast cancer.

8.2. Survivin

Based on the above studies, it was determined that Notch expression is correlated with survival outcome; however, the downstream pathways that enable such aggressive behavior are still under investigation. One of the candidate effector molecules is survivin, which may function as a direct transcriptional target of Notch-1 by controlling mitotic transition and resistance to apoptosis in breast cancer. Elevated Notch-1 and Jagged-1 are associated with increased expression of survivin, which has been implicated in stem cell viability (Raouf et al., 2008; van Es et al., 2005). A subsequent study by Lee, Simin, et al. (2008) demonstrated that the expression of Notch-1 and survivin by immunohistochemistry is associated with clinically aggressive and recurrence-prone basal breast cancer.

9. THERAPEUTIC STRATEGIES IN TNBC

TNBC is considered sensitive to chemotherapy in the adjuvant setting; however, there is no evidence from randomized trials that TNBC have a different sensitivity to specific chemotherapy compared with other molecular subtypes (Berrada, Delaloge, & Andre, 2010). Additionally, ER-targeted and HER-2-based therapies are not effective against TNBC. Neoadjuvant chemotherapy has comprised the gold standard of treatment for TNBC and is associated with high efficacy. Rouzier et al. (2005) determined that TNBC was associated with a high likelihood of pathologic complete response to neoadjuvant chemotherapy and better outcome. Additionally, Conforti et al. (2007) demonstrated that adjuvant chemotherapy was associated with an adjusted hazard ratio for relapse or death of 0.54 (95% confidence interval 0.27–1.08) in patients with a basal-like phenotype. However, the population of TNBC patients who are refractory to chemotherapy demonstrates early relapse and poor outcome, with a peak of metastases occurring at 1 year and a median survival of 2.3 years after metastatic relapse (Liedtke et al., 2008). Although several potential approaches for TNBC treatment have been suggested (Tan & Swain, 2008), the pathogenesis of TNBC is still largely unknown, which inhibits the development of therapies specific for this subtype of breast cancer. Developing a better understanding of the pathology, new molecular signatures and their prospective validation are essential for designing optimal treatment for TNBC (Chen & Russo, 2009). Although there are several signaling pathways, chemokines, miRNA signatures, enzymes involved in nucleotide excision repair, and adhesion molecules currently under investigation for therapeutic targets for TNBC (Miele, 2008), this chapter focuses on therapies associated with the Notch signaling pathway.

9.1. γ-Secretase inhibitors

The γ-secretase complex catalyzes the intramembranous proteolysis of Notch derivatives to generate Notch intracellular domain (Kim, Yin, Li, & Sisodia, 2004), which is necessary for Notch activation. Since aberrant Notch signaling can induce mammary carcinomas in transgenic mice and high expression levels of Notch receptors and ligands correlate with overall poor clinical outcomes, inhibiting γ-secretase with small molecules may be a promising approach for breast cancer treatment (Han, Ma, Hendzel, & Allalunis-Turner, 2009). Lee, Simin, et al. (2008) investigated this theory and found that targeting Notch signaling with a GSI suppressed survivin levels, induced apoptosis, abolished colony formation in soft agar, and inhibited metastatic tumor growth in mice. Additionally, studies in ER-negative breast cancer cell lines have shown arrested growth after treatment with a GSI (van Es et al., 2005). In a series of preclinical and clinical studies, Chang et al. (2009) used triple-negative xenograft lines and patient samples to demonstrate that treatment with a GSI inhibited mammosphere formation and mammosphere-forming efficiency and tumor-initiating capacity, respectively. It appears that GSIs may arrest growth and reduce the number of tumorigenic cancer cells remaining after chemotherapy in TNBC patients. Unfortunately, GSIs have been associated with gastrointestinal toxicity (Nakamura, Tsuchiya, & Watanabe, 2007; Okamoto, Tsuchiya, & Watanabe, 2007), so further study in human subjects is needed to not only establish the efficacy but also examine the side-effect profile of GSIs.

Recent research suggests multiple pathways through which γ-secretase may be exerting its therapeutic effects. Kondratyev et al. (2012) hypothesized that GSIs may specifically be inhibiting TICs or cancer stem cells and demonstrated that treatment with a GSI in mice eliminated tumor-resident TIC and resulted in rapid and durable tumor regression. In contrast, Kalen et al. (2011) hypothesized that GSIs are inhibiting Notch-induced angiogenesis driven by vascular endothelial growth factor A and showed that treatment with a GSI promotes abnormal blood vessel growth characterized by vessel occlusion, disrupted blood flow, and increased vascular leakage.

GSI may also play a role in ER-negative, PR-negative, and HER-2-positive tumors. Although ErbB-2-positive cells have low Notch transcriptional activity compared with nonoverexpressing cells, Osipo et al. (2008) demonstrated that Trastuzumab or a dual EGFR/ErbB-2 TKI increased Notch activity by two- to sixfold and that the activity was abrogated by a GSI or Notch-1 siRNA.

9.2. Polyomavirus enhancer activator 3

There are also several factors that regulate Notch receptor transcription that may be important targets for therapy. One of the most investigated factors, polyomavirus enhancer activator 3 (PEA3/E1AF/ETV4) and its activators, is a member of the ETS family of transcription factors, which also includes ERM and ER-81. PEA3 is overexpressed in metastatic breast carcinomas, particularly triple-negative breast tumors (Trimble et al., 1993). PEA3 regulates critical genes involved in inflammation and invasion, such as IL-8 (Iguchi et al., 2000), cyclooxygenase-2 (COX-2; Subbaramaiah, Norton, Gerald, & Dannenberg, 2002), and matrix metalloproteases (MMPs; Benbow & Brinckerhoff, 1997; Hida et al., 1997; Kapila, Xie, & Wang, 2009; Tower, Coon, Belguise, Chalbos, & Brinckerhoff, 2003). A dominant-negative form of PEA3 reduced tumor onset and growth in a MMTV/neu-transgenic model of breast cancer in vivo (Shepherd, Kockeritz, Szrajber, Muller, & Hassell, 2001). PEA3 contains an ETS-winged helix–turn–helix DNA-binding motif (Graves & Petersen, 1998) that binds to the canonical sequence GGAA/T on target genes (Sharrocks, 2001). The affinity of binding relies on proximal sequences surrounding the ETS binding site which aids in transcriptional control based on context (Oikawa & Yamada, 2003). Phosphorylation of serine and threonine residues by the mitogen-activating protein kinase cascade activates PEA3 and is negatively regulated by the ubiquitin–proteasome pathway as well as by sumoylation (Bojovic & Hassell, 2008; Takahashi et al., 2005; Wasylyk, Hagman, & Gutierrez-Hartmann, 1998).

The transcriptional activity of PEA3 is dependent on other activators to regulate gene transcription and is commonly partnered with AP-1 to regulate genes such as MMP-1, MMP-3, MMP-7, and MMP-9; urokinase-type plasminogen activator (Evans, Stapp, Dall'Era, Juarez, & Yang, 2001); COX-2; and ErbB-2 (Matsui et al., 2006). AP-1 is a dimeric complex consisting of the Fos (c-FOS, FosB, Fra-1, and Fra-2) and Jun (c-JUN, JunB, and JunD) families (Curran & Franza, 1988). Depending on the cellular context, AP-1 cooperates with other proteins including, but not limited to, NFκB, CBP/p300, Rb, and PEA3 (Hesselbrock, Kurpios, Hassell, Watson, & Fleming, 2005; Matthews, Colburn, & Young, 2007). The functional role of AP-1 is to recruit and direct appropriate factors to regulate gene expression and promote proliferation, differentiation, inflammation, and/or apoptosis (Angel & Karin, 1991).

Previous investigations have determined that overexpression of Notch-1 and Notch-4 plays a critical role in breast tumorigenesis (Brou et al., 2000) and that PEA3 overexpression is associated with aggressive breast cancers, particularly the triple-negative subtype (Bieche et al., 2004; Davidson et al., 2004; Discenza, Vaz, Hassell, & Pelletier, 2004; Firlej et al., 2008; Kinoshita et al., 2002; Xia et al., 2006). PEA3 has been shown to be a transcriptional activator of Notch-1 and Notch-4 and a repressor of Notch-2 in MDA-MB-231 cells, an example of triple-negative breast cancer cells (Clementz, Rogowski, Pandya, Miele, & Osipo, 2011). PEA3-mediated Notch-1 transcription is AP-1 independent, while Notch-4 transcription requires both PEA3 and c-JUN. PEA3 and/or Notch signaling are essential for proliferation, survival, and tumor growth of MDA-MB-231 cells. Furthermore, PEA3 is a transcriptional activator of both Notch-1 and Notch-4 in other breast cancer cell subtypes.

Clementz et al. (2011) demonstrated evidence for the transcriptional regulation of Notch by PEA3 in breast cancer. Additionally, they showed that inhibition of Notch signaling via a GSI and knockdown of PEA3 arrested growth of breast cancer cell lines in the G_1 phase, decreased both anchorage-dependent and anchorage-independent growth and significantly increased apoptotic cells *in vitro*.

Targeting of the PEA3 and/or Notch pathways might provide a new therapeutic strategy for triple-negative breast cancer as well as possibly other breast cancer subtypes where PEA3 regulates Notch-1 and/or Notch-4. Additionally, the severe side effects associated with GSI treatment could possibly be avoided if inhibition of PEA3 is able to inhibit several growth- and metastases-promoting signaling pathways.

9.3. Notch-1 siRNA

siRNA, sometimes known as short interfering RNA or silencing RNA, is a class of double-stranded RNA molecules, 20–25 nucleotides in length, that play a variety of roles in biology. Among its many roles, siRNA is involved in the RNA interference pathway (Elbashir et al., 2001), where it interferes with the expression of a specific gene. Zang et al. (2010) investigated the role of Notch-1 siRNA in human breast cancer cells. They downregulated the expression of the Notch-1 receptor by siRNA, which caused increased chemosensitivity. Their results suggest that Notch signaling by siRNA may be a promising target for breast cancer treatment.

9.4. Notch-1 and delta-like ligand 4 monoclonal antibodies

Overexpression of Notch receptors and ligands has been associated with TNBC, making Notch a potential therapeutic target monoclonal antibody (mAb) therapy. There are few studies addressing the therapeutic potential of mAbs directed toward Notch-1. However, a study by Sharma, Paranjape, Rangarajan, and Dighe (2012) demonstrated that the inhibition of Notch-1 by mAbs (1) inhibited ligand-dependent expression of downstream target genes of Notch such as HES-1, HES-5, and HEY-L in the breast cancer cell line MDA-MB-231; (2) decreased cell proliferation and induced apoptotic cell death; (3) reduced CD44(Hi)/CD24(Low) subpopulation (cancer stem-like population) in MDA-MB-231 cells; (4) irreversibly decreased the primary, secondary, and tertiary mammosphere formation efficiency of the cells; and (5) modulated expression of genes associated with stemness and epithelial–mesenchymal transition.

Delta-like ligand 4 (DLL4) is a Notch ligand that is predominantly expressed in the endothelium of breast cancer and lactating breast as well as a statistically significant multivariate adverse prognostic factor in breast cancer (Jubb et al., 2010). A study by Ridgway et al. (2006) demonstrated that neutralizing DLL4 with a DLL4-selective antibody (1) rendered endothelial cells hyperproliferative; (2) caused defective cell fate specification or differentiation both *in vitro* and *in vivo*; and (3) inhibited tumor growth in several tumor models. A subsequent study by Hoey et al. (2009) in colon cancer demonstrated that selectively inhibiting DLL4 signaling in human tumor cells with anti-hDLL4 21M18 leads to a decrease in tumor growth, a delay in tumor recurrence after chemotherapeutic treatment, and a decrease in the percentage of tumorigenic cells. Yen, Fischer, Lewicki, Gurney, & Hoey (2009) examined DLL4 mAb therapy in TNBC patients and found that (1) anti-DLL4 was efficacious as a single agent and in combination with paclitaxel (Taxol) against triple-negative breast tumors; (2) gene expression analysis showed that anti–DLL4 affected vascular-related genes in the stroma and Notch target genes in the tumor and stroma; (3) inclusion of anti–DLL4 delayed breast tumor recurrence following termination of paclitaxel treatment; and (4) treatment with anti–DLL4 decreased cancer stem cell frequency, whereas paclitaxel alone was ineffective. Further studies in humans on this subject are needed, as Dll4 mAbs may serve as an important therapeutic target as well as a potential vaccine.

REFERENCES

Al-Hajj, M., Wicha, M. S., Benito-Hernandez, A., Morrison, S. J., & Clarke, M. F. (2003). Prospective identification of tumorigenic breast cancer cells. *Proceedings of the National Academy of Sciences of the United States of America*, *100*(7), 3983–3988. http://dx.doi.org/10.1073/pnas.0530291100.

Alimirah, F., Panchanathan, R., Davis, F. J., Chen, J., & Choubey, D. (2007). Restoration of p53 expression in human cancer cell lines upregulates the expression of Notch1: Implications for cancer cell fate determination after genotoxic stress. *Neoplasia*, *9*(5), 427–434.

Allred, D. C., Harvey, J. M., Berardo, M., & Clark, G. M. (1998). Prognostic and predictive factors in breast cancer by immunohistochemical analysis. *Modern Pathology: An Official Journal of the United States and Canadian Academy of Pathology, Inc.*, *11*(2), 155–168.

Angel, P., & Karin, M. (1991). The role of Jun, Fos and the AP-1 complex in cell-proliferation and transformation. *Biochimica et Biophysica Acta*, *1072*(2–3), 129–157.

Bauer, K. R., Brown, M., Cress, R. D., Parise, C. A., & Caggiano, V. (2007). Descriptive analysis of estrogen receptor (ER)-negative, progesterone receptor (PR)-negative, and HER2-negative invasive breast cancer, the so-called triple negative phenotype. *Cancer*, *109*(9), 1721–1728.

Benbow, U., & Brinckerhoff, C. E. (1997). The AP-1 site and MMP gene regulation: What is all the fuss about? *Matrix Biology: Journal of the International Society for Matrix Biology*, *15*(8–9), 519–526.

Berrada, N., Delaloge, S., & Andre, F. (2010). Treatment of triple-negative metastatic breast cancer: Toward individualized targeted treatments or chemosensitization? (Review). *Annals of Oncology: Official Journal of the European Society for Medical Oncology/ESMO*, *21*(Suppl. 7), vii30–vii35. http://dx.doi.org/10.1093/annonc/mdq279.

Beverly, L. J., Felsher, D. W., & Capobianco, A. J. (2005). Suppression of p53 by Notch in lymphomagenesis: Implications for initiation and regression. *Cancer Research*, *65*(16), 7159–7168. http://dx.doi.org/10.1158/0008-5472.CAN-05-1664.

Bieche, I., Tozlu, S., Girault, I., Onody, P., Driouch, K., Vidaud, M., et al. (2004). Expression of PEA3/E1AF/ETV4, an Ets-related transcription factor, in breast tumors: Positive links to MMP2, NRG1 and CGB expression. *Carcinogenesis*, *25*(3), 405–411. http://dx.doi.org/10.1093/carcin/bgh024.

Blaumueller, C. M., & Artiavanis-Tsakonas, S. (1997). Comparative aspects of Notch signaling in lower and higher eukaryotes. *Perspectives on Developmental Neurobiology*, *4*, 325–343.

Bojovic, B. B., & Hassell, J. A. (2008). The transactivation function of the Pea3 subfamily Ets transcription factors is regulated by sumoylation. *DNA and Cell Biology*, *27*(6), 289–305. http://dx.doi.org/10.1089/dna.2007.0680.

Bolton, J. L., & Thatcher, G. R. (2008). Potential mechanisms of estrogen quinone carcinogenesis. *Chemical Research in Toxicology*, *21*(1), 93–101. http://dx.doi.org/10.1021/tx700191p.

Bonnet, D., & Dick, J. E. (1997). Human acute myeloid leukemia is organized as a hierarchy that originates from a primitive hematopoietic cell. *Nature Medicine, 3*(7), 730–737.

Brennan, K., & Brown, A. M. (2003). Is there a role for Notch signalling in human breast cancer? *Breast Cancer Research: BCR, 5*(2), 69–75.

Brou, C., Logeat, F., Gupta, N., Bessia, C., LeBail, O., Doedens, J. R., et al. (2000). A novel proteolytic cleavage involved in Notch signaling: The role of the disintegrin-metalloprotease TACE. *Molecular Cell, 5*(2), 207–216.

Callahan, R., & Raafat, A. (2001). Notch signaling in mammary gland tumorigenesis. *Journal of Mammary Gland Biology and Neoplasia, 6*(1), 23–36 (Review).

Chang, E. C., Frasor, J., Komm, B., & Katzenellenbogen, B. S. (2006). Impact of estrogen receptor beta on gene networks regulated by estrogen receptor alpha in breast cancer cells. *Endocrinology, 147*(10), 4831–4842. http://dx.doi.org/10.1210/en.2006-0563.

Chang, J., Landis, M., Schott, A., Pavlick, A., Dobrolecki, L., Korkaya, H., et al. (2009). Targeting intrinsically-resistant breast cancer stem cells with gamma-secretase inhibitors. *Cancer Research, 69*(24). Supplement 3.

Cheang, M. C., Voduc, D., Bajdik, C., Leung, S., McKinney, S., Chia, S. K., et al. (2008). Basal-like breast cancer defined by five biomarkers has superior prognostic value than triple-negative phenotype. *Clinical Cancer Research: An Official Journal of the American Association for Cancer Research, 14*(5), 1368–1376. http://dx.doi.org/10.1158/1078-0432. CCR-07-1658.

Chen, Y., Fischer, W. H., & Gill, G. N. (1997). Regulation of the ERBB-2 promoter by RBPJkappa and NOTCH. *The Journal of Biological Chemistry, 272*(22), 14110–14114.

Chen, J. Q., & Russo, J. (2009). ERalpha-negative and triple negative breast cancer: Molecular features and potential therapeutic approaches. *Biochimica et Biophysica Acta, 1796*(2), 162–175. http://dx.doi.org/10.1016/j.bbcan.2009.06.003.

Clementz, A. G., Rogowski, A., Pandya, K., Miele, L., & Osipo, C. (2011). NOTCH-1 and NOTCH-4 are novel gene targets of PEA3 in breast cancer: Novel therapeutic implications. *Breast Cancer Research: BCR, 13*(3), R63. http://dx.doi.org/10.1186/bcr2900.

Colditz, G. A., & Rosner, B. (2000). Cumulative risk of breast cancer to age 70 years according to risk factor status: Data from the Nurses' Health Study. *American Journal of Epidemiology, 152*(10), 950–964.

Conforti, R., Boulet, T., Tomasic, G., Taranchon, E., Arriagada, R., Spielmann, M., et al. (2007). Breast cancer molecular subclassification and estrogen receptor expression to predict efficacy of adjuvant anthracyclines-based chemotherapy: A biomarker study from two randomized trials. *Annals of Oncology: Official Journal of the European Society for Medical Oncology/ESMO, 18*(9), 1477–1483. http://dx.doi.org/10.1093/annonc/mdm209.

Curran, T., & Franza, B. R., Jr. (1988). Fos and Jun: The AP-1 connection. *Cell, 55*(3), 395–397 (Review).

Davidson, B., Goldberg, I., Tell, L., Vigdorchik, S., Baekelandt, M., Berner, A., et al. (2004). The clinical role of the PEA3 transcription factor in ovarian and breast carcinoma in effusions. *Clinical & Experimental Metastasis, 21*(3), 191–199.

Dent, R., Trudeau, M., Pritchard, K. I., Hanna, W. M., Kahn, H. K., Sawka, C. A., et al. (2007). Triple-negative breast cancer: clinical features and patterns of recurrence. *Clinical Cancer Research, 13*, 4429–4434.

Diaz, L. K., Cryns, V. L., Symmans, W. F., & Sneige, N. (2007). Triple negative breast - carcinoma and the basal phenotype: From expression profiling to clinical practice. *Advances in Anatomic Pathology, 14*(6), 419–430. http://dx.doi.org/10.1097/PAP. 0b013e3181594733.

Dickson, B. C., Mulligan, A. M., Zhang, H., Lockwood, G., O'Malley, F. P., Egan, S. E., et al. (2007). High-level JAG1 mRNA and protein predict poor outcome in breast cancer. *Modern Pathology: An Official Journal of the United States and Canadian Academy of Pathology, Inc., 20*(6), 685–693. http://dx.doi.org/10.1038/modpathol.3800785.

Discenza, M. T., Vaz, D., Hassell, J. A., & Pelletier, J. (2004). Activation of the WT1 tumor suppressor gene promoter by Pea3. *FEBS Letters, 560*(1–3), 183–191. http://dx.doi.org/10.1016/S0014-5793(04)00104-8.

Dotzlaw, H., Leygue, E., Watson, P. H., & Murphy, L. C. (1999). Estrogen receptor-beta messenger RNA expression in human breast tumor biopsies: Relationship to steroid receptor status and regulation by progestins. *Cancer Research, 59*(3), 529–532.

Dunnwald, L. K., Rossing, M. A., & Li, C. I. (2007). Hormone receptor status, tumor characteristics, and prognosis: A prospective cohort of breast cancer patients. *Breast Cancer Research: BCR, 9*(1), R6. http://dx.doi.org/10.1186/bcr1639.

Dunwoodie, S. L., Henrique, D., Harrison, S. M., & Beddington, R. S. (1997). Mouse Dll3: a novel divergent Delta gene which may compliment the function of other Delta homologues during early pattern formation in the mouse embryo. *Development, 124*, 3065–3076.

Elbashir, S. M., Harborth, J., Lendeckel, W., Yalcin, A., Weber, K., & Tuschl, T. (2001). Duplexes of 21-nucleotide RNAs mediate RNA interference in cultured mammalian cells. *Nature, 411*(6836), 494–498. http://dx.doi.org/10.1038/35078107.

Evans, C. P., Stapp, E. C., Dall'Era, M. A., Juarez, J., & Yang, J. C. (2001). Regulation of u-PA gene expression in human prostate cancer. *International Journal of Cancer. Journal International Du Cancer, 94*(3), 390–395.

Farnie, G., & Clarke, R. B. (2007). Mammary stem cells and breast cancer—Role of Notch signalling. *Stem Cell Reviews, 3*(2), 169–175 (Review).

Fasano, J., & Muggia, F. (2009). Breast cancer arising in a BRCA-mutated background: therapeutic implications from an animal model and drug development. *Annals of Oncology, 20*, 609–614.

Firlej, V., Ladam, F., Brysbaert, G., Dumont, P., Fuks, F., de Launoit, Y., et al. (2008). Reduced tumorigenesis in mouse mammary cancer cells following inhibition of Pea3- or Erm-dependent transcription. *Journal of Cell Science, 121*(Pt 20), 3393–3402. http://dx.doi.org/10.1242/jcs.027201.

Fortini, M. E. (2001). Notch and presenilin: A proteolytic mechanism emerges. *Current Opinion in Cell Biology, 13*(5), 627–634.

Fujita, T., Kobayashi, Y., Wada, O., Tateishi, Y., Kitada, L., Yamamoto, Y., et al. (2003). Full activation of estrogen receptor alpha activation function-1 induces proliferation of breast cancer cells. *The Journal of Biological Chemistry, 278*(29), 26704–26714. http://dx. doi.org/10.1074/jbc.M301031200.

Fuqua, S. A., Schiff, R., Parra, I., Moore, J. T., Mohsin, S. K., Osborne, C. K., et al. (2003). Estrogen receptor beta protein in human breast cancer: Correlation with clinical tumor parameters. *Cancer Research, 63*(10), 2434–2439.

Graham, J. D., Mote, P. A., Salagame, U., van Dijk, J. H., Balleine, R. L., Huschtscha, L. I., et al. (2009). DNA replication licensing and progenitor numbers are increased by progesterone in normal human breast. *Endocrinology, 150*(7), 3318–3326. http://dx.doi.org/10.1210/en.2008-1630.

Graves, B. J., & Petersen, J. M. (1998). Specificity within the ets family of transcription factors. *Advances in Cancer Research, 75*, 1–55.

Hall, J. M., Couse, J. F., & Korach, K. S. (2001). The multifaceted mechanisms of estradiol and estrogen receptor signaling. *The Journal of Biological Chemistry, 276*(40), 36869–36872. http://dx.doi.org/10.1074/jbc.R100029200 (Review).

Hammond, M. E., Hayes, D. F., Dowsett, M., Allred, D. C., Hagerty, K. L., Badve, S., et al. (2010). American society of clinical oncology/College Of American Pathologists guideline recommendations for immunohistochemical testing of estrogen and progesterone receptors in breast cancer. *Journal of Clinical Oncology: Official Journal of the American Society of Clinical Oncology, 28*(16), 2784–2795. http://dx.doi.org/10.1200/JCO.2009.25.6529 (Review).

Han, J., Ma, I., Hendzel, M. J., & Allalunis-Turner, J. (2009). The cytotoxicity of gamma-secretase inhibitor I to breast cancer cells is mediated by proteasome inhibition, not by gamma-secretase inhibition. *Breast Cancer Research: BCR, 11*(4), R57. http://dx.doi.org/10.1186/bcr2347.

Harrison, H., Farnie, G., Howell, S. J., Rock, R. E., Stylianou, S., Brennan, K. R., et al. (2010). Regulation of breast cancer stem cell activity by signaling through the Notch4 receptor. *Cancer Research, 70*(2), 709–718. http://dx.doi.org/10.1158/0008-5472.CAN-09-1681.

Harvey, J. M., Clark, G. M., Osborne, C. K., & Allred, D. C. (1999). Estrogen receptor status by immunohistochemistry is superior to the ligand-binding assay for predicting response to adjuvant endocrine therapy in breast cancer. *Journal of Clinical Oncology: Official Journal of the American Society of Clinical Oncology, 17*(5), 1474–1481.

Haughian, J. M., Pinto, M. P., Harrell, J. C., Bliesner, B. S., Joensuu, K. M., Dye, W. W., et al. (2012). Maintenance of hormone responsiveness in luminal breast cancers by suppression of Notch. *Proceedings of the National Academy of Sciences of the United States of America, 109*(8), 2742–2747. http://dx.doi.org/10.1073/pnas.1106509108.

Helguero, L. A., Faulds, M. H., Gustafsson, J. A., & Haldosen, L. A. (2005). Estrogen receptors alfa (ERalpha) and beta (ERbeta) differentially regulate proliferation and apoptosis of the normal murine mammary epithelial cell line HC11. *Oncogene, 24*(44), 6605–6616. http://dx.doi.org/10.1038/sj.onc.1208807.

Herynk, M. H., & Fuqua, S. A. (2004). Estrogen receptor mutations in human disease. *Endocrine Reviews, 25*(6), 869–898. http://dx.doi.org/10.1210/er.2003-0010.

Hesselbrock, D. R., Kurpios, N., Hassell, J. A., Watson, M. A., & Fleming, T. P. (2005). PEA3, AP-1, and a unique repetitive sequence all are involved in transcriptional regulation of the breast cancer-associated gene, mammaglobin. *Breast Cancer Research and Treatment, 89*(3), 289–296. http://dx.doi.org/10.1007/s10549-004-2622-z.

Hida, K., Shindoh, M., Yasuda, M., Hanzawa, M., Funaoka, K., Kohgo, T., et al. (1997). Antisense E1AF transfection restrains oral cancer invasion by reducing matrix metalloproteinase activities. *The American Journal of Pathology, 150*(6), 2125–2132.

Hoey, T., Yen, W. C., Axelrod, F., Basi, J., Donigian, L., Dylla, S., et al. (2009). DLL4 blockade inhibits tumor growth and reduces tumor-initiating cell frequency. *Cell Stem Cell, 5*(2), 168–177. http://dx.doi.org/10.1016/j.stem.2009.05.019.

Hopp, T. A., Weiss, H. L., Hilsenbeck, S. G., Cui, Y., Allred, D. C., Horwitz, K. B., et al. (2004). Breast cancer patients with progesterone receptor PR-A-rich tumors have poorer disease-free survival rates. *Clinical Cancer Research: An Official Journal of the American Association for Cancer Research, 10*(8), 2751–2760.

Horwitz, K. B., Dye, W. W., Harrell, J. C., Kabos, P., & Sartorius, C. A. (2008). Rare steroid receptor-negative basal-like tumorigenic cells in luminal subtype human breast cancer xenografts. *Proceedings of the National Academy of Sciences of the United States of America, 105*(15), 5774–5779. http://dx.doi.org/10.1073/pnas.0706216105.

Hsich, J. J., Zhou, S., Chen, L., Young, D. B., & Hayward, S. D. (1999). CIR, a corepressor linking the DNA binding factor CBF1 to the histone deacetylase complex. *Proceedings of the National Academy of Sciences of the United States of America, 96*(1), 23–28.

Hu, C., Dievart, A., Lupien, M., Calvo, E., Tremblay, G., & Jolicoeur, P. (2006). Overexpression of activated murine Notch1 and Notch3 in transgenic mice blocks mammary gland development and induces mammary tumors. *The American Journal of Pathology, 168*(3), 973–990. http://dx.doi.org/10.2353/ajpath.2006.050416.

Iguchi, A., Kitajima, I., Yamakuchi, M., Ueno, S., Aikou, T., Kubo, T., et al. (2000). PEA3 and AP-1 are required for constitutive IL-8 gene expression in hepatoma cells. *Biochemical and Biophysical Research Communications, 279*(1), 166–171. http://dx.doi.org/10.1006/bbrc.2000.3925.

Iwao, K., Miyoshi, Y., Egawa, C., Ikeda, N., & Noguchi, S. (2000). Quantitative analysis of estrogen receptor-beta mRNA and its variants in human breast cancers. *International Journal of Cancer. Journal International Du Cancer, 88*(5), 733–736.

Iwao, K., Miyoshi, Y., Egawa, C., Ikeda, N., Tsukamoto, F., & Noguchi, S. (2000). Quantitative analysis of estrogen receptor-alpha and -beta messenger RNA expression in breast carcinoma by real-time polymerase chain reaction. *Cancer, 89*(8), 1732–1738. http://dx. doi.org/10.1002/1097-0142(20001015)89:8<1732::AID-CNCR13>3.0.CO;2-2.

Jarvinen, T. A., Pelto-Huikko, M., Holli, K., & Isola, J. (2000). Estrogen receptor beta is coexpressed with ERalpha and PR and associated with nodal status, grade, and proliferation rate in breast cancer. *The American Journal of Pathology, 156*(1), 29–35.

Jensen, E. V., Cheng, G., Palmieri, C., Saji, S., Makela, S., Van Noorden, S., et al. (2001). Estrogen receptors and proliferation markers in primary and recurrent breast cancer. *Proceedings of the National Academy of Sciences of the United States of America, 98*(26), 15197–15202. http://dx.doi.org/10.1073/pnas.211556298.

Jubb, A. M., Soilleux, E. J., Turley, H., Steers, G., Parker, A., Low, I., et al. (2010). Expression of vascular notch ligand delta-like 4 and inflammatory markers in breast cancer. *The American Journal of Pathology, 176*(4), 2019–2028. http://dx.doi.org/10.2353/ajpath.2010.090908.

Kabos, P., Haughian, J. M., Wang, X., Dye, W. W., Finlayson, C., Elias, A., et al. (2011). Cytokeratin 5 positive cells represent a steroid receptor negative and therapy resistant subpopulation in luminal breast cancers. *Breast Cancer Research and Treatment, 128*(1), 45–55. http://dx.doi.org/10.1007/s10549-010-1078-6.

Kalen, M., Heikura, T., Karvinen, H., Nitzsche, A., Weber, H., Esser, N., et al. (2011). Gamma-secretase inhibitor treatment promotes VEGF-A-driven blood vessel growth and vascular leakage but disrupts neovascular perfusion. *PLoS One, 6*(4), e18709. http://dx.doi.org/10.1371/journal.pone.0018709.

Kapila, S., Xie, Y., & Wang, W. (2009). Induction of MMP-1 (collagenase-1) by relaxin in fibrocartilaginous cells requires both the AP-1 and PEA-3 promoter sites. *Orthodontics & Craniofacial Research, 12*(3), 178–186. http://dx.doi.org/10.1111/j.1601-6343.2009.01451.x.

Keith, B., & Simon, M. C. (2007). Hypoxia-inducible factors, stem cells, and cancer. *Cell, 129*(3), 465–472. http://dx.doi.org/10.1016/j.cell.2007.04.019.

Key, T., Appleby, P., Barnes, I., & Reeves, G. (2002). Endogenous sex hormones and breast cancer in postmenopausal women: Reanalysis of nine prospective studies. *Journal of the National Cancer Institute, 94*(8), 606–616.

Kim, S. H., Yin, Y. I., Li, Y. M., & Sisodia, S. S. (2004). Evidence that assembly of an active gamma-secretase complex occurs in the early compartments of the secretory pathway. *The Journal of Biological Chemistry, 279*(47), 48615–48619. http://dx.doi.org/10.1074/jbc.C400396200.

Kinoshita, J., Kitamura, K., Tanaka, S., Sugimachi, K., Ishida, M., & Saeki, H. (2002). Clinical significance of PEA3 in human breast cancer. *Surgery, 131*(Suppl. 1), S222–S225.

Khalifeh, I. M., Albarracin, C., Diaz, L. K., Symmans, F. W., Edgerton, M. E., Hwang, R. F., et al. (2008). Clinical, histopatholigic, and immunohistochemical features of microglandular adenosis and transition into in situ and invasive carcinoma. *The American Journal of Surgical Pathology, 32*, 544–552.

Knowlden, J. M., Gee, J. M., Robertson, J. F., Ellis, I. O., & Nicholson, R. I. (2000). A possible divergent role for the oestrogen receptor alpha and beta subtypes in clinical breast cancer. *International Journal of Cancer. Journal International Du Cancer, 89*(2), 209–212.

Kondratyev, M., Kreso, A., Hallett, R. M., Girgis-Gabardo, A., Barcelon, M. E., Ilieva, D., et al. (2012). Gamma-secretase inhibitors target tumor-initiating cells in a mouse model of ERBB2 breast cancer. *Oncogene, 31*(1), 93–103. http://dx.doi.org/10.1038/onc.2011.212.

Korkaya, H., Paulson, A., Iovino, F., & Wicha, M. S. (2008). HER2 regulates the mammary stem/progenitor cell population driving tumorigenesis and invasion. *Oncogene, 27*(47), 6120–6130. http://dx.doi.org/10.1038/onc.2008.207.

Korkaya, H., & Wicha, M. S. (2007). Selective targeting of cancer stem cells: A new concept in cancer therapeutics. *BioDrugs: Clinical Immunotherapeutics, Biopharmaceuticals and Gene Therapy, 21*(5), 299–310.

Korkaya, H., & Wicha, M. S. (2009). HER-2, notch, and breast cancer stem cells: Targeting an axis of evil. *Clinical Cancer Research: An Official Journal of the American Association for Cancer Research*, *15*(6), 1845–1847. http://dx.doi.org/10.1158/1078-0432.CCR-08-3087.

Lange, C. A., & Yee, D. (2008). Progesterone and breast cancer. *Women's Health*, *4*(2), 151–162. http://dx.doi.org/10.2217/17455057.4.2.151 (Review).

Lindsell, C. E., Shawber, C. J., Boulter, J., & Weinmaster, G. (1995). Jagged: a mammalian ligand that activates Notch1. *Cell*, *80*, 909–917.

Lee, C. W., Raskett, C. M., Prudovsky, I., & Altieri, D. C. (2008). Molecular dependence of estrogen receptor-negative breast cancer on a notch-survivin signaling axis. *Cancer Research*, *68*(13), 5273–5281. http://dx.doi.org/10.1158/0008-5472.CAN-07-6673.

Lee, C. W., Simin, K., Liu, Q., Plescia, J., Guha, M., Khan, A., et al. (2008). A functional Notch-survivin gene signature in basal breast cancer. *Breast Cancer Research: BCR*, *10*(6), R97. http://dx.doi.org/10.1186/bcr2200.

Lehmann, B. D., Bauer, J. A., Chen, X., Sanders, M. E., Chakravarthy, A. B., Shyr, Y., et al. (2011). Identification of human triple-negative breast cancer subtypes and preclinical models for selection of targeted therapies. *Journal of Clinical Investigation*, *121*(7), 2750–2767.

Leygue, E., Dotzlaw, H., Watson, P. H., & Murphy, L. C. (1998). Altered estrogen receptor alpha and beta messenger RNA expression during human breast tumorigenesis. *Cancer Research*, *58*(15), 3197–3201.

Liedtke, C., Mazouni, C., Hess, K. R., Andre, F., Tordai, A., Mejia, J. A., et al. (2008). Response to neoadjuvant therapy and long-term survival in patients with triple-negative breast cancer. *Journal of Clinical Oncology: Official Journal of the American Society of Clinical Oncology*, *26*(8), 1275–1281. http://dx.doi.org/10.1200/JCO.2007.14.4147.

Lydon, J. P., DeMayo, F. J., Funk, C. R., Mani, S. K., Hughes, A. R., Montgomery, C. A., Jr., et al. (1995). Mice lacking progesterone receptor exhibit pleiotropic reproductive abnormalities. *Genes & Development*, *9*(18), 2266–2278.

Lydon, J. P., & Edwards, D. P. (2009). Finally! A model for progesterone receptor action in normal human breast. *Endocrinology*, *150*(7), 2988–2990. http://dx.doi.org/10.1210/en.2009-0383.

Magnifico, A., Albano, L., Campaner, S., Delia, D., Castiglioni, F., Gasparini, P., et al. (2009). Tumor-initiating cells of HER2-positive carcinoma cell lines express the highest oncoprotein levels and are sensitive to trastuzumab. *Clinical Cancer Research: An official Journal of the American Association for Cancer Research*, *15*(6), 2010–2021. http://dx.doi.org/10.1158/1078-0432.CCR-08-1327.

Maier, M. M., & Gessler, M. (2000). Comparative analysis of the human and mouse Hey1 promoter: Hey genes are new Notch target genes. *Biochemical and Biophysical Research Communications*, *275*(2), 652–660. http://dx.doi.org/10.1006/bbrc.2000.3354.

Mann, S., Laucirica, R., Carlson, N., Younes, P. S., Ali, N., Younes, A., et al. (2001). Estrogen receptor beta expression in invasive breast cancer. *Human Pathology*, *32*(1), 113–118. http://dx.doi.org/10.1053/hupa.2001.21506.

Matsui, K., Sugimori, K., Motomura, H., Ejiri, N., Tsukada, K., & Kitajima, I. (2006). PEA3 cooperates with c-Jun in regulation of HER2/neu transcription. *Oncology Reports*, *16*(1), 153–158.

Matthews, C. P., Colburn, N. H., & Young, M. R. (2007). AP-1 a target for cancer prevention. *Current Cancer Drug Targets*, *7*(4), 317–324.

Miele, L. (2008). Rational targeting of Notch signaling in breast cancer. *Expert Review of Anticancer Therapy*, *8*(8), 1197–1202. http://dx.doi.org/10.1586/14737140.8.8.1197.

Miele, L., Miao, H., & Nickoloff, B. J. (2006). NOTCH signaling as a novel cancer therapeutic target. *Current Cancer Drug Targets*, *6*, 313–323.

Miyoshi, Y., Taguchi, T., Gustafsson, J. A., & Noguchi, S. (2001). Clinicopathological characteristics of estrogen receptor-beta-positive human breast cancers. *Japanese Journal of Cancer Research: Gann*, *92*(10), 1057–1061.

Mote, P. A., Bartow, S., Tran, N., & Clarke, C. L. (2002). Loss of co-ordinate expression of progesterone receptors A and B is an early event in breast carcinogenesis. *Breast Cancer Research and Treatment, 72*(2), 163–172.

Mote, P. A., Graham, J. D., & Clarke, C. L. (2007). Progesterone receptor isoforms in normal and malignant breast. *Ernst Schering Foundation Symposium Proceedings, 2007*(1), 77–107 (Review).

Nakamura, T., Tsuchiya, K., & Watanabe, M. (2007). Crosstalk between Wnt and Notch signaling in intestinal epithelial cell fate decision. *Journal of Gastroenterology, 42*(9), 705–710. http://dx.doi.org/10.1007/s00535-007-2087-z.

Oikawa, T., & Yamada, T. (2003). Molecular biology of the Ets family of transcription factors. *Gene, 303,* 11–34.

Okamoto, R., Tsuchiya, K., & Watanabe, M. (2007). Regulation of epithelial cell differentiation and regeneration in IBD. *Nihon Shokakibyo Gakkai zasshi—The Japanese Journal of Gastro-Enterology, 104*(8), 1165–1171.

Omoto, Y., Inoue, S., Ogawa, S., Toyama, T., Yamashita, H., Muramatsu, M., et al. (2001). Clinical value of the wild-type estrogen receptor beta expression in breast cancer. *Cancer Letters, 163*(2), 207–212.

Omoto, Y., Kobayashi, S., Inoue, S., Ogawa, S., Toyama, T., Yamashita, H., et al. (2002). Evaluation of oestrogen receptor beta wild-type and variant protein expression, and relationship with clinicopathological factors in breast cancers. *European Journal of Cancer, 38*(3), 380–386.

O'Neill, C. F., Urs, S., Cinelli, C., Lincoln, A., Nadeau, R. J., Leon, R., et al. (2007). Notch2 signaling induces apoptosis and inhibits human MDA-MB-231 xenograft growth. *The American Journal of Pathology, 171*(3), 1023–1036. http://dx.doi.org/10.2353/ajpath.2007.061029.

Osborne, B. (2000). Role of Notch in regulating apoptosis in the mammary gland. *Taken from Annual Grant Report DAMD17-98-1-8314, U.S. Army Medical Research and Materiel Command, Fort Detrick, Maryland.*

Osipo, C., Patel, P., Rizzo, P., Clementz, A. G., Hao, L., Golde, T. E., et al. (2008). ErbB-2 inhibition activates Notch-1 and sensitizes breast cancer cells to a gamma-secretase inhibitor. *Oncogene, 27*(37), 5019–5032. http://dx.doi.org/10.1038/onc.2008.149.

Park, S. Y., Gonen, M., Kim, H. J., Michor, F., & Polyak, K. (2010). Cellular and genetic diversity in the progression of in situ human breast carcinomas to an invasive phenotype. *The Journal of Clinical Investigation, 120*(2), 636–644. http://dx.doi.org/10.1172/JCI40724.

Paruthiyil, S., Parmar, H., Kerekatte, V., Cunha, G. R., Firestone, G. L., & Leitman, D. C. (2004). Estrogen receptor beta inhibits human breast cancer cell proliferation and tumor formation by causing a G2 cell cycle arrest. *Cancer Research, 64*(1), 423–428.

Perou, C. M., Sorlie, T., Eisen, M. B., van de Rijn, M., Jeffrey, S. S., Rees, C. A., et al. (2000). Molecular portraits of human breast tumours. *Nature, 406*(6797), 747–752. http://dx.doi.org/10.1038/35021093.

Prat, A., Parker, J. S., Karginova, O., Fan, C., Livasy, C., Herschkowitz, J. I., et al. (2010). Phenotypic and molecular characterization of the claudin-low intrinsic subtype of breast cancer. *Breast Cancer Research: BCR, 12*(5), R68. http://dx.doi.org/10.1186/bcr2635.

Rakha, E. A., Elsheikh, S. E., Aleskandarany, M. A., Habashi, H. O., Green, A. R., Powe, D. G., et al. (2009). Triple-negative breast cancer: Distinguishing between basal and nonbasal subtypes. *Clinical Cancer Research: An Official Journal of the American Association for Cancer Research, 15*(7), 2302–2310. http://dx.doi.org/10.1158/1078-0432.CCR-08-2132.

Rakha, E. A., Reis-Filho, J. S., & Ellis, I. O. (2008). Basal-like breast cancer: A critical review. *Journal of Clinical Oncology: Official Journal of the American Society of Clinical Oncology, 26*(15), 2568–2581. http://dx.doi.org/10.1200/JCO.2007.13.1748 (Review).

Raouf, A., Zhao, Y., To, K., Stingl, J., Delaney, A., Barbara, M., et al. (2008). Transcriptome analysis of the normal human mammary cell commitment and differentiation process. Cell Stem Cell, 3(1), 109–118. http://dx.doi.org/10.1016/j.stem.2008.05.018.

Reedijk, M., Odorcic, S., Chang, L., Zhang, H., Miller, N., McCready, D. R., et al. (2005). High-level coexpression of JAG1 and NOTCH1 is observed in human breast cancer and is associated with poor overall survival. Cancer Research, 65(18), 8530–8537. http://dx. doi.org/10.1158/0008-5472.CAN-05-1069.

Reedijk, M., Pinnaduwage, D., Dickson, B. C., Mulligan, A. M., Zhang, H., Bull, S. B., et al. (2008). JAG1 expression is associated with a basal phenotype and recurrence in lymph node-negative breast cancer. Breast Cancer Research and Treatment, 111(3), 439–448. http://dx.doi.org/10.1007/s10549-007-9805-3.

Reis-Filho, J. S., & Tutt, A. N. (2008). Triple negative tumors: a critical review. Histopathology, 52, 108–118.

Ridgway, J., Zhang, G., Wu, Y., Stawicki, S., Liang, W. C., Chanthery, Y., et al. (2006). Inhibition of Dll4 signalling inhibits tumour growth by deregulating angiogenesis. Nature, 444(7122), 1083–1087. http://dx.doi.org/10.1038/nature05313.

Rizzo, P., Miao, H., D'Souza, G., Osipo, C., Song, L. L., Yun, J., et al. (2008). Cross-talk between notch and the estrogen receptor in breast cancer suggests novel therapeutic approaches. Cancer Research, 68(13), 5226–5235. http://dx.doi.org/10.1158/0008-5472.CAN-07-5744.

Roger, P., Sahla, M. E., Makela, S., Gustafsson, J. A., Baldet, P., & Rochefort, H. (2001). Decreased expression of estrogen receptor beta protein in proliferative preinvasive mammary tumors. Cancer Research, 61(6), 2537–2541.

Ronchini, C., & Capobianco, A. J. (2001). Induction of cyclin D1 transcription and CDK2 activity by Notch(ic): Implication for cell cycle disruption in transformation by Notch (ic). Molecular and Cellular Biology, 21(17), 5925–5934.

Ross, R. K., Paganini-Hill, A., Wan, P. C., & Pike, M. C. (2000). Effect of hormone replacement therapy on breast cancer risk: Estrogen versus estrogen plus progestin. Journal of the National Cancer Institute, 92(4), 328–332.

Rouzier, R., Perou, C. M., Symmans, W. F., Ibrahim, N., Cristofanilli, M., Anderson, K., et al. (2005). Breast cancer molecular subtypes respond differently to preoperative chemotherapy. Clinical Cancer Research: An Official Journal of the American Association for Cancer Research, 11(16), 5678–5685. http://dx.doi.org/10.1158/1078-0432.CCR-04-2421.

Saxena, M. T., Schroeter, E. H., Mumm, J. S., & Kopan, R. (2001). Murine notch homologs (N1–4) undergo presenilin-dependent proteolysis. The Journal of Biological Chemistry, 276(43), 40268–40273. http://dx.doi.org/10.1074/jbc.M107234200.

Scarpin, K. M., Graham, J. D., Mote, P. A., & Clarke, C. L. (2009). Progesterone action in human tissues: Regulation by progesterone receptor (PR) isoform expression, nuclear positioning and coregulator expression. Nuclear Receptor Signaling, 7, e009. http://dx. doi.org/10.1621/nrs.07009 (Review).

Schroeter, E. H., Kisslinger, J. A., & Kopan, R. (1998). Notch-1 signalling requires ligand-induced proteolytic release of intracellular domain. Nature, 393(6683), 382–386. http://dx.doi.org/10.1038/30756.

Sharma, V. M., Calvo, J. A., Draheim, K. M., Cunningham, L. A., Hermance, N., Beverly, L., et al. (2006). Notch1 contributes to mouse T-cell leukemia by directly inducing the expression of c-myc. Molecular and Cellular Biology, 26(21), 8022–8031. http://dx.doi.org/10.1128/MCB.01091-06.

Sharma, A., Paranjape, A. N., Rangarajan, A., & Dighe, R. R. (2012). A monoclonal antibody against human Notch1 ligand-binding domain depletes subpopulation of putative breast cancer stem-like cells. Molecular Cancer Therapeutics, 11(1), 77–86. http://dx.doi.org/10.1158/1535-7163.MCT-11-0508.

Sharrocks, A. D. (2001). The ETS-domain transcription factor family. Nature Reviews. Molecular Cell Biology, 2(11), 827–837. http://dx.doi.org/10.1038/35099076.

Shawber, C., Boulter, J., Lindsell, C. E., & Weinmaster, G. (1996). Jagged2: A serrate-like gene expressed during rat embryogenesis. *Developmental Biology, 180*(1), 370–376. http://dx.doi.org/10.1006/dbio.1996.0310.

Shepherd, T. G., Kockeritz, L., Szrajber, M. R., Muller, W. J., & Hassell, J. A. (2001). The pea3 subfamily ets genes are required for HER2/Neu-mediated mammary oncogenesis. *Current Biology, 11*(22), 1739–1748.

Skliris, G. P., Carder, P. J., Lansdown, M. R., & Speirs, V. (2001). Immunohistochemical detection of ERbeta in breast cancer: Towards more detailed receptor profiling? *British Journal of Cancer, 84*(8), 1095–1098. http://dx.doi.org/10.1054/bjoc.2001.1721.

Skliris, G. P., Leygue, E., Watson, P. H., & Murphy, L. C. (2008). Estrogen receptor alpha negative breast cancer patients: Estrogen receptor beta as a therapeutic target. *The Journal of Steroid Biochemistry and Molecular Biology, 109*(1–2), 1–10. http://dx.doi.org/10.1016/j.jsbmb.2007.12.010.

Skliris, G. P., Munot, K., Bell, S. M., Carder, P. J., Lane, S., Horgan, K., et al. (2003). Reduced expression of oestrogen receptor beta in invasive breast cancer and its re-expression using DNA methyl transferase inhibitors in a cell line model. *The Journal of Pathology, 201*(2), 213–220. http://dx.doi.org/10.1002/path.1436.

Slamon, D. J., Godolphin, W., Jones, L. A., Holt, J. A., Wong, S. G., Keith, D. E., et al. (1989). Studies of the HER-2/neu proto-oncogene in human breast and ovarian cancer. *Science, 244*(4905), 707–712.

Soares, R., Balogh, G., Guo, S., Gartner, F., Russo, J., & Schmitt, F. (2004). Evidence for the notch signaling pathway on the role of estrogen in angiogenesis. *Molecular Endocrinology, 18*(9), 2333–2343. http://dx.doi.org/10.1210/me.2003-0362.

Soares, R., Guo, S., Gartner, F., Schmitt, F. C., & Russo, J. (2003). 17 beta -estradiol-mediated vessel assembly and stabilization in tumor angiogenesis requires TGF beta and EGFR crosstalk. *Angiogenesis, 6*(4), 271–281. http://dx.doi.org/10.1023/B:AGEN.0000029413.32882.dd.

Sotiriou, C., Neo, S. Y., McShane, L. M., Korn, E. L., Long, P. M., Jazaeri, A., et al. (2003). Breast cancer classification and prognosis based on gene expression profiles from a population-based study. *Proceedings of the National Academy of Sciences of the United States of America, 100*(18), 10393–10398. http://dx.doi.org/10.1073/pnas.1732912100.

Sotiriou, C., & Pusztai, L. (2009). Gene-expression signatures in breast cancer. *The New England Journal of Medicine, 360*(8), 790–800. http://dx.doi.org/10.1056/NEJMra0801289.

Speirs, V., Parkes, A. T., Kerin, M. J., Walton, D. S., Carleton, P. J., Fox, J. N., et al. (1999). Coexpression of estrogen receptor alpha and beta: Poor prognostic factors in human breast cancer? *Cancer Research, 59*(3), 525–528.

Speiser, J., Foreman, K., Drinka, E., Godellas, C., Perez, C., Salhadar, A., et al. (2012). Notch-1 and Notch-4 biomarker expression in triple-negative breast cancer. *International Journal of Surgical Pathology, 20*(2), 139–145. http://dx.doi.org/10.1177/1066896911427035.

Strom, A., Hartman, J., Foster, J. S., Kietz, S., Wimalasena, J., & Gustafsson, J. A. (2004). Estrogen receptor beta inhibits 17beta-estradiol-stimulated proliferation of the breast cancer cell line T47D. *Proceedings of the National Academy of Sciences of the United States of America, 101*(6), 1566–1571. http://dx.doi.org/10.1073/pnas.0308319100.

Subbaramaiah, K., Norton, L., Gerald, W., & Dannenberg, A. J. (2002). Cyclooxygenase-2 is overexpressed in HER-2/neu-positive breast cancer: Evidence for involvement of AP-1 and PEA3. *The Journal of Biological Chemistry, 277*(21), 18649–18657. http://dx.doi.org/10.1074/jbc.M111415200.

Takahashi, A., Higashino, F., Aoyagi, M., Yoshida, K., Itoh, M., Kobayashi, M., et al. (2005). E1AF degradation by a ubiquitin-proteasome pathway. *Biochemical and Biophysical Research Communications, 327*(2), 575–580. http://dx.doi.org/10.1016/j.bbrc.2004.12.045.

Tan, A. R., & Swain, S. M. (2008). Therapeutic strategies for triple-negative breast cancer. *Cancer Journal, 14*(6), 343–351. http://dx.doi.org/10.1097/PPO.0b013e31818d839b (Review).

Tower, G. B., Coon, C. I., Belguise, K., Chalbos, D., & Brinckerhoff, C. E. (2003). Fra-1 targets the AP-1 site/2G single nucleotide polymorphism (ETS site) in the MMP-1 promoter. *European Journal of Biochemistry, 270*(20), 4216–4225.

Trimble, M. S., Xin, J. H., Guy, C. T., Muller, W. J., & Hassell, J. A. (1993). PEA3 is overexpressed in mouse metastatic mammary adenocarcinomas. *Oncogene, 8*(11), 3037–3042.

van Es, J. H., van Gijn, M. E., Riccio, O., van den Born, M., Vooijs, M., Begthel, H., et al. (2005). Notch/gamma-secretase inhibition turns proliferative cells in intestinal crypts and adenomas into goblet cells. *Nature, 435*(7044), 959–963. http://dx.doi.org/10.1038/nature03659.

Vona-Davis, L., Rose, D. P., Hazard, H., Howard-McNatt, M., Adkins, F., Partin, J., et al. (2008). Triple negative breast cancer and obesity in a rural Appalachian population. *Cancer Epidemiology, Biomarkers & Prevention, 17*, 3319–3324.

Wasylyk, B., Hagman, J., & Gutierrez-Hartmann, A. (1998). Ets transcription factors: Nuclear effectors of the Ras-MAP-kinase signaling pathway. *Trends in Biochemical Sciences, 23*(6), 213–216.

Weigelt, B., Baehner, F. L., & Reis-Filho, J. S. (2010). The contribution of gene expression profiling to breast cancer classification, prognostication, and prediction: a retrospective of the last decade. *The Journal of Pathology, 220*, 263–280.

Weijzen, S., Rizzo, P., Braid, M., Vaishnav, R., Jonkheer, S. M., Zlobin, A., et al. (2002). Activation of Notch-1 signaling maintains the neoplastic phenotype in human Ras-transformed cells. *Nature Medicine, 8*(9), 979–986. http://dx.doi.org/10.1038/nm754.

Weng, A. P., Millholland, J. M., Yashiro-Ohtani, Y., Arcangeli, M. L., Lau, A., Wai, C., et al. (2006). c-Myc is an important direct target of Notch1 in T-cell acute lymphoblastic leukemia/lymphoma. *Genes & Development, 20*(15), 2096–2109. http://dx.doi.org/10.1101/gad.1450406.

Wu, L., Aster, J. C., Blacklow, S. C., Lake, R., Artavanis-Tsakonas, S., & Griffin, J. D. (2000). MAML1, a human homologue of Drosophila mastermind, is a transcriptional co-activator for NOTCH receptors. *Nature Genetics, 26*(4), 484–489. http://dx.doi.org/10.1038/82644.

Wu, J., Iwata, F., Grass, J. A., Osborne, C. S., Elnitski, L., Fraser, P., et al. (2005). Molecular determinants of NOTCH4 transcription in vascular endothelium. *Molecular and Cellular Biology, 25*(4), 1458–1474. http://dx.doi.org/10.1128/MCB.25.4.1458-1474.2005.

Xia, W. Y., Lien, H. C., Wang, S. C., Pan, Y., Sahin, A., Kuo, Y. H., et al. (2006). Expression of PEA3 and lack of correlation between PEA3 and HER-2/neu expression in breast cancer. *Breast Cancer Research and Treatment, 98*(3), 295–301. http://dx.doi.org/10.1007/s10549-006-9162-7.

Yamaguchi, N., Oyama, T., Ito, E., Satoh, H., Azuma, S., Hayashi, M., et al. (2008). NOTCH3 signaling pathway plays crucial roles in the proliferation of ErbB2-negative human breast cancer cells. *Cancer Research, 68*(6), 1881–1888. http://dx.doi.org/10.1158/0008-5472.CAN-07-1597.

Yao, K., Rizzo, P., Rajan, P., Albain, K., Rychlik, K., Shah, S., et al. (2011). Notch-1 and notch-4 receptors as prognostic markers in breast cancer. *International Journal of Surgical Pathology, 19*(5), 607–613. http://dx.doi.org/10.1177/1066896910362080.

Yong, S. R., Pilarski, R. T., Donenberg, T., Shapiro, C., Hammond, L. S., Miller, J., et al. (2009). The prevalence of BRCA-1 mutations among young women with triple - negative breast cancer. *BMC Cancer, 9*, 86.

Yen, W., Fischer, M., Lewicki, J., Gurney, A., & Hoey, T. (2009). Targeting cancer stem cells and vasculature by a novel anti-delta-like 4 ligand (DLL4) antibody for treatment of triple negative breast cancer. *Cancer Research, 69*(24) Supplement 3.

Zang, S., Chen, F., Dai, J., Guo, D., Tse, W., Qu, X., et al. (2010). RNAi-mediated knockdown of Notch-1 leads to cell growth inhibition and enhanced chemosensitivity in human breast cancer. *Oncology Reports, 23*(4), 893–899.

CHAPTER TWELVE

ADAM22 as a Prognostic and Therapeutic Drug Target in the Treatment of Endocrine-Resistant Breast Cancer

Jarlath C. Bolger, Leonie S. Young[1]
Endocrine Oncology Research, Royal College of Surgeons in Ireland, Dublin 2, Ireland
[1]Corresponding author: e-mail address: lyoung@rcsi.ie

Contents

Abstract

The development of breast cancer resistance to endocrine therapies may result from an increase in cellular plasticity, permitting the emergence of a hormone-independent tumor. ADAM proteins are multidomain transmembrane proteins that have a diverse array of functions in both natural physiology and disease. A number of ADAM proteins have been implicated in the occurrence of breast cancer, including ADAM 9, ADAM12, ADAM15, ADAM17, ADAM22, and ADAM28. ADAM22 expression is driven by the coactivator protein SRC-1 in response to tamoxifen treatment in the resistant setting. ADAM22 is an ER-independent predictor of disease-free survival. LGI1 is a neuropeptide that binds ADAM22 in the nervous system. In addition to being a ligand for ADAM11, ADAM22, and ADAM23, LGI1 may play a role as a tumor suppressor. Furthermore, LGI1

Vitamins and Hormones, Volume 93
ISSN 0083-6729
http://dx.doi.org/10.1016/B978-0-12-416673-8.00014-9

may act to reduce cell migration and may impair proliferation. Therapies based on LGI1 may provide a building block for future therapies in ADAM22-positive breast cancer.

1. INTRODUCTION

In recent years, ADAM (a disintegrin and metalloproteinase) proteins have proven to be significant players in a number of neoplasia. The ADAMs and related ADAMTS (a disintegrin and metalloproteinase with thrombospondin motifs) proteins belong to the reprolysin family and may play key roles in regulating cell–cell signaling and the interaction of cells with their microenvironment (Murphy, 2008). All ADAMs are multidomain type 1 transmembrane proteins (Murphy, 2008), although soluble splice variants without the transmembrane and cytoplasmic domains have been described in the case of ADAM12 and ADAM33 (Deuss, Reiss, & Hartmann, 2008; Gilpin et al., 1998; Powell, Wicks, Holloway, Holgate, & Davies, 2004). The generalized structure of an ADAM protein consists of eight distinct regions: a signal domain, a prodomain, a metalloproteinase domain, a disintegrin- or integrin-binding domain, a cysteine-rich region, an EGF (epidermal growth factor)-like domain, a transmembrane sequence, and an intracellular C-terminal end (Duffy et al., 2011; Edwards, Handsley, & Pennington, 2008).

Table 12.1 A selection of ADAM proteins are listed with their potential *in vivo* functions in addition to their integrin-binding sites

Protein	Function	Integrin binding
ADAM9	Sheddase, cell migration, differentiation	$\alpha2\beta1$, $\alpha3\beta1$, $\alpha6\beta1$, $\alpha9\beta1$, $\alpha6\beta4$, $\alpha V\beta5$
ADAM12	Sheddase, adipogenesis, myogenesis	$\alpha4\beta1$, $\alpha7\beta1$, $\alpha9\beta1$
ADAM15	Cell–cell interactions	$\alpha4\beta1$, $\alpha5\beta1$, $\alpha9\beta1$, $\alpha V\beta3$
ADAM17	Sheddase, osteoclast recruitment	$\alpha5\beta1$
ADAM19	Sheddase, dendritic cell development	$\alpha4\beta1$, $\alpha5\beta1$
ADAM22	Cell migration, nervous system development	$\alpha6\beta1$, $\alpha9\beta1$, $\alpha V\beta3$
ADAM28	Immune surveillance	$\alpha4\beta1$, $\alpha4\beta7$, $\alpha9\beta1$
ADAM33	Linked to asthma	$\alpha4\beta1$, $\alpha5\beta1$, $\alpha9\beta1$

ADAMs are unique among cell-surface proteins in expressing a disintegrin domain (Blobel et al., 1992), and a number of ADAM disintegrin domains have subsequently been shown to regulate integrin-mediated cell adhesion (Table 12.1). Of the 21 human ADAMs described to date, 13 have intact metalloproteinase domains with the capacity for proteolytic activity (Murphy, 2008). Other mechanisms of biological action for ADAMs include cysteine-rich domains interacting with heparin sulfate proteoglycans which is important in protease-dependent biological responses *in vivo* (Smith et al., 2002), actions as sheddases, and the interactions of ADAM adhesive domains with extracellular matrix proteins including fibronectin and laminin (Gaultier, Cousin, Alfandari, & White, 2002). This chapter focuses on ADAM proteins in breast cancer, specifically on ADAM22. We look at the role of ADAM22 in endocrine-resistant breast cancer and focus on its potential as a biomarker and therapeutic target.

2. ADAM PROTEINS IN BREAST CANCER

A number of ADAM proteins have been identified in neoplastic processes, including brain, gastric, colon, prostate, and ovarian cancers. One of their best described roles, however, is in breast cancer.

ADAM17 has been shown to be an important regulator of mammary gland development and interacts with amphiregulin (AREG) and the epidermal growth factor receptor (EGFR) to regulate duct growth and differentiation (Sternlicht & Sunnarborg, 2008). It has been hypothesized that an aberrant reactivation of the ADAM17–EGFR axis may play a role in breast cancer. It has been shown that knockdown of ADAM17 suppresses AREG release and activity of downstream kinases. Furthermore, removal of ADAM17 from these breast epithelial-derived cells induces a malignant to nonmalignant conversion (Kenny & Bissell, 2007). ADAM17 also has a role in mediating release of membrane-bound proTNFa, thus playing a role in paracrine signaling (Sternlicht & Sunnarborg, 2008). ADAM17 overexpression produces increased migration and invasion in MCF-7 breast cancer cells, with the converse true when ADAM17 is knocked down in MDA-MB-435 cells (McGowan et al., 2008). Clinically, ADAM17 expression has been shown to correlate with high-grade, aggressive tumors and decreased disease-free survival (McGowan et al., 2008).

The ADAM9 family is a subgroup of ADAM proteins which includes ADAM12 and ADAM15. These also plays an active role in cleaving heparin-binding epidermal growth factor, Delta-like 1, a Notch ligand, as well as ADAM10 (Dyczynska et al., 2007; Izumi et al., 1998; Parkin & Harris, 2009; Tousseyn et al., 2009). There are a number of different isoforms of ADAM9 proteins, with some associated with node-positive disease, and some correlating with HER2 expression (O'Shea et al., 2003). Recent work, however, suggests that it may be a secreted form of ADAM9 which is involved in cell motility (Fry & Toker, 2010).

ADAM 12 is also an active metalloproteinase and has been implicated in insulin-like growth factor signaling and in EGFR pathways. There may also be a role for ADAM12 in interacting with integrins and syndecans to influence cell adhesion and cytoskeletal organization (Cao, Kang, & Zolkiewska, 2001). ADAM12 may also act as a signal transmitter itself, mediating cell signaling through its cytoplasmic tail domain which may interact with a number of protein–protein interactions important in intracellular signaling (Kveiborg, Albrechtsen, Couchman, & Wewer, 2008).

ADAM proteins have been implicated in a number of processes linked to cellular adhesion. Many of these are linked to proteolytic processes, solubilizing molecules such as L-selectin, L1-CAM, VCAM1, CD44, E-cadherin, and N-cadherin (Tousseyn, Jorissen, Reiss, & Hartmann, 2006). However, ADAMs may also exert adhesive properties through their noncatalytic disintegrin and cysteine-rich domains. There has been little study to date on the noncatalytic roles of ADAM proteins in cancer. ADAM22, the focus of this chapter, lacks an active metalloproteinase domain, and this chapter approaches it as a nonproteolytic cell surface protein which may be acting through its disintegrin domain.

3. ADAM22 AND BREAST CANCER

3.1. About ADAM22

ADAM22 was first described alongside ADAM23 in human and murine neural tissue, where they were hypothesized to have a role in development of the nervous system (Sagane, Ohya, Hasegawa, & Tanaka, 1998; Sagane, Yamazaki, Mizui, & Tanaka, 1999). ADAM22 and ADAM23 share highly homologous sequences in their extracellular domains, especially in their putative integrin-binding sequences located in the disintegrin domain (Sagane et al., 2005). ADAM22 also has highly conserved cysteine residues and shares certain sequence homology with ADAM2 and ADAM15, which are both known integrin ligands (Zhu et al., 2005).

ADAM22 has a four-leaf clover structure in its ectodomain (Liu, Shim, & He, 2009; Fig. 12.1). This structure may be common across a

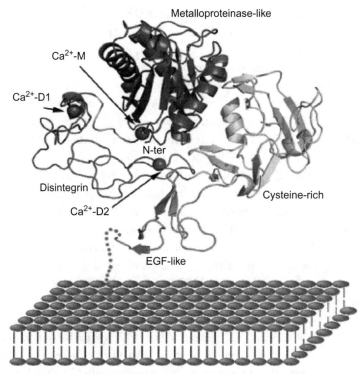

Figure 12.1 Ribbons diagram showing the topology of the ADAM22 ectodomain. The M, D, C, and E domains are shown in blue, magenta, yellow, and cyan, respectively. The three putative calcium ions are colored the same as their host domains. EGF, epidermal growth factor. *Taken from Liu et al. (2009).* (See Color Insert.)

number of ADAM proteins, both catalytic and noncatalytic members of the ADAM family. Binding of catalytic or noncatalytic ADAM proteins to substrates may induce conformational changes allowing either protein cleavage or adhesion functions.

Sagane et al. (2005) showed using a knockout mouse model that although ADAM22 is not essential for embryogenesis, mice lacking functional ADAM22 rapidly developed ataxia and died prematurely. Autopsy analysis showed that although there were no central nervous system abnormalities, there was a significant impairment of myelin formation in the peripheral nervous system. It appears that the mice were dying as a result of repeated convulsive seizures, suggesting a role for ADAM22 in the both central and peripheral nervous system.

Zhu et al. have described a role for ADAM22 in cell adhesion and spreading in conjunction with 14-3-3ζ. 14-3-3 family proteins are highly conserved proteins, ubiquitously expressed in eukaryotic cells. These proteins may operate as adapters, linkers, scaffolds, or coordinators in assembling signaling complexes (Jones, Ley, & Aitken, 1995). 14-3-3 proteins may also be associated with a number of signaling mechanisms including Raf-1, MEKK1, and PI3-kinase (Bonnefoy-Bérard et al., 1995; Fanger et al., 1998; McPherson et al., 1999). The cytoplasmic tail of ADAM22 can interact with 14-3-3ζ and 14-3-3β (Zhu et al., 2002, 2005). It has also been shown that ADAM22 interactions with 14-3-3 cells are crucial for cell adhesion and cell spreading on fibronectin-coated surfaces (Zhu et al., 2005). Although this has been described in an *in vitro* setting, the exact biological significance of these interactions remains unclear.

ADAM22 has been shown to interact with extracellular proteins to alter cellular processes. Leucine-rich, glioma-inactivated 1 (LGI1) has been shown to act as a ligand for ADAM22 and regulate synaptic transmission (Fukata et al., 2006). This demonstrated that LGI1 acted in a postsynaptic manner to regulate synaptic strength at excitatory synapses. The interactions between LGI1 and ADAM22 appear to stabilize AMPAR/stargazin complexes in regulating the strength of these postsynaptic responses. Further studies have shown that LGI-4 may also interact with ADAM22. In addition, LGI1 and LGI-4 may also interact with ADAM11 and ADAM23 at the cell surface (Sagane, Yasushi, & Sugimoto, 2008). Given the considerable structural homology between ADAM22 and ADAM23, this is not an unexpected finding.

3.2. SRC-1 regulates ADAM22 expression in breast cancer

Endocrine therapies such as tamoxifen in the premenopausal population and aromatase inhibitors in the postmenopausal population are the mainstay of treatment for estrogen receptor (ER)-positive tumors. Although many patients initially respond well to endocrine therapy, many will eventually relapse and develop recurrent and metastatic disease. Steroid receptor coactivator 1 (SRC-1) is a member of the p160 family of nuclear receptor coactivator proteins alongside SRC-2 and SRC-3. SRC-1 is an independent predictor of disease-free survival in both tamoxifen-treated and aromatase inhibitor-treated patients (McBryan et al., 2012; Redmond et al., 2009). Patients who develop resistance to endocrine treatments and subsequent disease recurrence show increased interactions between SRC-1 and ERα (Redmond et al., 2009). There is also increasing evidence, however, that SRC-1 may engage in transcriptional regulation independent of ER (McCartan et al., 2012).

ADAM22 has been identified as being transcriptionally regulated by SRC-1 using global sequencing experiments. Chromatin immunoprecipitation sequencing profiled SRC-1 targets in tamoxifen-resistant LY2 cells, which represent a luminal B breast cancer phenotype (McCartan et al., 2012). This identified a high number of functional peaks, in or near the transcriptional start site, the promoter region, or just upstream of the promoter. There was a significant difference in the numbers of peaks identified between the tamoxifen- and vehicle-treated samples. This evidence that tamoxifen may drive SRC-1-dependent gene transcription raises a clinical conundrum: if this observation remains consistent in patient populations, is continuing tamoxifen treatment in the setting of endocrine resistance driving their recurrent disease?

As SRC-1 is a defined ER coactivator, it is to be expected that a large number of SRC-1 peaks should contain an ERE-binding motif. McCartan et al. showed that 43% of the SRC-1 peaks identified contained an ERE. ADAM22 was one of those genes being regulated that did not contain an ERE-binding motif in its peak, raising the possibility that SRC-1-dependent ADAM22 expression may occur independent of ER. It was confirmed that ADAM22 expression is regulated independent of ER using siRNA against ER in cell line models.

ADAM22 regulation was confirmed using siRNA directed against SRC-1 *in vitro*, and *in vivo* using an SRC-1 knockout mouse model. Further bioinformatic analysis of the *ADAM22* promoter identified a potential binding site for the transcription factor Myb. Myb has been implicated in regulating a number of processes involved in cancer cell invasion, metastasis, and epithelial–mesenchymal transition (Cesi et al., 2011; Knopfová et al., 2012). Analysis of cell lines showed that there are increased interactions between SRC-1 and Myb following tamoxifen treatment, suggesting that SRC-1 is regulating ER-independent transcription at least in part through its interaction with Myb (McCartan et al., 2012). ChIP analysis showed that in endocrine-sensitive MCF7 cells, neither SRC-1 nor Myb is recruited to the *ADAM22* promoter, while there was significant recruitment in the resistant LY2 cells. This finding suggests that as breast cancer progresses, cellular adaptability may allow SRC-1 to regulate genes independent of ER.

3.3. ADAM22 predicts poor disease-free survival

SRC-1 has previously been established as a key mediator of disease recurrence in the endocrine-resistant phenotype. ADAM22 localizes to the cell membrane of tumor epithelial cells when expressed in breast cancer and has also been shown to be a strong predictor of disease recurrence in breast cancer patients and is indeed stronger than many classic clinicopathological predictors (Table 12.2; Fig. 12.2). Furthermore, ADAM22 strongly associates with both SRC-1 and poor disease-free survival. There is no relationship between ADAM22 expression and ER status. This supports molecular observations that SRC-1 may be working independent of ER to promote ADAM22 expression.

3.4. ADAM22 expression and tamoxifen treatment

The McCartan et al. paper raises the possibility that ADAM22 expression in endocrine-resistant breast cancer is, in fact, being driven by tamoxifen treatment. This suggests that cellular adaptability in the face of endocrine therapy may alter the expressed phenotype. In xenograft studies, treating endocrine-resistant tumors with tamoxifen may in fact drive tumor growth. As expected when endocrine-sensitive tumors are treated with tamoxifen, there is markedly reduced tumor growth. This was in stark contrast to resistant tumors: those treated with tamoxifen show significantly greater growth than the untreated control group. In addition, the resistant tumors treated with tamoxifen show significantly increased ADAM22 expression. There is no detectable expression of ADAM22 in the endocrine-sensitive

Table 12.2 Odds ratios for disease-free survival for clinicopathological variables in a cohort of 560 breast cancer patients

Predictor	OR	P	95% Confidence interval
ER	0.68	0.242	0.36–1.29
Grade	1.03	0.932	0.55–1.90
T stage	2.33	0.011	1.21–4.47
Nodal status	1.35	0.335	0.73–2.50
Adjuvant chemotherapy	1.18	0.605	0.63–2.22
SRC-1	2.18	0.014	1.17–4.05
ADAM22	2.40	0.005	1.31–4.14

From McCartan et al. (2012).

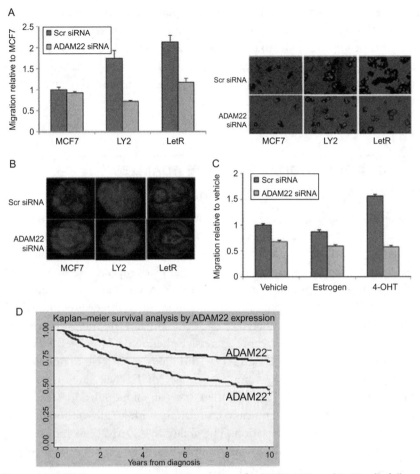

Figure 12.2 (A) Representative migration pattern for MCF7, LY2, and LetR cells follow-ing transient transfection with scrambled (Scr) siRNA or ADAM22 siRNA. Average migra-tion is given as a ratio of scr-siRNA in MCF7 cells. (B) Endocrine-resistant cells (LY2 and LetR) have reduced cellular differentiation as exemplified by their inability to form acni in three-dimensional culture in comparison with endocrine-sensitive MCF7 cells; this was restored by knockdown of ADAM22 with siRNA. (C) Migration in LY2 cells treated with estrogen and tamoxifen following ADAM22 knockdown with siRNA. (D) Kaplan–Meier estimates of disease-free survival according to ADAM22 in patients with breast cancer ($n = 560$; $P < 0.0001$). *Taken from McCartan et al. (2012).* (See Color Insert.)

xenografts (McCartan et al., 2012). This supports the notion that in treat-ment resistance, continuing with an endocrine treatment may be of little benefit and may in fact be driving disease progression. Unfortunately, there is no definitive clinical evidence yet to support this observation. Current protocols suggest that on disease recurrence, an alternative endocrine therapy with or without cytotoxic chemotherapy (depending on the extent of the disease) is the optimal treatment strategy. This approach may need reexamination if further preclinical evidence can support the observation that continued exposure of the tumor to endocrine therapy may drive tumor progression.

4. A FUNCTIONAL ROLE FOR ADAM22
4.1. ADAM22 and differentiation

As a protein which expresses both a cell surface component and a cytoplasmic tail that may interact with the cytoskeleton, there may be a role for ADAM22 in altering cell differentiation through interactions with the tumor microenvironment. Three-dimensional cell cultures allow the *in vitro* assessment of cell differentiation. When endocrine-sensitive cells (MCF7) and two endocrine-resistant cell lines (LY2 and LetR cells) are subjected to three-dimensional cell culture, the both LY2 and LetR cells form disorganized spheres, correlating with their less differentiated, more aggressive phenotype. However, following knockdown of ADAM22 using siRNA, the ability of the cells to polarize and form acinar-type structures, similar to the MCF7 cell line, is restored (McCartan et al., 2012; Fig. 12.2). In the patient population stained for ADAM22, there is no significant correlation with grade, although there was a trend toward an association. The ability to ADAM22 to induce a less differentiated phenotype may warrant further exploration, both on a cellular level and in clinical breast cancer patient populations.

4.2. ADAM22 and cell migration

ADAM proteins have been implicated in cell migration previously, but this is usually as a consequence of their interactions with other cell surface proteins and actions as sheddases. It has been suggested that ADAM22 may play a role in modulating cell migration (McCartan et al., 2012). As cell migration is a process central to the development of metastatic disease, ADAM22 may be influencing disease progression by promoting tumor metastasis.

The ability of breast cancer cell lines to migrate *in vitro* corresponds with the phenotype that represents. Luminal B-type endocrine-resistant cell lines, LY2 and LetR cells, are significantly more migratory at basal levels than the luminal A MCF7 cell line. This corresponds with the expected aggressiveness of these cell lines. Following knockdown of ADAM22 using siRNA, there is significant reduction in the ability of the LY2 and LetR cells to migrate, restoring their migratory pattern to one similar to MCF7s (McCartan et al., 2012; Fig. 12.2). This supports the hypothesis that ADAM22 may modulate aggressive disease by promoting tumor metastasis.

The migration of the resistant LY2 cells depends on tamoxifen treatment. Steroid-depleted cells subsequently treated with estrogen or tamoxifen for 24 h show altered cell migration patterns. Tamoxifen-treated cells are significantly more migratory than either vehicle-treated or estrogen-treated cells. When ADAM22 is knocked down using siRNA, the sensitivity of the cells to tamoxifen was restored, and there is a significant reduction in cellular migration (McCartan et al., 2012). This shows that at an *in vitro* level at least, knocking down ADAM22 may resensitize endocrine-resistant disease to endocrine treatment. This raises the possibility that in patients, if ADAM22 could be effectively inhibited, it may reduce the ability of cells to migrate in addition to helping to ensure patients remain sensitive to endocrine therapies.

5. ADAMs AS THERAPEUTIC TARGETS

5.1. ADAM proteins as therapeutic targets

Early experiences targeting metalloproteinases met with little success, as the inhibitors trialed were nonspecific, leading to ineffectual therapies with poor side-effect profiles (Murphy, 2008). Targeting ADAM proteins in future must focus on the use of agents that selectively target the proneoplastic elements of ADAM proteins. Most work in preclinical studies has focussed on the inhibition of TNFα in rheumatoid arthritis, although no drug has reached the market to date.

Other areas of interest, particularly in cancer, have focussed on the ability of ADAM proteins to modulate ERBB signaling. Early preclinical studies have shown that inhibition of ADAM10 and ADAM17 prevents cleavage of membrane-bound ERBB ligand precursors (Fridman et al., 2007; Kenny & Bissell, 2007). This may offer an effective therapeutic strategy in treating ERBB positive tumors in conjunction with more established inhibitors such as trastuzumab.

The integrin-binding properties of ADAM proteins in cancer have not been studied in great depth to date. However, this potential role in cellular adhesion may offer further therapeutic approaches.

5.2. ADAM22 as a therapeutic target

LGI1 is a neuronal protein that has been shown to be a specific extracellular ligand for ADAM22 in the central nervous system (Fukata et al., 2006). LGI1 may act as tumor suppressor for glioblastoma and neuroblastoma, and it has been shown that LGI1 may play a role in impairing proliferation and survival in HeLa cells (Gabellini & Masola, 2009; Gabellini et al., 2006; Kunapuli, Kasyapa, Hawthorn, & Cowell, 2004). The LGI1–ADAM22 ligand/receptor complex has been suggested as a potential therapeutic target in treating synaptic disorders in the nervous system. This also forms the rationale for targeting ADAM22 with LGI1 in breast cancer. Treatment of endocrine-resistant cells (either tamoxifen or letrozole resistant) with LGI1 significantly reduces cell migration, in line with effects seen following knockdown of ADAM22 with siRNA. Furthermore, this antimigratory effect is in line with the suppression of cell invasion seen in glioma cells following treatment with LGI1 (Kunapuli et al., 2004). LGI1 binds the extracellular domain of ADAM22 and may be functioning by inhibiting the disintegrin domain. It must be stressed, however, that LGI1 may also inhibit other cell surface proteins such as ADAM11 and ADAM23 (Sagane et al., 2008).

Although the specific mechanism of LGI1 inhibition of breast cancer cell migration remains unclear, it is plausible that this is at least in part through the inhibition of ADAM22. Much work remains to determine if LGI1 or its derivatives may form the basis for a viable therapeutic option in targeting ADAM22-positive breast cancer.

6. CONCLUSIONS

ADAM proteins are a biologically diverse group of proteins that play numerous different roles in cell interactions with the surrounding microenvironment. Many ADAM proteins have been implicated in neoplastic processes. Work outlined here shows that ADAM22 may play a role in resistance to endocrine therapy in breast cancer. ADAM22 is a target of the coactivator protein SRC-1 and is regulated in an ER-independent manner. ADAM22 predicts poor disease-free survival and may play a significant functional role: it may functions in cell differentiation and migration. Furthermore, inhibition of ADAM22 may be advantageous in restoring sensitivity of cells to endocrine treatment in addition to reducing the metastatic potential of breast tumors. Although much work remains to be done,

ADAM22 offers exciting potential as a novel biomarker and therapeutic target in endocrine-resistant breast cancer.

REFERENCES

Blobel, C. P., Wolfsberg, T. G., Turck, C. W., Myles, D. G., Primakoff, P., & White, J. M. (1992). A potential fusion peptide and an integrin ligand domain in a protein active in sperm-egg fusion. *Nature, 356,* 248–252.

Bonnefoy-Bérard, N., Liu, Y. C., von Willebrand, M., Sung, A., Elly, C., Mustelin, T., et al. (1995). Inhibition of phosphatidylinositol 3-kinase activity by association with 14–3–3 proteins in T cells. *Proceedings of the National Academy of Sciences United States of America, 92*(22), 10142–10146.

Cao, Y., Kang, Q., & Zolkiewska, A. (2001). Metalloprotease-disintegrin ADAM 12 interacts with alpha-actinin-1. *The Biochemical Journal, 357*(Pt 2), 353–361.

Cesi, V., Casciati, A., Sesti, F., Tanno, B., Calabretta, B., & Raschellà, G. (2011). TGFβ-induced c-Myb affects the expression of EMT-associated genes and promotes invasion of ER+ breast cancer cells. *Cell Cycle, 10*(23), 4149–4161.

Deuss, M., Reiss, K., & Hartmann, D. (2008). Part-time α-secretases: The functional biology of ADAM 9, 10 and 17. *Current Alzheimer Research, 5,* 187–201.

Duffy, M. J., Mullooly, M., O'Donovan, N., Sukor, S., Crown, J., Pierce, A., et al. (2011). The ADAMs family of proteases: New biomarkers and therapeutic targets for cancer? *Clinical Proteomics, 9,* 8–9.

Dyczynska, E., Sun, D., Yi, H., Sehara-Fujisawa, A., Blobel, C. P., & Zolkiewska, A. (2007). Proteolytic processing of delta-like 1 by ADAM proteases. *The Journal of Biological Chemistry, 282*(1), 436–444.

Edwards, D. R., Handsley, M. M., & Pennington, C. J. (2008). The ADAM metalloproteinases. *Molecular Aspects of Medicine, 29,* 258–259.

Fanger, G. R., Widmann, C., Porter, A. C., Sather, S., Johnson, G. L., Vaillancourt, R. R. (1998). 14–3–3 proteins interact with specific MEK kinases. *Journal of Biological Chemistry, 273*(6), 3476–3483.

Fridman, J. S., Caulder, E., Hansbury, M., Liu, X., Yang, G., Wang, Q., et al. (2007). Selective inhibition of ADAM metalloproteases as a novel approach for modulating ErbB pathways in cancer. *Clinical Cancer Research, 13*(6), 1892–1902.

Fry, J. L., & Toker, A. (2010). Secreted and membrane-bound isoforms of protease ADAM9 have opposing effects on breast cancer cell migration. *Cancer Research, 70*(20), 8187–8198.

Fukata, Y., Adesnik, H., Iwanaga, T., Bredt, D. S., Nicoll, R. A., & Fukata, M. (2006). Epilepsy-related ligand/receptor complex LGI1 and ADAM22 regulate synaptic transmission. *Science, 313*(5794), 1792–1795.

Gabellini, N., & Masola, V. (2009). Expression of LGI1 impairs proliferation and survival of HeLa cells. *International Journal of Cell Biology, 2009,* 417197.

Gabellini, N., Masola, V., Quartesan, S., Oselladore, B., Nobile, C., Michelucci, R., et al. (2006). Increased expression of LGI1 gene triggers growth inhibition and apoptosis of neuroblastoma cells. *Journal of Cellular Physiology, 207,* 711–721.

Gaultier, A., Cousin, H., Alfandari, D., & White, J. M. (2002). ADAM13 disintegrin and cysteine-rich domains bind to the second heparin-binding domain of fibronectin. *The Journal of Biological Chemistry, 277,* 23336–23344.

Gilpin, B. J., Loechel, F., Mattei, M. G., Engvall, E., Albrechtsen, R., & Wewer, U. M. (1998). A novel secreted form of human ADAM12 (Meltrin a) provokes myogenesis in vivo. *The Journal of Biological Chemistry, 273,* 157–166.

Izumi, Y., Hirata, M., Hasuwa, H., Iwamoto, R., Umata, T., Miyado, K., et al. (1998). A metalloprotease-disintegrin, MDC9/meltrin-gamma/ADAM9 and PKCdelta are involved in TPA-induced ectodomain shedding of membrane-anchored heparin-binding EGF-like growth factor. *The EMBO Journal*, *17*(24), 7260–7272.

Jones, D. H., Ley, S., & Aitken, A. (1995). Isoforms of 14-3-3 protein can form homo- and heterodimers *in vivo* and *in vitro*: Implications for function as adapter proteins. *FEBS Letters*, *368*, 55–58.

Kenny, P. A., & Bissell, M. J. (2007). Targeting TACE-dependent EGFR ligand shedding in breast cancer. *The Journal of Clinical Investigation*, *117*(2), 337–345.

Knopfová, L., Beneš, P., Pekarčíková, L., Hermanová, M., Masařík, M., Pernicová, Z., et al. (2012). c-Myb regulates matrix metalloproteinases 1/9, and cathepsin D: Implications for matrix-dependent breast cancer cell invasion and metastasis. *Molecular Cancer*, *11*, 15.

Kunapuli, P., Kasyapa, C. S., Hawthorn, L., & Cowell, J. K. (2004). LGI1, a putative tumour metastasis suppressor gene, controls *in vitro* invasiveness and expression of matrix metalloproteinase in glioma cells through the ERK1/2 pathway. *The Journal of Biological Chemistry*, *279*, 23151–23157.

Kveiborg, M., Albrechtsen, R., Couchman, J. R., & Wewer, U. M. (2008). Cellular roles of ADAM12 in health and disease. *The International Journal of Biochemistry & Cell Biology*, *40*(9), 1685–1702.

Liu, H., Shim, A. H., & He, X. (2009). Structural characterization of the ectodomain of a disintegrin and metalloproteinase-22 (ADAM22), a neural adhesion receptor instead of metalloproteinase: Insights on ADAM function. *The Journal of Biological Chemistry*, *284*(42), 29077–29086.

McBryan, J., Theissen, S. M., Byrne, C., Hughes, E., Cocchiglia, S., Sande, S., et al. (2012). Metastatic progression with resistance to aromatase inhibitors is driven by the steroid receptor coactivator SRC-1. *Cancer Research*, *72*(2), 548–559.

McCartan, D., Bolger, J. C., Fagan, A., Byrne, C., Hao, Y., Qin, L., et al. (2012). Global characterization of the SRC-1 transcriptome identifies ADAM22 as an ER-independent mediator of endocrine-resistant breast cancer. *Cancer Research*, *72*(1), 220–229.

McGowan, P. M., McKiernan, E., Bolster, F., Ryan, B. M., Hill, A. D., McDermott, E. W., et al. (2008). ADAM-17 predicts adverse outcome in patients with breast cancer. *Annals of Oncology*, *19*(6), 1075–1081.

McPherson, R. A., Harding, A., Roy, S., Lane, A., & Hancock, J. F. (1999). Interactions of c-Raf-1 with phosphatidylserine and 14-3-3. *Oncogene*, *18*(26), 3862–3869.

Murphy, G. (2008). The ADAMs: Signalling scissors in the tumour microenvironment. *Nature Reviews. Cancer*, *8*(12), 929–941.

O'Shea, C., McKie, N., Buggy, Y., Duggan, C., Hill, A. D., McDermott, E., et al. (2003). Expression of ADAM-9 mRNA and protein in human breast cancer. *International Journal of Cancer*, *105*(6), 754–761.

Parkin, E., & Harris, B. (2009). A disintegrin and metalloproteinase (ADAM)-mediated ectodomain shedding of ADAM10. *Journal of Neurochemistry*, *108*(6), 1464–1479.

Powell, R. M., Wicks, J., Holloway, J. W., Holgate, S. T., & Davies, D. E. (2004). The splicing and fate of ADAM33 transcripts in primary human airway fibroblasts. *American Journal of Respiratory Cell and Molecular Biology*, *31*, 13–21.

Redmond, A. M., Bane, F. T., Stafford, A. T., McIlroy, M., Dillon, M. F., Crotty, T. B., et al. (2009). Coassociation of estrogen receptor and p160 proteins predicts resistance to endocrine treatment; SRC-1 is an independent predictor of breast cancer recurrence. *Clinical Cancer Research*, *15*(6), 2098–2106.

Sagane, K., Hayakawa, K., Kai, J., Hirohashi, T., Takahashi, E., Miyamoto, N., et al. (2005). Ataxia and peripheral nerve hypomyelination in ADAM22-deficient mice. *BMC Neuroscience*, *6*, 33.

Sagane, K., Ohya, Y., Hasegawa, Y., & Tanaka, I. (1998). Metalloproteinase-like, disintegrin-like, cysteine-rich proteins MDC2 and MDC3: Novel human cellular disintegrins highly expressed in the brain. *The Biochemical Journal, 334*(Pt 1), 93–98.

Sagane, K., Yamazaki, K., Mizui, Y., & Tanaka, I. (1999). Cloning and chromosomal mapping of mouse ADAM11, ADAM22 and ADAM23. *Gene, 236*(1), 79–86.

Sagane, K., Yasushi, Y., & Sugimoto, H. (2008). LGI1 and LGI4 bind to ADAM22, ADAM23 and ADAM11. *International Journal of Biological Sciences, 4,* 387–396.

Smith, K. M., Gaultier, A., Cousin, H., Alfandari, D., White, J. M., & DeSimone, D. W. (2002). The cysteine-rich domain regulates ADAM protease function in vivo. *The Journal of Cell Biology, 159,* 893–902.

Sternlicht, M. D., & Sunnarborg, S. W. (2008). The ADAM17-amphiregulin-EGFR axis in mammary development and cancer. *Journal of Mammary Gland Biology and Neoplasia, 13*(2), 181–194.

Tousseyn, T., Jorissen, E., Reiss, K., & Hartmann, D. (2006). Make stick and cut loose–disintegrin metalloproteases in development and disease. *Birth Defects Research. Part C, Embryo Today: Review, 78*(1), 24–46.

Tousseyn, T., Thathiah, A., Jorissen, E., Raemaekers, T., Konietzko, U., Reiss, K., et al. (2009). ADAM10, the rate-limiting protease of regulated intramembrane proteolysis of Notch and other proteins, is processed by ADAMS-9, ADAMS-15, and the gamma-secretase. *The Journal of Biological Chemistry, 284*(17), 11738–11747.

Zhu, P., Sang, Y., Xu, R., Zhao, J., Li, C., & Zhao, S. (2002). The interaction between ADAM22 and 14-3-3beta. *Science in China. Series C, Life Sciences, 45*(6), 577–582.

Zhu, P., Sang, Y., Xu, H., Zhao, J., Xu, R., Sun, Y., et al. (2005). ADAM22 plays an important role in cell adhesion and spreading with the assistance of 14-3-3. *Biochemical and Biophysical Research Communications, 331*(4), 938–946.

CHAPTER THIRTEEN

Alpha-Actinin 4 and Tumorigenesis of Breast Cancer

Kuo-Sheng Hsu, Hung-Ying Kao[1]

Department of Biochemistry, School of Medicine, Case Western Reserve University (CWRU),
The Comprehensive Cancer Center of CWRU, Cleveland, Ohio, USA
[1]Corresponding author: e-mail address: hxk43@cwru.edu

Contents

Abstract

Alpha-actinins (ACTNs) were originally identified as cytoskeletal proteins which cross-link filamentous actin to establish cytoskeletal architect that protects cells from mechanical stress and controls cell movement. Notably, unlike other ACTNs, alpha-actinin 4 (ACTN4) displays unique characteristics in signaling transduction, nuclear translocation, and gene expression regulation. Initial reports indicated that ACTN4 is part of the breast cancer cell motile apparatus and is highly expressed in the nucleus. These results imply that ACTN4 plays a role in breast cancer tumorigenesis. While several observations in breast cancer and other cancers support this hypothesis, little direct evidence links the tumorigenic phenotype with ACTN4-mediated pathological mechanisms. Recently, several studies have demonstrated that in addition to its role in coordinating cytoskeleton, ACTN4 interacts with signaling mediators, chromatin remodeling factors, and transcription factors including nuclear receptors. Thus, ACTN4 functions as a versatile promoter for breast cancer tumorigenesis and appears to be an ideal drug target for future therapeutic development.

1. INTRODUCTION

Alpha-actinins (ACTNs) are ubiquitously expressed proteins known to be cross-linked with filamentous actin (F-actin) to maintain cytoskeletal integrity and to control cell movement (Sjöblom, Salmazo, & Djinović-Carugo, 2008). ACTNs localize to cell–cell and cell–matrix contact sites, cellular protrusions, and stress fiber-dense regions and regulate diverse signaling pathways by linking membrane receptors with the cytoskeleton (Edlund, Lotano, & Otey, 2001; Otey & Carpen, 2004; Pavalko, Otey, Simon, & Burridge, 1991). Four ACTN family members, numbered 1–4, are present in humans (Beggs et al., 1992; Honda et al., 1998) and highly conserved in other mammals (Arimura et al., 1988; Fyrberg, Kelly, Ball, Fyrberg, & Reedy, 1990). ACTNs can be categorized as "muscle" or "non-muscle" due to their tissue-specific function and expression patterns (Oikonomou, Zachou, & Dalekos, 2011). ACTN2 and ACTN3 are muscle specific and are major components of contractile machinery connecting with actin filaments at Z lines in striated muscles or at dense bodies in smooth muscle cells (Mills et al., 2001). In contrast, ACTN1 and alpha-actinin 4 (ACTN4) are ubiquitously expressed. ACTN1 and ACTN4 share 80% and about 90% similarity in nucleotide and amino acid sequence, respectively (Honda et al., 1998). Despite the high level of similarity in their protein sequences, ACTN1 and ACTN4 are found in different subcellular compartments and are function distinct (Honda et al., 1998; Quick & Skalli, 2010). ACTN1 localizes with stress fibers and is present in adherent junctions, suggesting a major function in cytoskeleton regulation. By contrast, ACTN4 is more widely distributed in the cell compared to ACTN1 (Honda et al., 1998). In addition to stress fibers, ACTN4 is found in membrane ruffles and inhibition of PI3 kinase (PI3K) promotes ACTN4 nuclear translocation in breast cancer and several cancer cell lines (Araki, Hatae, Yamada, & Hirohashi, 2000; Honda et al., 1998). These observations strongly implicate ACTN4 as a mediator of signal transduction and a regulator of gene expression. Indeed, histological analyses of cancer tissues show a strong correlation between ACTN4 expression and tumorigenesis in several types of cancers, though the detailed mechanism is still elusive (Honda et al., 2005; Welsch et al., 2009; Yamamoto et al., 2007). It was demonstrated that ACTN4 functions as a transcriptional coactivator of nuclear receptors and interacts with other DNA binding transcription factors (Fig. 13.2; Babakov et al., 2008; Hayashida et al., 2005; Jasavala et al., 2007; Khurana, Chakraborty, Cheng, Su, & Kao, 2011; Khurana et al., 2012). Additionally, elevated expression of ACTN4 in cancer cells has been suggested as a biomarker for malignant cell invasion and drug resistance (Fellenberg, Dechant, Ewerbeck, & Mau, 2003; He et al., 2011; Kikuchi et al., 2008; Zhou et al., 2012). In this chapter, we focus on the function of ACTN4 in intracellular signal transduction, especially related to breast cancer tumorigenesis.

2. OVERVIEW OF ACTNs

2.1. The evolutionarily conserved domain organization

All four ACTN family members, ACTN1–4, share a similar structural organization and are known to cross-link F-actin to maintain cell morphology and control cell movement (Otey & Carpen, 2004). The first member of ACTN, ACTN1, was identified 40 years ago because of its abundance in the striated muscle contractile apparatus (Maruyama & Ebashi, 1965). In humans, ACTN2 is preferentially expressed in cardiac and oxidative muscle fiber with some expression in brain, while ACTN3 is mainly detected in type II (fast) muscle fibers (Mills et al., 2001). In contrast, ACTN1 and ACTN4 are ubiquitously expressed with distinct tissue expression patterns, subcellular localizations, and biological functions from the muscle ACTNs (Edlund et al., 2001; Honda et al., 1998; Otey & Carpen, 2004). Although the major biological functions of muscle and nonmuscle ACTNs are different, their overall functional domain organization and F-actin attachment characteristics are conserved (Sheterline, Clayton, & Sparrow, 1995). The full-length protein structure has not been solved, but a schematic depiction of ACTNs can be created based on known structures of the individual domains (Fig. 13.1A; Atkinson et al., 2001; Djinović-Carugo, Young, Gautel, & Saraste, 1999; Franzot, Sjöblom, Gautel, & Djinović Carugo, 2005; Sjöblom et al., 2008; Tang, Taylor, & Taylor, 2001). Each ACTN is composed of three major structural domains, an N-terminal calponin-homology (CH) repeat, a central region consisting of four spectrin repeats (SR), followed by a C-terminal calmodulin (CaM)-like domain consisting of two EF-hand motifs (Sjöblom et al., 2008). The functional F-actin-associated ACTN unit is composed of two antiparallel 90° twisted single

A

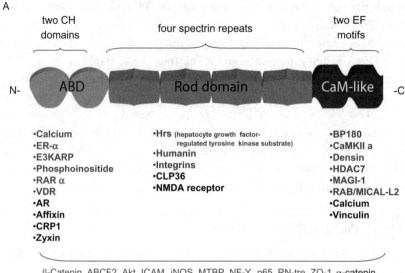

two CH domains

four spectrin repeats

two EF motifs

N-   ABD   Rod domain   CaM-like   -C

•Calcium
•ER-α
•E3KARP
•Phosphoinositide
•RAR α
•VDR
•AR
•Affixin
•CRP1
•Zyxin

•Hrs (hepatocyte growth factor-
      regulated tyrosine kinase substrate)
•Humanin
•Integrins
•CLP36
•NMDA receptor

•BP180
•CaMKII a
•Densin
•HDAC7
•MAGI-1
•RAB/MICAL-L2
•Calcium
•Vinculin

β-Catenin, ABCF2, Akt, ICAM, iNOS, MTBP, NF-Y, p65, RN-tre, ZO-1, α-catenin, A2A, ADAM12, ADIP, PI3K, FAK, Gp1b-IX, L-selectin, MEKK1, Palladin, Rabphilin 3A, Syndecan 4

B

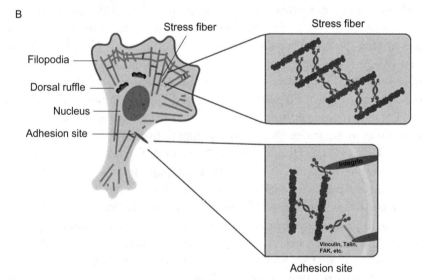

Filopodia
Dorsal ruffle
Nucleus
Adhesion site

Stress fiber
Stress fiber

Integrin

Vinculin, Talin, FAK, etc.

Adhesion site

Figure 13.1 (A) A schematic representation of the structural domains of ACTN. The N-terminal CH repeat constitutes a functional actin-binding domain (ABD), which can also bind to phosphoinositide and calcium. Following the ABD, four SRs form a rod-shaped structure that connects to the EF motif-integrated CaM-like domain. A list of ACTN binding partners is also shown under the corresponding domains. Among these binding partners, the proteins annotated in red are validated ACTN4 binding partners. Shown at the bottom are ACTN binding partners of which the interaction domains were not mapped. (B) A cartoon depicting a moving cell demonstrating the detailed localization of ACTN4 in stress fiber and adhesion sites. F-actin is shown in green and ACTN4

peptides (Ylänne, Scheffzek, Young, & Saraste, 2001). Actin-binding domain (ABD) at both ends can bind F-actin. The middle SR domain links the N-terminal ABD domain and C-terminal CaM-like domain to build a complete rod-shaped molecule by two mediate flexible neck structures (Atkinson et al., 2001; Djinovic-Carugo, Gautel, Ylänne, & Young, 2002; Djinović-Carugo et al., 1999; Franzot et al., 2005; Sjöblom et al., 2008). The SR domain typically consists of four SR motifs, named after their homology to the actin-binding spectrin family (Djinovic-Carugo et al., 2002). These provide structural elasticity and mechanical strength for ACTNs (Kusunoki, MacDonald, & Mondragón, 2004; Otey & Carpen, 2004). In addition to its physical function in cytoskeletal architecture, the SR repeats also serve as a protein–protein interaction platform and provide ACTN member-specific functions in signal transduction (Oikonomou et al., 2011; Trulsson et al., 2011; Ylänne et al., 2001). Notably, the conserved negatively charged surface of the ACTN rod has the potential to interact with membrane phospholipids and the cytoplasmic domains of various transmembrane receptors (Fig. 13.1A; Fraley, Pereira, Tran, Singleton, & Greenwood, 2005; Fukami, Sawada, Endo, & Takenawa, 1996; Otey, Pavalko, & Burridge, 1990; Ylänne et al., 2001).

2.2. Tissue expression and subcellular distribution

In muscle cells, ACTN2 and ACTN3 are predominantly localized in sarcomeric Z-discs (Masaki, Endo, & Ebashi, 1967). They bind F-actin filaments and interact with sarcomeric proteins to cross-link adjacent sarcomeres and maintain the overall cytoskeletal organization during muscle contraction (Squire, 1997). In contrast, nonmuscle ACTN1 and ACTN4 are widely expressed. ACTN4 is expressed at a lower level than ACTN1 in most nonmuscle cells with the exception of kidney cells (Oikonomou et al., 2011). Interestingly, ACTN4 expression is higher in motile cells than in static cells (Araki et al., 2000; Honda et al., 1998). In general, both ACTN1 and ACTN4 localize in stress fibers and focal adhesions. In stress fiber, nonmuscle ACTNs cross-link with F-actin to organize filamentous frame networks which provide a mechanical platform in maintaining cell

---

is shown as a brown line or a twisted cherry-like shape. Inside the cells, ACTN4 cross-links with F-actin to form stress fibers or locates in other motile apparatus components or in the nucleus. Close to the focal adhesion sites, ACTN4 directly links integrins with F-actin or other adhesion molecules, such as vinculin or talin. (See Color Insert.)

shape (Fig. 13.1B; Edlund et al., 2001; Pavalko & Burridge, 1991). In focal adhesion sites, the rod-shaped ACTNs cooperate with membrane-associated cytoskeletal proteins including vinculin, talin, tensin, and zyxin to link actin filaments with membrane-bound integrin receptors (Otey & Carpen, 2004; Pavalko et al., 1991, 1995). Although ACTN1 and ACTN4 share approximately 80% and 86% similarity in DNA and protein sequence, respectively, they exhibit different characteristics and functions (Honda et al., 1998). For example, ACTN4 harbors fewer calcium (Ca^{2+})-binding motifs than ACTN1 and hence the interaction between ACTN1 and F-actin is more sensitive to Ca^{2+} (Imamura et al., 1994; Nikolopoulos et al., 2000). Additionally, although both ACTN1 and ACTN4 localize in stress fibers and focal contacts, ACTN1 is concentrated in adhesion junctions, whereas ACTN4 predominantly accumulates at dorsal circular ruffles and also can be found in the nucleus (Fig. 13.1B; Araki et al., 2000; Honda et al., 1998; Knudsen, Soler, Johnson, & Wheelock, 1995). This suggests that these two nonmuscle ACTNs may function in distinct signaling and cellular processes.

2.3. ACTN4 regulation and function

The subcellular distribution and binding partners of ACTN1 and ACTN4 strongly suggest that they link signaling and gene regulation to cell movement, the cell cycle, and cell proliferation (Honda et al., 1998; Khurana et al., 2011; Kumeta, Yoshimura, Harata, & Takeyasu, 2010; Otey & Carpen, 2004). The activity of nonmuscle ACTNs is controlled by four major mechanisms, processing by calpain protease, phosphorylation by kinases, binding to phosphatidylinositol intermediates, and Ca^{2+} binding (Otey & Carpen, 2004).

Calpain, a Ca^{2+}-sensitive protease, predominantly localizes in focal adhesions where it cleaves various focal adhesion proteins, including ACTNs (Carragher, Fincham, Riley, & Frame, 2001; Carragher, Levkau, Ross, & Raines, 1999; Sprague, Fraley, Jang, Lal, & Greenwood, 2008). The calpain-mediated ACTN proteolysis has been implicated in focal contact protein disassembly, which triggers sequential rear adhesion detachment for cell migration (Dourdin et al., 2001; Laukaitis, Webb, Donais, & Horwitz, 2001). Several kinases, including tyrosine receptor kinases and cytoplasmic serine/threonine kinases, interact with ACTNs and phosphorylate it at different sites for various functions (Sjöblom et al., 2008). MEKK1 colocalizes with and binds to ACTNs in stress fibers and focal adhesions to facilitate calpain-mediated ACTNs proteolysis (Christerson, Vanderbilt, & Cobb, 1999; Cuevas et al., 2003). The regulatory subunit of PI3K, p85, also directly binds to ACTNs (Shibasaki, Fukami, Fukui, & Takenawa, 1994). Instead of direct targeting, activated PI3K disrupts ACTN:actin and ACTN:integrin interactions and promotes cytoskeletal remodeling (Fraley et al., 2005; Greenwood, Theibert, Prestwich, & Murphy-Ullrich, 2000). Furthermore, the PI3K downstream kinase, Akt, also interacts with ACTN4 (Ding et al., 2006; Vandermoere et al., 2007). This interaction is required for Akt activation and Akt-mediated cell survival through recruiting Akt to membrane ruffles (Fig. 13.2; Ding et al., 2006). In addition to serine/threonine kinases, integrin-activated focal adhesion kinase (FAK) phosphorylates Y12 on the ABD of ACTN, thereby reducing its affinity with F-actin (Izaguirre et al., 2001). Moreover, phosphorylation of ACTN4 at Y4 and Y31 by an epithelial growth factor (EGF) downstream kinase also reduces ACTN4:F-actin interaction (Fig. 13.2; Shao, Wu, & Wells, 2010). These observations indicate that extracellular signals are capable of regulating cytoskeletal architect by modulating ACTN4:F-actin interaction.

Two intracellular secondary messengers, phosphatidylinositol and Ca^{2+}, bind to ACTN4 via the ABD and EF-hand motifs, respectively (Fukami et al., 1996; Nikolopoulos et al., 2000). Binding of phosphatidylinositol 3,4,5-trisphosphate (PIP3) or phosphatidylinositol 4,5-diphosphate (PIP2) also regulates the susceptibility of ACTNs to calpain-1 and -2-mediated proteolysis (Sprague et al., 2008). However, binding of Ca^{2+} to ACTN4 blocks its actin-binding activity. Differential Ca^{2+} sensitivity between ACTN1 and ACTN4 may play a role in tuning ACTN-mediated cytoskeleton organization (Nikolopoulos et al., 2000). Increasing PIP3 production by PDGF-activated PI3K blocks the ACTN4:integrin interaction, thereby disassembling focal adhesion structures (Greenwood et al., 2000). A further study suggested that the abundant PIP2 functions as a regulator to control the dynamics of ACTN:F-actin interaction. However, PI3K transiently produces PIP3 and regulates local ACTN:integrin binding, hence facilitating reorganization of focal adhesions (Fraley et al., 2005; Greenwood et al., 2000).

In addition to its well-established cytoplasmic function, ACTN4 is also found in the nucleus in some types of cells (Honda et al., 1998). Notably, inhibition of PI3K or depolymerization of actin filaments promotes ACTN4 nuclear accumulation, indicating that cytoplasmic signaling controls ACTN4 nuclear translocation and function. In tumor necrosis factor alpha (TNF-α) and EGF-treated epithelial carcinoma, the nuclear translocation of

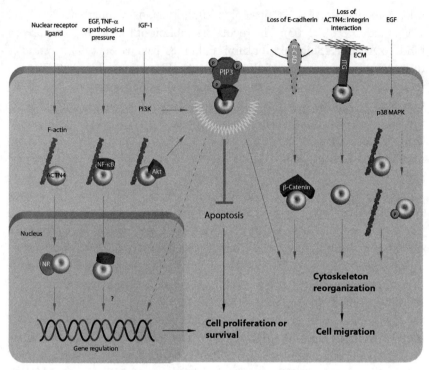

Figure 13.2 A summary of key ACTN4-associated oncogenic pathways. In the nucleus, ACTN4 functions as a transcriptional coactivator to potentiate expression of nuclear receptor target genes, some of which promote cancer cell proliferation and survival. ACTN4 also interacts with NF-κB and chromatin remodeling factors, but the functional significance of these associations is currently not clear. In the cytosol, activated PI3K induces an association between ACTN4, Akt, and PIP3. Once anchored to PIP3, Akt is activated, thereby inhibiting apoptosis and promoting cell proliferation and migration. As a cytoskeletal protein, the interactions of ACTN4 and its cytoskeletal binding partners are subject to regulation by several signals. For example, loss of E-cadherin in colorectal cancer results in an increase in an ACTN4:β catenin interaction which subsequently facilitates cytoskeletal reorganization and cancer cell migration. Similarly, disruption of the ACTN4:integrin or ACTN4:F-actin interactions results in acceleration of cytoskeletal reorganization and subsequent increases in cell migration. (See Color Insert.)

ACTN4 occurs with NF-κB, although the biological significance of this interaction remains elusive (Fig. 13.2; Babakov et al., 2008). Recently, Kumeta et al. (2010) found that the central SR domain of ACTN4 facilitates its nuclear translocation through the nuclear pore complex, whereas the chromosome region maintenance-1 promotes ACTN4 nuclear export. The distribution of cytoplasmic and nuclear ACTN4 is altered during cell cycle progression (Kumeta et al., 2010). In the nucleus, ACTN4 interacts with the INO80 complex and the rRNA transcriptional machinery to regulate a subset cell cycle-related genes (Kumeta et al., 2010). This suggests that ACTN4 also plays a role in cell cycle progression. In addition, ACTN4 is capable of interacting and cooperating with nuclear receptors, including vitamin D receptor, retinoic acid receptor alpha, estrogen receptor alpha (ER-α), and androgen receptor (AR) (Fig. 13.1A; Jasavala et al., 2007; Khurana et al., 2011, 2012).

3. THE FUNCTION OF ACTN4 IN BREAST CANCER

Breast cancer is a complex disease because it can be genetically heterogeneous and contains a variety of cell types. For a number of years, breast cancer researchers have tried to categorize these diverse tumors into different classes and identify distinct biomarkers in each subtype for clinical prognosis and therapeutic targets. Based on their responses to hormones and receptor status, breast cancer can be broadly classified into four major subtypes: (1) luminal A and (2) B breast cancer subtypes that are estrogen receptor (ER)-positive but distinct from different genetic mutation backgrounds; (3) human epidermal growth factor receptor 2 (HER2)-positive breast cancer; (4) basal-like breast cancer that is ER-, HER2-, and progesterone receptor (PR)-triple negative (Perou et al., 2000). Based on this molecular portrait of breast cancer and subsequent studies (Brenton, Carey, Ahmed, & Caldas, 2005; Kao et al., 2009; Perou et al., 2000), ER and HER2 have been considered the two major therapeutic targets for the treatment of breast cancer. The former is a hormone-responsive nuclear receptor that regulates specific genes involved in mammary cell proliferation and survival. Upon estrogen binding to ER in the cytoplasm, it translocates to the nucleus where it binds DNA sequence called estrogen response elements. This ligand-bound ER then recruits coregulators to turn on or off the expression of genes that promote mammary cell differentiation and proliferation. HER2 is a membrane-bound tyrosine kinase receptor possessing mitogenic activity that promotes mammary cell proliferation. Notably, ACTN4 has been shown to potentiate ER transcription activity (Khurana et al., 2011), while the HER2 activator, EGF, is known to modulate ACTN4 function (Shao, Wu, et al., 2010).

ACTN4 was first discovered based on its association with cell motility and breast cancer invasion (Honda et al., 1998). The same report showed that ACTN4 is ubiquitously expressed and was found in virtually every carcinoma they examined (Honda et al., 1998), suggesting that ACTN4 may play an important role in tumorigenesis. In contrast to ACTN1 localization, ACTN4 not only colocalizes in stress fibers but also is dispersed in the cytoplasm and the nucleus in fibroblasts (Fig. 13.1B; Honda et al., 1998). In some cancer cells that lack stress fibers, ACTN4 is distributed in the cytoplasm and accumulates at the edge of cell extended filopodia (Honda et al., 1998). Furthermore, β-catenin, a key oncogenic protein in colorectal cancer tumorigenesis, can bind ACTN4 and their colocalization in cytoplasm is elevated in the infiltrative colorectal cancer (Hayashida et al., 2005). The location, the expression pattern, and the ability of ACTN4 to enhance cell movement imply a function in cancer cell migration and metastasis. Importantly, ACTN4 was found exclusively in the nucleus of several breast and other cancer cell lines (Honda et al., 1998). Nuclear ACTN4 is regulated by PI3K and its abundance in the nucleus correlates with the malignant grade of breast cancer. Indeed, Khurana et al. demonstrated that ACTN4 is a transcriptional coactivator of ER-α, a critical nuclear hormone receptor in breast cancer tumorigenesis (Khurana et al., 2011). Since ACTN4 has a dual function in regulating gene expression and cytoskeletal organization, in this section, we will discuss the detailed mechanisms by which ACTN4 is regulated in breast cancer cells and how it promotes breast cancer proliferation and metastasis, respectively (Fig. 13.2).

3.1. ACTN4 promotes breast cancer proliferation

3.1.1 ACTN4 is a transcriptional coactivator of ER-α

The early observation that ACTN4 was also found in the nucleus of breast cancer cells suggested a role of ACTN4 in the nucleus. The first evidence that ACTN4 plays a role in transcriptional regulation was suggested by the findings that ACTN4 interacts with class II histone deacetylases (HDACs) and myocyte enhancer factor 2s (MEF2s) and functions as a coactivator for MEF2s (Chakraborty et al., 2006). Through sequence analyses, Khurana et al. further demonstrated that ACTN4 harbors a functional nuclear receptor interacting motif (or NR box), LXXLL, within its CH1 domain (Khurana et al., 2011). The ability of ACTN4 to activate ER-α reporter activity and ER-α target gene expression depends on the NR box. In ER-α positive MCF-7 breast cancer cells, estradiol (E2) promotes recruitment of ACTN4 to the promoter of *pS2*, an ER-α target gene (Khurana et al., 2011).

The fact that ACTN4 regulates ER-α-mediated transcriptional activation suggested that ACTN4 may also play a role in E2-mediated regulation of cell proliferation. Indeed, knockdown of ACTN4 in MCF-7 breast cancer cells significantly decreased E2-mediated induction of ER-α target genes, such as *pS2* and *PR*, and abolished estrogen-mediated cancer cell proliferation (Khurana et al., 2011). Therefore, at least in some breast cancer subtypes, ACTN4 functions as a transcriptional coactivator to potentiate ER-α-mediated gene expression and cell proliferation. Together, these findings established a critical role of ACTN4 in transcriptional regulation and cell proliferation by ER-α.

3.1.2 Histone deacetylase 7 (HDAC7) and ACTN4 in breast cancer proliferation

Through a yeast-two hybrid screen, Chakraborty et al. (2006) isolated ACTN4 as a novel interacting protein bound to transcriptional corepressor HDAC7. HDAC7 belongs to class IIa HDACs known to mediate repression activity of MEF2s, a family of master transcription factors implicated in heart development, blood vessel development, neuron differentiation, and muscle differentiation (Dressel et al., 2001). Further domain-mapping studies indicated that there is a reciprocal protein–protein interaction between, MEF2, HDAC7, and ACTN4. Chakraborty et al. (2006) showed that the N-terminal MADS domain of MEF2s is capable of interacting with HDAC7 or ACTN4, while amino acids 72–172 of HDAC7 interacts with MEF2 or ACTN4. Similarly, the C-terminal CaM-like domain of ACTN4 is required to bind HDAC7 and MEF2. Indeed, a point mutant, L112A in HDAC7 abolished its ability to bind MEF2 and ACTN4 (Chakraborty et al., 2006). Functionally, ectopic expression of wild-type ACTN4, but not the mutant defective in MEF2A or HDAC7 binding, disrupts the association between HDAC7 and MEF2 and abolishes HDAC7-mediated transcription repression on MEF2 target genes (Chakraborty et al., 2006). These data suggest that ACTN4 and MEF2 binding sites on HDAC7 largely overlap. ACTN4 in the nucleus may compete with HDAC7 for MEF2 binding, thereby further relieving the repressive effect of HDAC7 on MEF2-stimulated genes (Chakraborty et al., 2006). MEF2-bound ACTN4 functions as a coactivator to potentiate MEF2-mediated transcription activation. Taken together, these data support a model in which ACTN4 antagonizes HDAC7-mediated MEF2 repression activity by competing with HDAC7 for MEF2 binding. This Ying-Yang effect is reminiscent of corepressor and coactivator action in signal-dependent transcriptional regulation. Indeed, the interplay between HDAC7 and ACTN4 in MEF2 target gene regulation is recapitulated in E2-mediated transcriptional regulation and breast cancer cell proliferation. In MCF-7 breast cancer cells,

HDAC7 and ACTN4 associate with ER-α target gene promoters in a largely mutual exclusive pattern such that HDAC7 and ACTN4 do not associate with ER-α target genes simultaneously (Khurana et al., 2011). In contrast to the outcome following ACTN4 knockdown, knockdown of HDAC7 enhances MCF-7 cell growth, releases repression, and further promotes E2 activity for MCF-7 cell proliferation (Khurana et al., 2011). These data provide a model that accounts for elevated expression of ACTN4 observed in some breast cancers. It facilitates the switch from HDAC7-bound ER-α to ACTN4-bound ER-α and thereby contributes to increased cell proliferation.

3.1.3 NF-κB and ACTN4 in breast cancer cell proliferation

The Rel family of transcription factors includes the heterodimeric NF-κB that mediates the activity of multiple signaling pathways regulating cell proliferation, survival, and drug resistance (Ahmed, Cao, & Li, 2006; Piva, Belardo, & Santoro, 2006). Under nonstimulated conditions, the inhibitor of kappa B (I-κB) sequesters NF-κB in the cytoplasm. Signal-induced activation of the I-κB-kinase (IKK) complex promotes ubiquitination-dependent degradation of I-κB, releasing cytoplasmic NF-κB to translocate to the nucleus and bind specific DNA sequences that activate target gene expression (Karin & Ben-Neriah, 2000). In breast cancer, aberrant NF-κB activation has been observed predominantly in ER-α-negative breast cancer cell lines compared to ER-α-positive breast cancer cell lines (Nakshatri, Bhat-Nakshatri, Martin, Goulet, & Sledge, 1997; Pratt et al., 2003). Other studies suggest that NF-κB activation promotes ER-α-negative breast cancer survival, while inhibition of NF-κB in these cells inhibits cancer cell proliferation and induces apoptosis (Biswas et al., 2004; Liu et al., 2003). Although the role of NF-κB in ER-α-positive breast cancer is controversial, ablation of NF-κB activity in ER-α-positive or ER-α-negative breast cancer could be a plausible therapeutic approach for endocrine treatment-resistant breast cancer in the future.

In the cytoplasm, F-actin colocalizes with NF-κB, suggesting a potential mechanism for the regulation of NF-κB nuclear translocation following cytoskeletal alternations (Are, Galkin, Pospelova, & Pinaev, 2000; Rosette & Karin, 1995). ACTN4 colocalizes with p65/RelA subunit of NF-κB in stress fibers and membrane lamellae in unstimulated epithelial carcinoma cells (Babakov et al., 2008). Upon TNF-α and EGF stimulation, a majority of ACTN4 and p65/RelA cotranslocates into the nucleus (Fig. 13.2; Babakov et al., 2008). Additionally, disassembly of p65/RelA- and

ACTN4-associated actin filaments by cytochalasin D also results in nuclear translocation of p65/RelA and ACTN4 (Babakov et al., 2008). While it was proposed that cytoplasmic ACTN4 regulates p65/RelA activity and its nuclear translocation, experimental evidence is still lacking to support this hypothesis.

Since intratumoral and intravascular stress promote cancer cell survival, angiogenesis, and metastasis, Downey et al. proposed that ACTN4, as a stress-sensitive cytoskeletal component, senses the extracellular stress to facilitate malignant cancer cell progression. Indeed, depletion of ACTN4 significantly reduces experimental pressure-induced cell proliferation (Downey, Craig, & Basson, 2011). Furthermore, the experimental pressure enhances ACTN4 and NF-κB association, implying that this interaction has the potential to respond to pathological pressure and promote cancer cell proliferation (Downey et al., 2011). Interestingly, depletion of ACTN4 by siRNA did not block pressure-induced NF-κB activation. In summary, these observations suggest that ACTN4 interacts with NF-κB in response to extracellular stimuli, but the functional significance of this interaction in tumorigenesis warrants further investigation.

3.1.4 ACTN4 and AKT-1 in breast cancer cell proliferation

Akt is a serine/threonine kinase originally identified through its similarity to retroviral oncogene *v-Akt* (Staal, Hartley, & Rowe, 1977). Overexpression of Akt is often found in breast cancer but not in normal mammary epithelial cells (Stål et al., 2003). A major pathway to activate Akt is through PI3K–Akt axis. Upon extracellular stimuli, activated membrane-bound receptor tyrosine kinases induce PI3K activation and subsequent PIP3 production. The latter is a second lipid messenger that promotes Akt recruitment to cell membranes for activation (Castaneda, Cortes-Funes, Gomez, & Ciruelos, 2010). As described earlier, binding of PIP3 to ACTNs increases their susceptibility to calpain-1 and -2-mediated proteolysis (Sprague et al., 2008). Aberrant activation of Akt is a well-known mechanism for initiating tumorigenesis and subsequent cancer cell survival, and hence targeting Akt is a potential therapy for cancer treatment (Luo, Manning, & Cantley, 2003).

Through a retrovirus-based protein-fragment complementation assay, ACTN4 was shown to interact with Akt1 in mammalian cells (Ding et al., 2006). Under starvation conditions, the ACTN4–Akt complex is dispersed throughout the cytoplasm. Upon serum stimulation in HeLa cells, the complex surrounds nucleus with some preference for membrane ruffles (Ding et al., 2006). The serum-dependent ACTN4–Akt complex membrane translocation requires the presence of the PI3K downstream signal mediator, PIP3 (Fig. 13.2). Interestingly, knockdown of ACTN4 largely reduces Akt membrane translocation and phosphorylation and further enhances the abundance of the cyclin-dependent kinase inhibitor, p27^{Kip1}, which is negatively regulated by Akt (Ding et al., 2006). These observations suggest a sequential signaling relay between PI3K and Akt via ACTN4. The overall effect of ACTN4 depletion results in reduced cell proliferation, at least partially because of a loss of ACTN4-mediated Akt activation. Using a proteomic approach, ACTN4 was also shown to coimmunoprecipitate with Akt by anti-Akt antibodies in MCF-7 breast cancer cells, suggesting that ACTN4–Akt complex-mediated cell growth and survival in HeLa cells can be recapitulated in an ER-α-positive breast cancer cell line (Vandermoere et al., 2007).

3.2. ACTN4 enhances breast cancer metastasis

As an actin-binding protein, it is not surprising that ACTN4 regulates cell motility and cancer metastasis. Histological investigations of ACTN4 expression levels in staged malignant cancers demonstrate a strong correlation between cytoplasmic ACTN4 expression and tumor grade (Honda et al., 1998, 2005; Kikuchi et al., 2008; Koizumi et al., 2010; Yamamoto et al., 2007). In invasive cancers, ACTN4 largely accumulates at the leading edge of invasive front. Knockdown of ACTN4 in several invasive cancers significantly attenuates their migration and metastatic ability (Barbolina et al., 2008; Koizumi et al., 2010; Yamada et al., 2010). Conversely, constitutive expression of ACTN4 in colorectal cancer enhances cell motility and promotes metastasis in a mouse model (Honda et al., 2005). These data support the hypothesis that high ACTN4 expression and its distinct pattern of cytoplasmic accumulation contribute toward a gain in metastatic potential.

In most malignant carcinoma cell lines, including epithelial A431 and invasive breast carcinoma R27, ACTN4 is diffusively distributed in the cytoplasm and cannot be detected in stress fibers since most malignant carcinomas lose substantial cytoskeletal fiber structure (Honda et al., 1998). Accumulation of ACTN4 in focal clusters was observed when cells exhibited an extended morphology poised for movement (Honda et al., 1998). Comparing ER-α-positive MCF-7 and R27, a tamoxifen-resistant MCF-7 subcell type, ACTN4 exhibited a different subcellular distribution pattern in which ACTN4 was detected in the nucleus in MCF-7 and in the cytoplasm in R27 (Honda et al., 1998). However, we observed ACTN4 in both nucleus and cytoplasm in MCF-7 cells (Khurana et al., 2011). Further clinical investigation indicates that ACTN4 predominantly localizes in the nucleus of low-infiltrative breast cancer and shows an exclusively cytoplasmic distribution in invasive mammary lobular carcinoma (Honda et al., 1998). Based on these observations, it was proposed that ACTN4 potentially contributes to cancer metastatic progression and a poor survival rate in patients with breast cancer of the nonnuclear ACTN4 subtype (Honda et al., 1998).

A clear picture of how cytoplasmic ACTN4 controls breast cancer migration and the nature of the upstream stimuli that trigger ACTN4-mediated breast cancer metastasis is still not well established. Metastasis is a complicated process in which distal tumor dissemination occurs after cancer cells in the primary tumor experience epithelial–mesenchymal transition (EMT) to disrupt intercellular junctions, reorganize the actin cytoskeleton, and increase cell motility for initial cancer cell spreading (Sarrió et al., 2008). Several stromal and endocrine growth factors, including insulin-like growth factor I (IGF-1), fibroblast growth factor, EGF, and angiogenin (ANG), regulate ACTN or ACTN4 binding to its cytoskeletal working partners and hence result in cell morphological changes and cytoskeletal reorganization, both of which may facilitate the metastatic process (Guvakova, Adams, & Boettiger, 2002; Shao, Wu, et al., 2010; Vandermoere et al., 2007; Wei, Gao, Du, Su, & Xu, 2011). In most breast cancers, the separation of invasive carcinoma from nearby adherent epithelium is an early step for metastases. Short-term IGF-1 stimulation in MCF-7 breast cancer cells causes cell morphological changes, loss of cell–cell contacts, and subsequent induction of cell separation (Guvakova et al., 2002). In the early transition state, IGF-1 treatment activates IGF-1R downstream PI3K, which disassembles stress fibers and facilitates ACTN and actin reorganization in a PIP3-dependent manner (Fig. 13.2; Guvakova et al., 2002). Both ACTNs and actin accumulate in the newly formed microspike structures at the border of separating cell–cell adherent regions. The scenario of IGF-1-induced ACTN reorganization in breast cancer cell separation resembles the accumulation of cytoplasmic ACTN4 in the protrusion edge of other metastatic cancer cells (Guvakova et al., 2002; Honda et al., 1998, 2005). Upon disruption of cell–cell adhesion, the subsequent cellular cytoskeletal reassembly promotes forward filopodia formation and rear detachment, both of which enhance cell migration. In normal macrophages and highly motile cells, ACTN4 accumulates in circular dorsal ruffles and extended filopodia to trigger cell forward movement (Fig. 13.1B; Araki et al., 2000; Shao, Wang, Pollak, & Wells, 2010). The same is true in mobile cancer cells. Downregulation of ACTN4 in fibroblasts and carcinomas blocks cell filopodia formation and contractility (Agarwal et al., 2013; Shao, Wang, et al., 2010), suggesting that ACTN4 not only increases cell forward spread but also assists cell detachment. Indeed, ACTN4 interacts with integrins, the major adherence receptors, and disruption of ACTN4:integrin interactions facilitates the motile cell detachment step (Kobayashi, Kamiie, Yasuno, Ogihara, & Shirota, 2011; Trulsson et al., 2011). In addition to its involvement in the detachment step in motile cells, the disassembly of ACTN4–integrin complexes may also play an important role in dissociation of cell–cell adhesion and cell–extracellular matrix junction in EMT. Integrins are key components that link extracellular matrix to intercellular contacts (Kobayashi et al., 2011; Pavalko et al., 1991). Along this line, in invasive colorectal cancer, downregulation of E-cadherin, a starting feature in the loss of intercellular contacts enhances β-catenin and ACTN4 interaction that results in their relocation in the protrusion region for cell movement (Fig. 13.2; Hayashida et al., 2005). The EGF induces ACTN4 phosphorylation and reduces its cross-link with actin to facilitate ACTN4-mediated cytoskeleton reorganization (Fig. 13.2; Shao, Wu, et al., 2010). Recently, ANG was reported to interact with ACTN4 and regulate ACTN4-associated cytoskeleton reorganization, focal adhesion, and cell migration (Wei et al., 2011). Taken together, ACTN4 can be viewed as a motility promoter, causing reorganization in the motile apparatus following growth factor exposure, resulting in enhanced cell migration and metastasis.

3.3. ACTN4 potentiates drug resistance for breast cancer therapy

Recent studies suggest that ACTN4 plays a role in drug resistance in cancer therapy. Using a proteomic approach to analyze samples prepared from 39 HER2-positive and triple-negative chemo-resistant breast cancer (TNCBC) patients, He and his colleague found elevated ACTN4 in TNCBC. They proposed that ACTN4 is one of the top 30 proteins associated with neoadjuvant chemotherapy resistance in docetaxel and carboplatin-treated TNCBC (He et al., 2011). Misregulation of ER-α-associated coregulators has been shown to enhance ER-α-positive breast cancer resistance to adjuvant endocrine therapy (Smith, Nawaz, & O'Malley, 1997; Stanya, Liu, Means, & Kao, 2008; Su et al., 2008). In another study, using high-performance liquid chromatography Mass spectrometry, Zhou et al. found that ACTN4 had higher expression levels in tamoxifen-resistant MCF-7 than the parental cells, suggesting that ACTN4 may promote cell mobility or enhance transcription activity to enhance tumor survival against tamoxifen therapy (Zhou et al., 2012).

Induction of several NF-κB target genes enhances cancer survival against radio-, chemo-, and endocrine therapy (Ahmed et al., 2006; Zhou, 2005). For example, activated NF-κB induces the expression of MnSOD, an antioxidant enzyme, to promote radiation-induced adaptive responses in radioresistant MCF-7 cells (Guo et al., 2003). The HER2–PI3K–Akt axis has been shown to potentiate multiple drug resistance in breast cancer cells (Knuefermann et al., 2003), in part, by activating the antiapoptotic Bcl-2 family (Datta et al., 1997; Stål et al., 2003). Notably, overexpression of oncogenic HER2 enhances NF-κB activity via PI3K–Akt by a non-canonical, IKK-independent pathway in mammary gland tumors (Pianetti, Arsura, Romieu-Mourez, Coffey, & Sonenshein, 2001). Inhibition of either PI3K–Akt or NF-κB activity significantly enhances sensitivity of breast cancer cells to small molecule drugs or radiotherapy (Guo et al., 2003; Liang et al., 2003). As mentioned earlier, ACTN4 potentiates Akt function and promotes Akt-mediated cell survival by recruiting Akt to membrane ruffles (Ding et al., 2006; Vandermoere et al., 2007). Moreover, ACTN4 may regulate NF-κB-mediated stress responses (Babakov et al., 2008; Downey et al., 2011). In summary, these observations strongly support the notion that ACTN4 is a potential candidate for drug targeting for the treatment of adjuvant therapy-resistant breast cancer.

4. ACTN4 AND OTHER CANCERS

In addition to breast cancer, ACTN4 is also found aberrantly expressed in many other types of cancers (Table 13.1). Recent studies further suggest its role in the initiation of tumors and subsequent malignancy. The contribution of ACTN4 in other cancers is similar to that described in breast cancer. It enhances cancer cell proliferation, survival, migration, and metastasis. In this section, we discuss ACTN4 in several other cancers. Table 13.1 lists the major findings on oncogenic activity of ACTN4 in ovarian, prostate, colorectal, and pancreas cancers.

4.1. Colorectal cancer

By histochemical analyses, it was found that 70% of tested colorectal cancers showed higher ACTN4 expression compared to normal intestinal

Table 13.1 A summary of known ACTN4 function in various cancers

Cancer type	Associated oncogenic factor	Observations and proposed function	References
Breast	ER Akt	Transcriptional coactivator; promote cell proliferation, survival, and metastasis	Honda et al. (1998), Khurana et al. (2011), and Vandermoere et al. (2007)
Bladder	N.D.	High ACTN4 mRNA and protein levels are found in bladder cancer; knockdown of ACTN4 attenuates bladder cancer invasive ability	Koizumi et al. (2010)
Colorectal cancer	β–Catenin	Increased ACTN4 found in 70% of colon cancer; overexpression of ACTN4 elevates colon cancer cell migration and metastasis; loss of epithelial marker, β–cadherin, in colon cancer increases β–catenin–ACTN4 association which may contribute to metastasis	Downey et al. (2011), Hayashida et al. (2005), and Honda et al. (2005)
Epithelial carcinoma	NF-κB	NF-κB and ACTN4 interact in the cytoplasm of epithelial cancer; translocate into nucleus upon EGF and TNF-D stimuli	Bolshakova et al. (2007)
Esophageal and oral cancer	N.D.	High expression of ACTN4 is found in advanced oral and neck cancers; knockdown of ACTN4 decreases oral carcinoma invasive ability; ACTN4 serves as a metastasis biomarker	Fu et al. (2007), Hatakeyama et al. (2006), and Yamada et al. (2010)
Hepatocellular carcinoma	CD81-PI4KIIβ	CD81-PI4KIIβ axis lowers hepatocellular carcinoma cell motility via sequestering ACTN4 in CD81 enriched vesicle	Mazzocca et al. (2008)

Table 13.1 A summary of known ACTN4 function in various cancers—cont'd

Cancer type	Associated oncogenic factor	Observations and proposed function	References
Glioblastoma	N.D.	Knockdown of ACTN4 alters cytoskeleton organization and reduces glioma motility	Henry et al. (2011) and Sen et al. (2009)
Neuroblastoma	N.D.	*Overexpression of ACTN4 in BE(2)-C human neuroblastoma cell line suppresses colony formation, tumor suppressor	*Nikolopoulos et al. (2000)
Lung carcinoma	N.D.	*Overexpression of ACTN4 (K122N) in lung carcinoma loses ACTN4 tumor suppression ability	*Menez et al. (2004)
Small cell lung cancer	N.D.	Expression of a spliced isoform of ACTN4 is found in patient with small cell lung cancer; may be considered as a diagnostic biomarker	Honda et al. (2004)
Ovary	N.D.	High expression of ACTN4 is found in advanced ovary cancer; knockdown of ACTN4 in ovary cancer reduces cell migration ability	Barbolina et al. (2008) and Yamamoto et al. (2007, 2009)
Pancreas	N.D.	High expression of ACTN4 correlates with advanced pancreatic cancer; knockdown of ACTN4 in pancreatic cancer reduces cancer invasive growth ability	Kikuchi et al. (2008) and Pan et al. (2009)

In this table, the reported ACTN4-associated cancers are updated. Asterisks mark the studies in which ACTN4 is proposed to be a tumor suppressor. ACTN4 binding partners, which have been shown to facilitate ACTN4-mediated tumorigenesis, are listed.

epithelium (Honda et al., 2005). Most ACTN4-associated colorectal cancers harbor an aggressive propensity due to their lack of the epithelial marker E-cadherin and differentiated glandular structure (Honda et al., 2005). To further determine the role of ACTN4 in colorectal cancer malignancy, a stable colorectal cancer cell line expressing ACTN4 was established and showed higher extended morphology and migration activity (Honda et al., 2005). Using an animal model and clinical specimens, it was concluded that elevated expression of ACTN4 facilitates colon cancer EMT and promotes metastasis via lymph node colonization (Honda et al., 2005). In a later report, it was shown that the association of ACTN4 and β-catenin is regulated by E-cadherin (Hayashida et al., 2005). In E-cadherin-positive non-infiltrative colorectal cancer, the colocalization of ACTN4 and β-catenin was mainly observed in the nucleus. However, it was localized to membrane ruffles when E-cadherin was knocked down (Hayashida et al., 2005). In addition, elevated ACTN4 increased β-catenin colocalization at the leading edge of protrusion in DLD-1 colorectal cancer (Hayashida et al., 2005). In clinical colorectal cancer tissues, the subcellular distribution of β-catenin and ACTN4 was similar to those observed in aggressive cancer cell lines and showed overlap around membrane ruffles in the leading invasive border (Hayashida et al., 2005). In summary, ACTN4 plays an important role in the promotion of colorectal cancer cell migration through E-cadherin- and β-catenin-associated pathways. It may control cell proliferation by affecting β-catenin's subcellular localization and function.

4.2. Ovarian cancer

Ovarian epithelial carcinoma is a major type of ovary cancer that shows a poor prognosis and outcome for patient therapy (Shih & Kurman, 2004). Increased expression of cytoplasmic ACTN4 has been observed in high-grade ovarian cancer in tissue microarray analyses (Yamamoto et al., 2007). Similar to those described in breast cancer, predominant nuclear ACTN4 is found in low-grade ovarian tumor (Yamamoto et al., 2007). These data imply that the role of ACTN4 in cytoskeleton assembly is highly correlated with ovarian cancer metastasis. Knockdown of ACTN4 in epithelial ovarian carcinoma resulted in significantly decreased cell migration (Barbolina et al., 2008). It was hypothesized that high expression of ACTN4 in ovarian cancer may result from the duplicated amplicon including *ACTN4* in chromosome 19 of those advanced cancer cells (Yamamoto et al., 2009). In summary, current data support a role of ACTN4 in ovarian cancer metastasis, but the direct link and detailed mechanisms require further investigation.

4.3. Pancreatic cancer

Pancreatic cancer causes a higher mortality compared to other types of cancer but shows a better survival rate when surgery or other interventions are executed at an early stage. The etiology of this indocile tumor is still mysterious. Therefore, it is important to establish biomarkers to serve as early prognostic indicators. Histological and proteomic studies have indicated that ACTN4 is highly expressed in malignant pancreatic tissue and the surrounding stroma (Kikuchi et al., 2008; Pan et al., 2009). The increased expression of ACTN4 in pancreatic tumors is, in part, caused by the amplification of *ACTN4* gene on chromosome 19 (Kikuchi et al., 2008). Injection of BxPC3 pancreatic cancer cells after ACTN4 knockdown in nude mice showed lower invasive growth compared to the control group (Kikuchi et al., 2008), indicating a role of ACTN4 in promoting pancreatic cancer invasiveness and proliferation. In total, these findings provide a strong rationale to understand ACTN4's function in pancreatic tumorigenesis as a potential prognostic marker and for drug development.

4.4. Prostate cancer

Two groups have reported opposite activity of ACTN4 in the regulation of prostate cancer cells. In a study by Hara et al. (2007), ACTN4 expression was found to be lower in most prostate cancers than in normal prostate epithelial cells. Using a colony formation assay, they observed that overexpression of ACTN4 in androgen-independent prostate cancers, such as 22RV1 and PC-3, decreased colony formation, indicating that ACTN4 possesses tumor suppressor activity in these cells. These authors proposed that ACTN4 tumor suppression activity is related to its ability to regulate endocytosis. Surprisingly, Jasavala et al. (2007) found that ACTN4 showed high expression in malignant prostate tissue and exhibited distinct cytoplasmic and nuclear localization patterns during tumor progression. They further demonstrated that ACTN4 interacts with AR, a major nuclear receptor critical for prostate development and tumorigenesis, and functions as a coregulator to control AR transactivation activity (Jasavala et al., 2007). Therefore, it is likely that ACTN4 contributes to prostate tumorigenesis due to its coactivator function in AR-dependent transcriptional regulation. Whether the conflicting conclusions on ACTN4 in prostate cancer are due to the examinations in different prostate cancer types requires further experiments.

5. CONCLUSION AND FUTURE DIRECTION

Breast cancer is the most common cancer among women and ranked as the second leading cause of death in women among all cancers, except lung cancer (http://www.cdc.gov/cancer/breast/). While intensive efforts have been devoted to developing therapeutic agents targeting known breast cancer oncoproteins, such as ER-α and HER2, it is well established that some patients will develop resistance to these drugs (Osborne & Schiff, 2011; Pohlmann, Mayer, & Mernaugh, 2009). Therefore, identifying new drug targets and understanding the mechanisms underlying drug resistance are critical to combat drug-resistant breast cancer. ACTN4 seems to be one such drug target.

Since ACTN4 has the ability to bind ER-α, oncogenic transcription factors and chromatin remodeling factors (Fig. 13.1A; Babakov et al., 2008; Chakraborty et al., 2006; Downey et al., 2011; Jasavala et al., 2007; Khurana et al., 2011), it may function as a transcription coactivator to promote cell proliferation via induction of antiapoptotic, proproliferation, and prosurvival genes (Fig. 13.2). Transcriptional coactivators in breast cancer are known to play a role in adjuvant endocrine therapy resistance (Smith et al., 1997; Stanya et al., 2008; Su et al., 2008). Therefore, it might be beneficial in cancer therapy if one can identify ACTN4 binding partners related to breast cancer and exploit these interactions. There is substantial evidence that knockdown of ACTN4 decreases cancer cell migration and lowers cancer metastasis (Table 13.1; Barbolina et al., 2008; Koizumi et al., 2010; Yamada et al., 2010). However, few reports identify upstream signals in breast cancer that are important for stimulating ACTN4 activity to increase cell migration. To this end, the PI3K–Akt axis has been shown to induce ACTN4-mediated cytoskeletal reorganization which subsequently facilitates cell migration (Fig. 13.2; Honda et al., 1998; Sprague et al., 2008). Additionally, FAK or EGF downstream kinases may regulate the ACTN4:F-actin interaction to increase cell migration (Izaguirre et al., 2001; Shao, Wu, et al., 2010). Although these two pathways are known to promote ACTN4-mediated cell migration, the upstream signaling in breast cancer cells that drives this process still needs validation.

While several studies have proposed that ACTN4 participates in cancer resistance to adjuvant therapy (He et al., 2011; Zhou et al., 2012), direct evidence of its role in cancer cell survival is still missing. Further investigation into the function of ACTN4 in cell survival may help the development of therapeutic agents that alleviate drug resistance.

In summary, ACTN4 has dual functions that may contribute to cancer cell proliferation and migration due to its localization in both the nucleus and cytoplasm. Histologic data suggest that accumulation of ACTN4 in the leading edge of cancer cell protrusion coincides with cancer malignant transition (Hayashida et al., 2005; Honda et al., 1998, 2005). Along this line, we hypothesize a role of nuclear ACTN4 as an initiator of early benign tumor formation and that shuttling to the cytoplasm facilitates late malignant stages such as metastasis. As such, understanding the mechanisms underlying nucleocytoplasmic shuttling of ACTN4 is of particular importance.

Finally, although the majority of studies indicate that ACTN4 is a proto-oncogene (Table 13.1), several reports have suggested that ACTN4 suppresses tumor formation. This is particularly true in prostate cancer and neuroblastoma (Hara et al., 2007; Nikolopoulos et al., 2000). This issue requires an in-depth investigation in order to clarify these conflicting conclusions.

ACKNOWLEDGMENTS

We thank Dr. Samols for discussion and Sandy Gu for her assistance in graphic art. This work was supported by National Institutes of Health, RO1 DK078965, and HL093269 to H. -Y. K.

REFERENCES

Agarwal, N., Adhikari, A. S., Iyer, S. V., Hekmatdoost, K., Welch, D. R., & Iwakuma, T. (2013). MTBP suppresses cell migration and filopodia formation by inhibiting ACTN4. *Oncogene*, *32*, 462–470.

Ahmed, K. M., Cao, N., & Li, J. J. (2006). HER-2 and NF-κB as the targets for therapy-resistant breast cancer. *Anticancer Research*, *26*, 4235–4243.

Araki, N., Hatae, T., Yamada, T., & Hirohashi, S. (2000). Actinin-4 is preferentially involved in circular ruffling and macropinocytosis in mouse macrophages: Analysis by fluorescence ratio imaging. *Journal of Cell Science*, *113*, 3329–3340.

Are, A. F., Galkin, V. E., Pospelova, T. V., & Pinaev, G. P. (2000). The p65/RelA subunit of NF-kappaB interacts with actin-containing structures. *Experimental Cell Research*, *256*, 533–544.

Arimura, C., Suzuki, T., Yanagisawa, M., Imamura, M., Hamada, Y., & Masaki, T. (1988). Primary structure of chicken skeletal muscle and fibroblast alpha-actinins deduced from cDNA sequences. *European Journal of Biochemistry*, *177*, 649–655.

Atkinson, R. A., Joseph, C., Kelly, G., Muskett, F. W., Frenkiel, T. A., Nietlispach, D., et al. (2001). Ca2+-independent binding of an EF-hand domain to a novel motif in the alpha-actinin-titin complex. *Nature Structural Biology*, *8*, 853–857.

Babakov, V. N., Petukhova, O. A., Turoverova, L. V., Kropacheva, I. V., Tentler, D. G., Bolshakova, A. V., et al. (2008). RelA/NF-κB transcription factor associates with α-actinin-4. *Experimental Cell Research*, *314*, 1030–1038.

Barbolina, M. V., Adley, B. P., Kelly, D. L., Fought, A. J., Scholtens, D. M., Shea, L. D., et al. (2008). Motility-related actinin alpha-4 is associated with advanced and metastatic ovarian carcinoma. *Laboratory Investigation*, *88*, 602–614.

Beggs, A. H., Byers, T. J., Knoll, J. H., Boyce, F. M., Bruns, G. A., & Kunkel, L. M. (1992). Cloning and characterization of two human skeletal muscle alpha-actinin genes located on chromosomes 1 and 11. *Journal of Biological Chemistry, 267*, 9281–9288.

Biswas, D. K., Shi, Q., Baily, S., Strickland, I., Ghosh, S., Pardee, A. B., et al. (2004). NF-κB activation in human breast cancer specimens and its role in cell proliferation and apoptosis. *Proceedings of the National Academy of Sciences of the United States of America, 101*, 10137–10142.

Bolshakova, A., Petukhova, O., Turoverova, L., Tentler, D., Babakov, V., Magnusson, K.-E., et al. (2007). Extra-cellular matrix proteins induce re-distribution of alpha-actinin-1 and alpha-actinin-4 in A431 cells. *Cell Biology International, 31*, 360–365.

Brenton, J. D., Carey, L. A., Ahmed, A. A., & Caldas, C. (2005). Molecular classification and molecular forecasting of breast cancer: Ready for clinical application? *Journal of Cell Oncology, 23*, 7350–7360.

Carragher, N. O., Fincham, V. J., Riley, D., & Frame, M. C. (2001). Cleavage of focal adhesion kinase by different proteases during src-regulated transformation and apoptosis. Distinct roles for calpain and caspases. *Journal of Biological Chemistry, 276*, 4270–4275.

Carragher, N. O., Levkau, B., Ross, R., & Raines, E. W. (1999). Degraded collagen fragments promote rapid disassembly of smooth muscle focal adhesions that correlates with cleavage of pp125^{FAK}, Paxillin, and Talin. *The Journal of Cell Biology, 147*, 619–630.

Castaneda, C., Cortes-Funes, H., Gomez, H., & Ciruelos, E. (2010). The phosphatidyl inositol 3-kinase/AKT signaling pathway in breast cancer. *Cancer and Metastasis Reviews, 29*, 751–759.

Chakraborty, S., Reineke, E. L., Lam, M., Li, X., Liu, Y., Gao, C., et al. (2006). α-Actinin 4 potentiates myocyte enhancer factor-2 transcription activity by antagonizing histone deacetylase 7. *Journal of Biological Chemistry, 281*, 35070–35080.

Christerson, L. B., Vanderbilt, C. A., & Cobb, M. H. (1999). MEKK1 interacts with α-actinin and localizes to stress fibers and focal adhesions. *Cell Motility and the Cytoskeleton, 43*, 186–198.

Cuevas, B. D., Abell, A. N., Witowsky, J. A., Yujiri, T., Johnson, N. L., Kesavan, K., et al. (2003). MEKK1 regulates calpain-dependent proteolysis of focal adhesion proteins for rear-end detachment of migrating fibroblasts. *EMBO Journal, 22*, 3346–3355.

Datta, S. R., Dudek, H., Tao, X., Masters, S., Fu, H., Gotoh, Y., et al. (1997). Akt phosphorylation of BAD couples survival signals to the cell-intrinsic death machinery. *Cell, 91*, 231–241.

Ding, Z., Liang, J., Lu, Y., Yu, Q., Songyang, Z., Lin, S.-Y., et al. (2006). A retrovirus-based protein complementation assay screen reveals functional AKT1-binding partners. *Proceedings of the National Academy of Sciences of the United States of America, 103*, 15014–15019.

Djinovic-Carugo, K., Gautel, M., Ylänne, J., & Young, P. (2002). The spectrin repeat: A structural platform for cytoskeletal protein assemblies. *FEBS Letters, 513*, 119–123.

Djinović-Carugo, K., Young, P., Gautel, M., & Saraste, M. (1999). Structure of the alpha-actinin rod: Molecular basis for cross-linking of actin filaments. *Cell, 98*, 537–546.

Dourdin, N., Bhatt, A. K., Dutt, P., Greer, P. A., Arthur, J. S. C., Elce, J. S., et al. (2001). Reduced cell migration and disruption of the actin cytoskeleton in calpain-deficient embryonic fibroblasts. *Journal of Biological Chemistry, 276*, 48382–48388.

Downey, C., Craig, D. H., & Basson, M. D. (2011). Isoform-specific modulation of pressure-stimulated cancer cell proliferation and adhesion by α-actinin. *American Journal of Surgery, 202*, 520–523.

Dressel, U., Bailey, P. J., Wang, S.-C. M., Downes, M., Evans, R. M., & Muscat, G. E. O. (2001). A dynamic role for HDAC7 in MEF2-mediated muscle differentiation. *Journal of Biological Chemistry, 276*, 17007–17013.

Edlund, M., Lotano, M. A., & Otey, C. A. (2001). Dynamics of α-actinin in focal adhesions and stress fibers visualized with α-actinin-green fluorescent protein. *Cell Motility and the Cytoskeleton, 48*, 190–200.

Fellenberg, J., Dechant, M. J., Ewerbeck, V., & Mau, H. (2003). Identification of drug-regulated genes in osteosarcoma cells. *International Journal of Cancer, 105,* 636–643.

Fraley, T. S., Pereira, C. B., Tran, T. C., Singleton, C., & Greenwood, J. A. (2005). Phosphoinositide binding regulates α-actinin dynamics. Mechanism for modulating cytoskeletal remodeling. *Journal of Biological Chemistry, 280,* 15479–15482.

Franzot, G., Sjöblom, B., Gautel, M., & Djinović Carugo, K. (2005). The crystal structure of the actin binding domain from alpha-actinin in its closed conformation: Structural insight into phospholipid regulation of alpha-actinin. *Journal of Molecular Biology, 348,* 151–165.

Fu, L., Qin, Y. R., Xie, D., Chow, H. Y., Ngai, S. M., Kwong, D. L. W., et al. (2007). Identification of alpha-actinin 4 and 67 kDa laminin receptor as stage-specific markers in esophageal cancer via proteomic approaches. *Cancer, 110,* 2672–2681.

Fukami, K., Sawada, N., Endo, T., & Takenawa, T. (1996). Identification of a phosphatidylinositol 4,5-bisphosphate-binding site in chicken skeletal muscle α-actinin. *Journal of Biological Chemistry, 271,* 2646–2650.

Fyrberg, E., Kelly, M., Ball, E., Fyrberg, C., & Reedy, M. C. (1990). Molecular genetics of Drosophila alpha-actinin: Mutant alleles disrupt Z disc integrity and muscle insertions. *The Journal of Cell Biology, 110,* 1999–2011.

Greenwood, J. A., Theibert, A. B., Prestwich, G. D., & Murphy-Ullrich, J. E. (2000). Restructuring of focal adhesion plaques by Pi 3-kinase regulation by PtdIns (3,4,5-P) 3 binding to α-actinin. *The Journal of Cell Biology, 150,* 627–642.

Guo, G., Yan-Sanders, Y., Lyn-Cook, B. D., Wang, T., Tamae, D., Ogi, J., et al. (2003). Manganese superoxide dismutase-mediated gene expression in radiation-induced adaptive responses. *Molecular and Cellular Biology, 23,* 2362–2378.

Guvakova, M. A., Adams, J. C., & Boettiger, D. (2002). Functional role of α-actinin, PI 3-kinase and MEK1/2 in insulin-like growth factor I receptor kinase regulated motility of human breast carcinoma cells. *Journal of Cell Science, 115,* 4149–4165.

Hara, T., Honda, K., Shitashige, M., Ono, M., Matsuyama, H., Naito, K., et al. (2007). Mass spectrometry analysis of the native protein complex containing actinin-4 in prostate cancer cells. *Molecular & Cellular Proteomics, 6,* 479–491.

Hatakeyama, H., Kondo, T., Fujii, K., Nakanishi, Y., Kato, H., Fukuda, S., et al. (2006). Protein clusters associated with carcinogenesis, histological differentiation and nodal metastasis in esophageal cancer. *Proteomics, 6,* 6300–6316.

Hayashida, Y., Honda, K., Idogawa, M., Ino, Y., Ono, M., Tsuchida, A., et al. (2005). E-Cadherin regulates the association between β-Catenin and Actinin-4. *Cancer Research, 65,* 8836–8845.

He, J., Whelan, S. A., Lu, M., Shen, D., Chung, D. U., Saxton, R. E., et al. (2011). Proteomic-based biosignatures in breast cancer classification and prediction of therapeutic response. *International Journal of Proteomics, 2011,* 1–16.

Henry, W. I., Dubois, J., & Quick, Q. A. (2011). The microtubule inhibiting agent epothilone B antagonizes glioma cell motility associated with reorganization of the actin-binding protein α-actinin 4. *Oncology Reports, 25,* 887–893.

Honda, K., Yamada, T., Endo, R., Ino, Y., Gotoh, M., Tsuda, H., et al. (1998). Actinin-4, a novel actin-bundling protein associated with cell motility and cancer invasion. *The Journal of Cell Biology, 140,* 1383–1393.

Honda, K., Yamada, T., Seike, M., Hayashida, Y., Idogawa, M., Kondo, T., et al. (2004). Alternative splice variant of actinin-4 in small cell lung cancer. *Oncogene, 23,* 5257–5262.

Honda, K., Yamada, T., Hayashida, Y., Idogawa, M., Sato, S., Hasegawa, F., et al. (2005). Actinin-4 increases cell motility and promotes lymph node metastasis of colorectal cancer. *Gastroenterology, 128,* 51–62.

Imamura, M., Sakurai, T., Ogawa, Y., Ishikawa, T., Goto, K., & Masaki, T. (1994). Molecular cloning of low-Ca(2+)-sensitive-type non-muscle alpha-actinin. *European Journal of Biochemistry, 223,* 395–401.

Izaguirre, G., Aguirre, L., Hu, Y.-P., Lee, H. Y., Schlaepfer, D. D., Aneskievich, B. J., et al. (2001). The cytoskeletal/non-muscle isoform of α-actinin is phosphorylated on its actin-binding domain by the focal adhesion kinase. *Journal of Biological Chemistry, 276,* 28676–28685.

Jasavala, R., Martinez, H., Thumar, J., Andaya, A., Gingras, A.-C., Eng, J. K., et al. (2007). Identification of putative androgen receptor interaction protein modules cytoskeleton and endosomes modulate androgen receptor signaling in prostate cancer cells. *Molecular & Cellular Proteomics, 6,* 252–271.

Kao, J., Salari, K., Bocanegra, M., Choi, Y.-L., Girard, L., Gandhi, J., et al. (2009). Molecular profiling of breast cancer cell lines defines relevant tumor models and provides a resource for cancer gene discovery. *PLoS One, 4,* e6146.

Karin, M., & Ben-Neriah, Y. (2000). Phosphorylation meets ubiquitination: The control of NF-κB activity. *Annual Review of Immunology, 18,* 621–663.

Khurana, S., Chakraborty, S., Cheng, X., Su, Y.-T., & Kao, H.-Y. (2011). The actin-binding protein, actinin alpha 4 (ACTN4), is a nuclear receptor coactivator that promotes proliferation of MCF-7 breast cancer cells. *Journal of Biological Chemistry, 286,* 1850–1859.

Khurana, S., Chakraborty, S., Lam, M., Liu, Y., Su, Y.-T., Zhao, X., et al. (2012). Familial focal segmental glomerulosclerosis (FSGS)-linked α-actinin 4 (ACTN4) protein mutants lose ability to activate transcription by nuclear hormone receptors. *Journal of Biological Chemistry, 287,* 12027–12035.

Kikuchi, S., Honda, K., Tsuda, H., Hiraoka, N., Imoto, I., Kosuge, T., et al. (2008). Expression and gene amplification of actinin-4 in invasive ductal carcinoma of the pancreas. *Clinical Cancer Research, 14,* 5348–5356.

Knudsen, K. A., Soler, A. P., Johnson, K. R., & Wheelock, M. J. (1995). Interaction of alpha-actinin with the cadherin/catenin cell-cell adhesion complex via alpha-catenin. *The Journal of Cell Biology, 130,* 67–77.

Knuefermann, C., Lu, Y., Liu, B., Jin, W., Liang, K., Wu, L., et al. (2003). HER2/PI-3K/ Akt activation leads to a multidrug resistance in human breast adenocarcinoma cells. *Oncogene, 22,* 3205–3212.

Kobayashi, R., Kamiie, J., Yasuno, K., Ogihara, K., & Shirota, K. (2011). Expression of nephrin, podocin, α-actinin-4 and α3-integrin in canine renal glomeruli. *Journal of Comparative Pathology, 145,* 220–225.

Koizumi, T., Nakatsuji, H., Fukawa, T., Avirmed, S., Fukumori, T., Takahashi, M., et al. (2010). The role of actinin-4 in bladder cancer invasion. *Urology, 75,* 357–364.

Kumeta, M., Yoshimura, S. H., Harata, M., & Takeyasu, K. (2010). Molecular mechanisms underlying nucleocytoplasmic shuttling of actinin-4. *Journal of Cell Science, 123,* 1020–1030.

Kusunoki, H., MacDonald, R. I., & Mondragón, A. (2004). Structural insights into the stability and flexibility of unusual erythroid spectrin repeats. *Structure, 12,* 645–656.

Laukaitis, C. M., Webb, D. J., Donais, K., & Horwitz, A. F. (2001). Differential dynamics of α5 integrin, paxillin, and α-actinin during formation and disassembly of adhesions in migrating cells. *The Journal of Cell Biology, 153,* 1427–1440.

Liang, K., Jin, W., Knuefermann, C., Schmidt, M., Mills, G. B., Ang, K. K., et al. (2003). Targeting the phosphatidylinositol 3-kinase/Akt pathway for enhancing breast cancer cells to radiotherapy1. *Molecular Cancer Therapeutics, 2,* 353–360.

Liu, H., Lee, E.-S., Gajdos, C., Pearce, S. T., Chen, B., Osipo, C., et al. (2003). Apoptotic action of 17β-estradiol in raloxifene-resistant MCF-7 cells in vitro and in vivo. *Journal of the National Cancer Institute, 95,* 1586–1597.

Luo, J., Manning, B. D., & Cantley, L. C. (2003). Targeting the PI3K-Akt pathway in human cancer: Rationale and promise. *Cancer Cell, 4,* 257–262.

Maruyama, K., & Ebashi, S. (1965). α Actinin, a new structural protein from striated muscle II. Action on actin. *Journal of Biochemistry, 58,* 13–19.

Masaki, T., Endo, M., & Ebashi, S. (1967). Localization of 6S component of a alpha-actinin at Z-band. *Journal of Biochemistry, 62,* 630–632.

Mazzocca, A., Liotta, F., & Carloni, V. (2008). Tetraspanin CD81-regulated cell motility plays a critical role in intrahepatic metastasis of hepatocellular carcinoma. *Gastroenterology, 135,* 244–256. e1.

Menez, J., Chansac, B. L. M., Dorothée, G., Vergnon, I., Jalil, A., Carlier, M.-F., et al. (2004). Mutant alpha-actinin-4 promotes tumorigenicity and regulates cell motility of a human lung carcinoma. *Oncogene, 23,* 2630–2639.

Mills, M., Yang, N., Weinberger, R., Woude, D. L. V., Beggs, A. H., Easteal, S., et al. (2001). Differential expression of the actin-binding proteins, α-actinin-2 and -3, in different species: Implications for the evolution of functional redundancy. *Human Molecular Genetics, 10,* 1335–1346.

Nakshatri, H., Bhat-Nakshatri, P., Martin, D. A., Goulet, R. J., & Sledge, G. W. (1997). Constitutive activation of NF-kappaB during progression of breast cancer to hormone-independent growth. *Molecular and Cellular Biology, 17,* 3629–3639.

Nikolopoulos, S. N., Spengler, B. A., Kisselbach, K., Evans, A. E., Biedler, J. L., & Ross, R. A. (2000). The human non-muscle alpha-actinin protein encoded by the ACTN4 gene suppresses tumorigenicity of human neuroblastoma cells. *Oncogene, 19,* 380–386.

Oikonomou, K. G., Zachou, K., & Dalekos, G. N. (2011). Alpha-actinin: A multidisciplinary protein with important role in B-cell driven autoimmunity. *Autoimmunity Reviews, 10,* 389–396.

Osborne, C. K., & Schiff, R. (2011). Mechanisms of endocrine resistance in breast cancer. *Annual Review of Medicine, 62,* 233–247.

Otey, C. A., & Carpen, O. (2004). α-Actinin revisited: A fresh look at an old player. *Cell Motility and the Cytoskeleton, 58,* 104–111.

Otey, C. A., Pavalko, F. M., & Burridge, K. (1990). An interaction between alpha-actinin and the beta 1 integrin subunit in vitro. *The Journal of Cell Biology, 111,* 721–729.

Pan, S., Chen, R., Reimel, B. A., Crispin, D. A., Mirzaei, H., Cooke, K., et al. (2009). Quantitative proteomics investigation of pancreatic intraepithelial neoplasia. *Electrophoresis, 30,* 1132–1144.

Pavalko, F. M., & Burridge, K. (1991). Disruption of the actin cytoskeleton after microinjection of proteolytic fragments of alpha-actinin. *The Journal of Cell Biology, 114,* 481–491.

Pavalko, F. M., Otey, C. A., Simon, K. O., & Burridge, K. (1991). Alpha-actinin: A direct link between actin and integrins. *Biochemical Society Transactions, 19,* 1065–1069.

Pavalko, F. M., Walker, D. M., Graham, L., Goheen, M., Doerschuk, C. M., & Kansas, G. S. (1995). The cytoplasmic domain of L-selectin interacts with cytoskeletal proteins via alpha-actinin: Receptor positioning in microvilli does not require interaction with alpha-actinin. *The Journal of Cell Biology, 129,* 1155–1164.

Perou, C. M., Sørlie, T., Eisen, M. B., van de Rijn, M., Jeffrey, S. S., Rees, C. A., et al. (2000). Molecular portraits of human breast tumours. *Nature, 406,* 747–752.

Pianetti, S., Arsura, M., Romieu-Mourez, R., Coffey, R. J., & Sonenshein, G. E. (2001). Her-2/neu overexpression induces NF-kappaB via a PI3-kinase/Akt pathway involving calpain-mediated degradation of IkappaB-alpha that can be inhibited by the tumor suppressor PTEN. *Oncogene, 20,* 1287–1299.

Piva, R., Belardo, G., & Santoro, M. G. (2006). NF-kappaB: A stress-regulated switch for cell survival. *Antioxidants & Redox Signaling, 8,* 478–486.

Pohlmann, P. R., Mayer, I. A., & Mernaugh, R. (2009). Resistance to trastuzumab in breast cancer. *Clinical Cancer Research, 15,* 7479–7491.

Pratt, M. A. C., Bishop, T. E., White, D., Yasvinski, G., Ménard, M., Niu, M. Y., et al. (2003). Estrogen withdrawal-induced NF-κB activity and Bcl-3 expression in breast cancer cells: Roles in growth and hormone independence. *Molecular and Cellular Biology, 23,* 6887–6900.

Quick, Q., & Skalli, O. (2010). α-Actinin 1 and α-actinin 4: Contrasting roles in the survival, motility, and RhoA signaling of astrocytoma cells. *Experimental Cell Research, 316,* 1137–1147.

Rosette, C., & Karin, M. (1995). Cytoskeletal control of gene expression: Depolymerization of microtubules activates NF-kappa B. *The Journal of Cell Biology, 128,* 1111–1119.

Sarrió, D., Rodriguez-Pinilla, S. M., Hardisson, D., Cano, A., Moreno-Bueno, G., & Palacios, J. (2008). Epithelial-mesenchymal transition in breast cancer relates to the basal-like phenotype. *Cancer Research, 68,* 989–997.

Sen, S., Dong, M., & Kumar, S. (2009). Isoform-Specific Contributions of α-Actinin to Glioma Cell Mechanobiology. *PLoS One, 4,* e8427.

Shao, H., Wang, J. H., Pollak, M. R., & Wells, A. (2010). α-Actinin-4 is essential for maintaining the spreading, motility and contractility of fibroblasts. *PLoS One, 5,* e13921.

Shao, H., Wu, C., & Wells, A. (2010). Phosphorylation of α-actinin 4 upon epidermal growth factor exposure regulates its interaction with actin. *Journal of Biological Chemistry, 285,* 2591–2600.

Sheterline, P., Clayton, J., & Sparrow, J. (1995). Actin. *Protein Profile, 2,* 1–103.

Shibasaki, F., Fukami, K., Fukui, Y., & Takenawa, T. (1994). Phosphatidylinositol 3-kinase binds to alpha-actinin through the p85 subunit. *Biochemical Journal, 302,* 551–557.

Shih, I.-M., & Kurman, R. J. (2004). Ovarian tumorigenesis: A proposed model based on morphological and molecular genetic analysis. *American Journal of Pathology, 164,* 1511–1518.

Sjöblom, B., Salmazo, A., & Djinović-Carugo, K. (2008). Alpha-actinin structure and regulation. *Cellular and Molecular Life Sciences, 65,* 2688–2701.

Smith, C. L., Nawaz, Z., & O'Malley, B. W. (1997). Coactivator and corepressor regulation of the agonist/antagonist activity of the mixed antiestrogen, 4-hydroxytamoxifen. *Molecular Endocrinology, 11,* 657–666.

Sprague, C. R., Fraley, T. S., Jang, H. S., Lal, S., & Greenwood, J. A. (2008). Phosphoinositide binding to the substrate regulates susceptibility to proteolysis by calpain. *Journal of Biological Chemistry, 283,* 9217–9223.

Squire, J. M. (1997). Architecture and function in the muscle sarcomere. *Current Opinion in Structural Biology, 7,* 247–257.

Staal, S. P., Hartley, J. W., & Rowe, W. P. (1977). Isolation of transforming murine leukemia viruses from mice with a high incidence of spontaneous lymphoma. *Proceedings of the National Academy of Sciences of the United States of America, 74,* 3065–3067.

Stål, O., Pérez-Tenorio, G., Akerberg, L., Olsson, B., Nordenskjöld, B., Skoog, L., et al. (2003). Akt kinases in breast cancer and the results of adjuvant therapy. *Breast Cancer Research, 5,* R37–R44.

Stanya, K. J., Liu, Y., Means, A. R., & Kao, H.-Y. (2008). Cdk2 and Pin1 negatively regulate the transcriptional corepressor SMRT. *The Journal of Cell Biology, 183,* 49–61.

Su, Q., Hu, S., Gao, H., Ma, R., Yang, Q., Pan, Z., et al. (2008). Role of AIB1 for tamoxifen resistance in estrogen receptor-positive breast cancer cells. *Oncology, 75,* 159–168.

Tang, J., Taylor, D. W., & Taylor, K. A. (2001). The three-dimensional structure of alpha-actinin obtained by cryoelectron microscopy suggests a model for Ca(2+)-dependent actin binding. *Journal of Molecular Biology, 310,* 845–858.

Trulsson, M., Yu, H., Gisselsson, L., Chao, Y., Urbano, A., Aits, S., et al. (2011). HAMLET binding to α-actinin facilitates tumor cell detachment. *PLoS One, 6,* e17179.

Vandermoere, F., Yazidi-Belkoura, I. E., Demont, Y., Slomianny, C., Antol, J., Lemoine, J., et al. (2007). Proteomics exploration reveals that actin is a signaling target of the kinase Akt. *Molecular & Cellular Proteomics, 6,* 114–124.

Wei, S., Gao, X., Du, J., Su, J., & Xu, Z. (2011). Angiogenin enhances cell migration by regulating stress fiber assembly and focal adhesion dynamics. *PLoS One, 6,* e28797.

Welsch, T., Keleg, S., Bergmann, F., Bauer, S., Hinz, U., & Schmidt, J. (2009). Actinin-4 expression in primary and metastasized pancreatic ductal adenocarcinoma. *Pancreas, 38,* 968–976.

Yamada, S., Yanamoto, S., Yoshida, H., Yoshitomi, I., Kawasaki, G., Mizuno, A., et al. (2010). RNAi-mediated down-regulation of α-actinin-4 decreases invasion potential in oral squamous cell carcinoma. *International Journal of Oral and Maxillofacial Surgery, 39*, 61–67.

Yamamoto, S., Tsuda, H., Honda, K., Kita, T., Takano, M., Tamai, S., et al. (2007). Actinin-4 expression in ovarian cancer: A novel prognostic indicator independent of clinical stage and histological type. *Modern Pathology, 20*, 1278–1285.

Yamamoto, S., Tsuda, H., Honda, K., Onozato, K., Takano, M., Tamai, S., et al. (2009). Actinin-4 gene amplification in ovarian cancer: A candidate oncogene associated with poor patient prognosis and tumor chemoresistance. *Modern Pathology, 22*, 499–507.

Ylänne, J., Scheffzek, K., Young, P., & Saraste, M. (2001). Crystal structure of the alpha-actinin rod reveals an extensive torsional twist. *Structure, 9*, 597–604.

Zhou, Y. (2005). The NFκB pathway and endocrine-resistant breast cancer. *Endocrine-Related Cancer, 12*, S37–S46.

Zhou, C., Zhong, Q., Rhodes, L. V., Townley, I., Bratton, M. R., Zhang, Q., et al. (2012). Proteomic analysis of acquired tamoxifen resistance in MCF-7 cells reveals expression signatures associated with enhanced migration. *Breast Cancer Research, 14*, R45.

CHAPTER FOURTEEN

Adherence Rates and Correlates in Long-term Hormonal Therapy

Julia Dunn, Carolyn Gotay[1]

School of Population and Public Health, University of British Columbia, Vancouver, British Columbia, Canada
[1]Corresponding author: e-mail address: carolyn.gotay@ubc.ca

Contents

Abstract

Breast cancer outcomes have improved markedly in the past few decades, due in part to the use of adjuvant hormonal therapy. To receive the optimal benefits of adjuvant therapies such as tamoxifen and aromatase inhibitors (AIs), patients need to take these agents orally each day for 5 years. Current evidence indicates that nonadherence is considerable and increases over time and the side effect profiles for tamoxifen and AIs present considerable barriers to optimal adherence. Interventions, both pharmacologic and nonpharmacologic, hold potential to treat adjuvant hormonal treatment side effects and improve adherence. More research and approaches to intervention to enhance the adherence need to be developed and tested.

1. INTRODUCTION

According to the World Health Organization, breast cancer is the most common cancer in women, accounting for 16% of all cancer cases and almost 520,000 deaths worldwide in 2004 (WHO, 2012). In North America and much of the developed world, breast cancer survival rates have increased markedly over the past several decades; in fact, current 5-year breast cancer survival rates in the United States are 90% (American Cancer Society, 2012). These positive outcomes can be attributed to a

Vitamins and Hormones, Volume 93
ISSN 0083-6729
http://dx.doi.org/10.1016/B978-0-12-416673-8.00003-4
353

number of influences, including more widespread use of mammography screening and more effective cancer treatments. Key among these treatment advances is the use of hormonal therapy following primary breast cancer surgery, often in combination with chemotherapy and/or radiation therapy.

Hormonal therapies for breast cancer adjuvant treatment are examples of targeted cancer therapies: that is, drugs or other substances that block the growth and spread of cancer by interfering with specific molecules involved in tumor growth and progression (National Cancer Institute, 2012). The hormone estrogen is responsible for stimulating breast cancer cell proliferation and growth that lead to the majority of invasive breast cancers, and targeted hormonal agents work by interfering with this activity. Two major classes of targeted agents—selective estrogen receptor modulators (SERMs) and aromatase inhibitors (AIs)—are used to prevent recurrence and new primary breast cancers.

The most commonly used SERM is tamoxifen, which has been part of standard breast cancer treatment for more than 30 years (Swaby, Sharma, & Jordan, 2007). More than 400,000 women are estimated to be alive today because of tamoxifen therapy, with millions experiencing palliation and extended disease-free survival due to tamoxifen treatment (Jordan, 2003). As an adjuvant following primary treatment of early-stage hormone-sensitive breast cancer, tamoxifen has been shown to prevent recurrence (Jordan, 2006) as well as the development of new breast cancer tumors. It is also used as a primary treatment for ductal carcinoma *in situ*, a noninvasive condition that may lead to the development of invasive breast cancer (Fisher et al., 1999). Tamoxifen also has other applications, including its use in primary prevention, where it has been shown to lead to an overall 49% reduction in invasive breast cancer (Fisher et al., 1998). Raloxifene is an example of another SERM often used in breast cancer.

The other class of targeted hormonal therapies for breast cancer, AIs, includes the agents anastrozole, exemestane, and letrozole. Similar to the SERMs, AIs have been found effective in the preventing recurrence as well as prevention of primary breast cancers and are used primarily in postmenopausal women. In fact, AIs have demonstrated significant benefits, comparable to or better than those seen with tamoxifen, and multiple international consensus panels recommend their use (Burstein et al., 2010; Carlson, Hudis, & Pritchard, 2006). Both SERMs and AIs require long-term administration in order for patients to receive their full benefits of therapy, involving patients taking a pill daily.

While both SERMs and AIs have demonstrated positive effects on disease-related outcomes, there are side effects associated with their use. A comprehensive review (Cella & Fallowfield, 2008) discusses the range of side effects that may occur, including vasomotor symptoms (hot flashes, cold sweats, night sweats, sleeping difficulties), neuropsychiatric symptoms (e.g., dizziness, headaches, mood swings, anxiety), gastrointestinal symptoms (e.g., weight gain, diarrhea, nausea), gynecological symptoms (e.g., vaginal bleeding, vaginal discharge, vaginal dryness, loss of libido), skeletal symptoms (e.g., bone loss, osteoporosis), arthralgia, and cognitive impairment. These side effects are not universally experienced, although certainly not unusual, for example, vasomotor symptoms were reported in up to 50% of women in the studies reviewed.

Given these side effect profiles and the need to take a daily medication for a long period, perhaps it is not surprising that adherence rates to long-term hormonal treatments may be less than 100%. However, nonadherence does result in higher mortality. Data show that women who adhere to tamoxifen less than fully (i.e., <80%) are more likely to die than women who are more adherent (Hackshaw et al., 2011; Hershman et al., 2011; McCowan et al., 2008). With the half-life of AIs being significantly shorter than that for tamoxifen, optimal adherence to AIs may be all the more crucial. The half-life of tamoxifen is 14 days, significantly longer than the 27-h half-life of exemestane or the 2-day half-life of letrozole and anastrozole (Fallowfield, 2009).

In addition to increased risk of mortality, there are other potential consequences of patient nonadherence. If a primary care physician is not aware that a patient is not taking the therapy prescribed, he or she may attribute progression of disease to a lack of efficacy and unnecessarily change the treatment. In some patient populations, nonadherence has also been shown to increase health-care use (Ruddy, Mayer, & Partridge, 2009).

Given the significant patient benefits associated with adjuvant hormonal therapies and, conversely, the negative outcomes associated with their absence, understanding the extent of adherence to endocrine therapies and factors that make adherence less and more likely need to be identified. This chapter provides a review of current literature reporting adherence rates and correlates of adherence to long-term hormonal adjuvant therapy for breast cancer. We also review ongoing research and suggest directions for future research and clinical practice.

2. NONADHERENCE IN CLINICAL PRACTICE

There has been a considerable increase in the literature regarding adherence to adjuvant hormonal therapies since Chlebowski and Geller's (2006) review of the literature up to that time, which included nine studies. This chapter updates a previous review by the authors (Gotay & Dunn, 2011). Using PubMed, clinicaltrials.gov, Google, and cross-reference checks, we searched for all papers (2007 to mid-2012) published in English that assessed adherence to SERMs or AIs for breast cancer adjuvant treatment in the context of clinical practice (rather than in clinical trials). We limited our review of adherence rates to publications with a sample size of at least 100. Additional papers that did not meet these criteria but which are relevant to the topic were also abstracted and will be discussed as appropriate.

Adherence was defined as "the extent to which a person's behavior—taking medication, following a diet, and/or executing lifestyle changes, corresponds with agreed recommendations from a health-care provider," based on the World Health Organization's definition (World Health Organization, 2003). As such, nonadherence may include irregular intermittent use, using other than the prescribed dosage (either more or less), and/or premature discontinuation. It should be noted that some studies in this review have been distinguished among different types of adherence, such as never filling the prescription, or levels of intermittent adherence (e.g., Kimmick et al., 2009; Neugut et al., 2011).

We identified 22 studies that met our requirements, 8 of which were published in 2011 and 3 published in 2012. Table 14.1 presents a summary of findings on adherence to tamoxifen (Barron, Connelly, Bennett, Feely, & Kennedy, 2007; Chan, Speers, O'Reilly, Pickering, & Chia, 2009; Cluze et al., 2011; Dezentjé et al., 2010; Kahn, Schneider, Malin, Adams, & Epstein, 2007; Kimmick et al., 2009; McCowan et al., 2008; Narod, 2010; Oguntola, Adeoti, & Akanbi, 2011; Owusu et al., 2008), and Table 14.2 on adherence to AIs with or without tamoxifen, including women who may have used both tamoxifen and one or more AIs (Chan et al., 2009; Guth, Myrick, Kilic, Eppenberger-Castori, & Schmid, 2012; Henry et al., 2012; Hershman et al., 2010; Huiart, Dell'Aniello, & Suissa, 2011; Nekhlyudov, Li, Ross-Degnan, & Wagner, 2011; Neugut et al., 2011; Partridge et al., 2008; Sedjo & Devine, 2011; van de Water et al., 2012; van Herk-Sukel et al., 2010; Ziller et al., 2009). (Interestingly, no

Table 14.1 Adherence to tamoxifen

First author (year)	Participant characteristics	Source of adherence data	Assessment of adherence	Period of observation	Outcomes	Correlates of nonadherence
Barron (2007)	>35 years Ireland N=2816 No racial data provided	Prescription records	≥180 days without supply	3.5 years	22% nonadherent at 1 year, 35% at 3.5 years	Older (>75) or younger (35–44), history of antidepressant use
Cluze (2011)	<40 years France N=196 No racial data provided	Prescription records	≥2-month nonrefill	28 months	42% "interrupted"	Early nonadherence: lack of information, low social support Later nonadherence: side effects, not fearing relapse, low social support, not enough questions asked, fewer treatment modalities
Dezentjé (2010)	<18 years The Netherlands N=1962 No racial data provided	Cancer registry and prescription records	Calculated by dividing the cumulative days covered by 365 days or event-free follow-up time exceeding 365 days	3 years	93% nonadherent at 1 year, 84% nonadherent after 3 years	Using strong CYP2D6 inhibitors; shorter event-free time

Continued

Table 14.1 Adherence to tamoxifen—cont'd

First author (year)	Participant characteristics	Source of adherence data	Assessment of adherence	Period of observation	Outcomes	Correlates of nonadherence
Kahn (2007)	Stages I–III 21–80 years The United States N=881 85% non-Hispanic white, 7% Black, 9% other	Patient survey, medical records	Self-report (yes/no)	4 years	21% nonadherent at 4 years	Nonadherence: low social support, less than preferred involvement in decision making, no doctor input in decision, not being told about side effects, older age, severity of side effects
Kimmick (2009)	Stages I–III Insured low income The United States N=1491 59% White 41% other	Cancer registry-Medicaid linked database	Prescription fill Adherence Persistence (absence of gaps in use)	1 year	64% filled prescriptions 60% adherence 80% persistence	Prescription nonfill: younger age, fewer other prescriptions, married, lower stage, unknown receptor status, chemotherapy, no radiation, large hospital Adherence and persistence: married
McCowan (2008)	Scotland N=1633 No racial data provided	Prescription records	>80%	5 years	51% nonadherent at 5 years	NI

Narod (2010)	BRCA1/BRCA2 mutation Canada, The United States, Poland $N=461$ Jewish$=95$ Polish$=104$ White$=221$ Other$=10$	Patient survey	Self-report of duration	5 years	63% adherent $\geq$4 years, 52% adherent $\geq$4.5 years	Better adherence: postmenopausal at diagnosis, of Jewish, French-Canadian or Polish ethnicity; having BRCA2 mutation
Oguntola (2011)	South-Western Nigeria $N=114$ 108 females, 6 males All participants were black African	Physician query	Nonuse of tamoxifen for up to a period of 1 week without physician consultation	1 year	25% nonadherence for $\geq$1 week in first year. 72% of nonadherence occurred during the first 6 months	Nonadherence: unbearable side effects (9 patients), financial constraints (6), spiritual Reasons (2), nonavailability (2), and presence of comorbidity (3)
Owusu (2008)	Stages I–IIB $\geq$65 years The United States $N=961$ White$=781$ Hispanic$=60$ African American$=84$ Other$=36$	Prescription records	Discontinuation $>$60 days	5 years	51% nonadherent at 5 years	Nonadherence (multivariate): older, more comorbidities, indeterminant ER status, breast conserving surgery without radiation therapy

ER, estrogen receptor.

Table 14.2 Adherence to aromatase inhibitors ± tamoxifen

First author (year)	Types of therapy	Participant characteristics	Source of adherence data	Assessment of adherence	Length of observation	Outcomes	Correlates of nonadherence
Chan (2009)	Tam/AI	Stages I–III Canada $N = 2414$ No racial data provided	Prescription records	Yes/no	3 years	Nonadherence Tam = 42%, AI = 37%	Nonadherence: older, better disease indicators, lower chemo; physician-specific rates ranged 16–67%
Guth (2012)	Tam, AI, or both	HR + disease Switzerland $N = 698$ ≤80 years No racial data provided	Medical records, patient telephone interview, physician report	Pts defined as "nonpersistent" if discontinuing therapy for reasons of choice, not medical need	3 years	13% nonpersistent	Younger, treated by general practitioner rather than oncologist
Henry (2012)	Exemestane/letrozole	Postmenopausal Stages 0–III HR + The United States $N = 503$ White = 441 Black = 46 Other = 13	Medical records	Persistence defined as continuation of second therapy postdiscontinuating first	2 years	32% discontinued initial AI therapy within 2 years due to adverse effects; 24% of these due to musculoskeletal effects	Treatment discontinuation: younger, taxane-based chemotherapy 39% of patients who chose to switch AIs continued the second AI for a median of 13.7 months

Study	Medication	Population	Data source	Adherence definition	Duration	Results	Nonadherence correlates
Hershman (2010)	Tam/AI/Both	Stages I–III The United States N=8769 White=6687 Black=488 Hispanic=630 Asian=964	Prescription records	Discontinuation: ≥180 days since refill ≥80%	4.5 years	32% discontinued at 4.5 years, 28% who continued were not fully adherent, 49% took full duration and dose. Tamoxifen discontinuation (30%) & nonadherence (30%); AI discontinuation (29%) & nonadherence (28%)	Nonadherence: African American, lumpectomy, unknown tumor size, lumpectomy, lymph node involvement, more comorbidity, being at age extreme (<40 or >75); positive adherence correlates: early year of diagnosis, married, longer prescription interval
Huiart (2011)	Tam/AI (anastrozole, letrozole, exemestane)	UK N=13,479 No racial data provided	Prescription records	≥80%	10 years	5-year nonadherence Tam=31%, AI=18.9%	Nonadherence: younger
Kirk (2008)	Tam/AI (anastrozole, letrozole, exemestane)	Online N=328 White=88%, Black=5%. Hispanic=3%, Other=4%	Self-reported internet survey	Adherence was construed as taking medication as directed	N/A	57.4% of respondents claimed to have not missed a single dose in the month prior	70% cited side effects as the reason for nonadherence, while 20% cited cost and 11% cited forgetfulness

Continued

Table 14.2 Adherence to aromatase inhibitors ± tamoxifen—cont'd

First author (year)	Types of therapy	Participant characteristics	Source of adherence data	Assessment of adherence	Length of observation	Outcomes	Correlates of nonadherence
Nekhlyudov (2011)	Tam/AI/ Both	≥18 The United States N=2207 No racial data provided	Prescription records	Length of gap: small (<60 days), large (>180 days)	5 years	1-year adherence, 79% ≤small gap, 85% ≤ large gap; 5 years, 27% and 29%	Nonadherence: older
Neugut (2011)	AIs	>50 years The United States N=22,160 Asian=400 Black=1048 Hispanic=673 White and other=19,836 Missing=203	Pharmacy and medical claims database	Nonpersistence: Gap >45 days without refill Nonadherence: having medication <80% of days	Data collected over a 2-year period	<65 years: 21% nonpersistent, 11% nonadherent ≥65 years: 25% nonpersistent, 9% nonadherent	Nonpersistence: older, more other prescriptions, having nononcologist write prescription Copayment >$90 affected both persistence and adherence: $30-89.99 impacted only younger women
Partridge (2008)	Anastrozole	Early stage The United States N=12,391 No racial data provided	Claims data drawn from three different health plans	≥80% adherent	3 years	1-year mean adherence=82-88%; for women with 3 years of data, adherence went from 78-86% to 62-79%	NI: varied across health plans

Study	Drug	Population	Data source	Adherence definition	Follow-up	Results	Predictors
Sedjo (2011)	Exemestane, anastrozole, letrozole tam	Health Insurance plans <65 years The United States N=13,593 No racial data provided	Claims data	≥80% adherent	1 year	23% nonadherent	Younger age, higher out of pocket costs, previous health-care utilization (i.e., lower pharmacy costs), mastectomy, more comorbidities
van Herk-Sukel (2010)	Tam/AIs (anastrozole, letrozole, and exemestane) or sequential therapy	Early stage The Netherlands N=1451 No racial data provided	PHARMO-ECR cohort, cancer registry	Calculated by dividing # units dispensed by # units to be used/day	5 years	The percentage of continuous users at 1, 2, 3, 4, and 5 years was 83%, 70%, 55%, 50%, and 40%, respectively	Older age, comorbidity
van de Water (2012)	Tam/exemestane	Postmenopausal Belgium, The Netherlands, UK, Ireland, The United States, Japan, Greece, Germany, France N=3142 No racial data provided	Physician query	Nonpersistence: discontinuation of endocrine therapy within 1 year of follow-up	5 years	8.1% discontinued therapy within 1 year of follow-up	Older age, adverse events

Continued

Table 14.2 Adherence to aromatase inhibitors ± tamoxifen—cont'd

First author (year)	Types of therapy	Participant characteristics	Source of adherence data	Assessment of adherence	Length of observation	Outcomes	Correlates of nonadherence
Ziller (2009)	Tam/ anastrozole	Postmenopausal Germany N=100 No racial data provided	Patient self-report Prescription records	≥80% adherent	NI	All women (100%) reported being adherent; prescription data showed adherence Tam = 80%, ANA = 69%	None

AIs, aromatase inhibitors; Tam, tamoxifen; NI, no information; ANA, anastrozole.

studies to date have yet reported adherence to the SERM raloxifene, an FDA-approved agent for breast cancer risk reduction.)

The studies varied considerably in their patient populations, the source of data, the assessment of adherence, the period over which adherence is observed, and the correlates that were measured. Nonetheless, in spite of these methodological differences, nonadherence was found in all studies. One-year adherence rates ranged from 74.5% to 93% (Barron et al., 2007; Chan et al., 2009; Dezentjé et al., 2010; Nekhlyudov et al., 2011; Oguntola et al., 2011; Partridge et al., 2008; Sedjo & Devine, 2011; van de Water et al., 2012); whereas studies reporting 4- to 5-year prescription-based adherence found rates between 21% and 64.7% (Chan et al., 2009; Hershman et al., 2010; Kahn et al., 2007; Narod, 2010; Nekhlyudov et al., 2011; van Herk-Sukel et al., 2010). Not surprisingly, then, adherence diminishes over time. These figures are very similar to Chlebowski and Geller's (2006) findings that 30–50% of patients in clinical practice were nonadherent by 4 years. Studies that used patient self-reports of adherence reported higher rates (Kahn et al., 2007; Narod, 2010; Oguntola et al., 2011; van de Water et al., 2012; Ziller et al., 2009). However, Ziller et al. (2009) found that whereas all 100 women in their study said that they adhered to their tamoxifen or AI regimen, prescription database information showed that actual adherence was likely to be 20–30% less. Guth et al. (2012) took a different approach to defining adherence and focused on women for whom adherence or discontinuation of therapy was a choice, as opposed to a medical necessity because of, for example, recurrence or other medical reasons. Using this definition, they reported that only 13% of patients were "nonpersistent." However, this rate is based on patient self-reports.

Studies reported a variety of different factors that were linked with adherence. To some degree, the variation reflects the different potential correlates measured in the study; but in other cases, different relationships were found. For example, age was investigated in most studies and was often found to be a significant correlate. However, the direction of the effect varied, with older age associated with less adherence in a number of studies (Barron et al., 2007; Chan et al., 2009; Hershman et al., 2010; Kahn et al., 2007; Nekhlyudov et al., 2011; Neugut et al., 2011; Owusu et al., 2008; van de Water et al., 2012; van Herk-Sukel et al., 2010); but younger age linked with lower adherence in some others (Barron et al., 2007; Chan et al., 2009; Guth et al., 2012; Henry et al., 2012; Hershman et al., 2010, Huiart et al., 2011; Kimmick et al., 2009; Sedjo & Devine, 2011) cohorts.

Perhaps, the safest conclusion to draw at present is that middle-aged women (e.g., aged 50–69 years) may be most adherent, with greater nonadherence at the age extremes. Less social support was associated with lower adherence in several studies (Cluze et al., 2011; Kahn et al., 2007), but being married was linked both with lower (Kimmick et al., 2009) and higher adherence (Hershman et al., 2010).

We were also interested in race/ethnicity as a possible correlate, given that this factor has been shown to be a strong predictor of adherence with medication for other chronic diseases such as hypertension (Ishisaka, Jukes, Romanelli, Wong, & Schiro, 2012). Of the 22 studies listed in Tables 14.1 and 14.2, 13 did not provide racial/ethnic information. Of the other nine, most had a large percentage of White participants, but no racial differences were found. Only two studies reported significant racial/ethnic differences, with Hershman et al. (2010) finding African-Americans were less adherent, and Narod (2010) reporting better adherence in women of Jewish, French-Canadian, or Polish ethnicity than in those with "white" race. It is worth paying special note to the Oguntola et al. (2011) study; not only is this the only study that has been reported from Africa (Nigeria specifically), but it is also one of the very few studies in the literature reporting adherence in male breast cancer patients. All patients in this study were Black and so no racial comparisons could be made. A recent paper on the initiation of adjuvant hormonal therapy reported a significant impact of race/ethnicity among insured women in the United States, such that Hispanic and Chinese women were less likely than non-Hispanic whites to fill their first tamoxifen or AI prescription (Livaudais et al., 2012). The further study of race, ethnicity, and cultural factors on the use of hormonal therapy is warranted.

Five studies identified side effects as a source of lower adherence (Cluze et al., 2011; Guth et al., 2012; Kahn et al., 2007; Oguntola et al., 2011; van de Water et al., 2012). Additional comorbid conditions were linked with lower adherence in a number of investigations (Hershman et al., 2010; Oguntola et al., 2011; Owusu et al., 2008; Sedjo & Devine, 2011; van Herk-Sukel et al., 2010). Guth et al. (2012) found that reason for nonpersistence varied according to age, but "lack of motivation" and general discomfort were the most prevalent reasons overall. Some reports assessed adherence to both tamoxifen and AIs, and these studies consistently found higher adherence with AIs (Chan et al., 2009; Huiart et al., 2011; Ziller et al., 2009). It should be noted that the women who received tamoxifen versus AIs differed in other important ways, such as menopausal status and age.

Additionally, four studies that did not meet our search criteria provide further insight into the correlates of adherence. Two studies point to possible biological mechanisms underlying drug activity and adherence: Schmid et al. (2012) study observed a correlation between high body mass index and higher levels of adherence, Rae et al. (2009) found that women with higher CYP2D6 activity were more likely to be nonadherent to tamoxifen. Visram, Kanji, and Dent (2010) observed adherence rates in men similar to those in women, with toxicity being very similar as well. Similarly, nonadherence rates were similar among women who took extended therapy (i.e., going for more than the 5 years currently recommended) on the recommendation of their physicians, as in standard care, with approximately 30% of women nonadherent (Myrick, Schmid, Kilic, & Güth, 2012).

3. PATIENT-REPORTED BARRIERS TO ADHERENCE TO ADJUVANT HORMONAL THERAPIES

This literature supports the prevalence of nonadherence to hormonal adjuvant treatments for breast cancer, as well as identifies some correlates of adherence and nonadherence. These data are enriched by studies that have collected patient-reported outcomes and qualitative information, particularly related to side effects and symptoms that affect patient quality of life.

In a mailed questionnaire study of 452 American women, 42% attributed not taking hormonal therapy to side effects, most frequently hot flashes, which were cited by 35% of tamoxifen and 30% of AI users; 22% of AI users also cited muscle aches (Garreau, DeLaMelena, Walts, Karamlou, & Johnson, 2006). Similarly, a clinical trial in which 503 women were enrolled observed that 32% of women discontinued AI therapy due to adverse effects, 24% attributed to muscle arthralgia (Henry et al., 2012). Qualitative studies also convey well the experience of some patients: the poignant title of a paper by Winters, Habin, Flanagan, and Cashavelly (2010)—"I Feel Like I'm 100 Years Old!"—vividly conveys the arthralgia experience of some AI patients and points to why nonadherence may be likely. Qualitative interviews conducted with 34 French AI users underscore this sentiment as women struggle with the paradox of taking a therapy that leads to better health outcomes while at the same time making them feel worse; as one woman described it, "It is a treatment which is tiring, aging and the same time you say, well, it saves your life" (Pellegrini et al., 2010, p. 476).

The Y-ME National Breast Cancer Organization conducted an Internet survey that was completed by 328 breast cancer patients who had been prescribed adjuvant hormonal therapy (Kirk & Hudis, 2008). Provider communication was cited as a primary contributor to nonadherence, and fewer than half of the respondents (44%) said that instructions about the importance of taking oral medication as directed were provided at each office visit. Only 57% of the women indicated that they had not missed a single dose during the previous month, and these women believed that they would adhere more consistently if they were better aware of the importance of their adherence for improved clinical outcomes (89%), and if their treatment-related side effects were managed more effectively (60%). Kahn et al. (2007) also found that adherence was affected by the physician's input into the treatment decision and being told about side effects. This conclusion was reinforced by a study that observed actual office encounters between community oncologists and breast cancer patients beginning or receiving hormonal therapy and found that possible challenges to long-term adherence were not discussed (Davidson, Vogel, & Wickerham, 2007). Guth et al. (2012) remark that individual patient decisions are complex and nuanced and require thoughtful patient: physician discussion.

As Miaskowski, Shockney, and Chlebowski . (2008) point out, factors related to the patient's attitudes and perceptions (e.g., their susceptibility to breast cancer recurrence, the severity of the disease, benefits of adjuvant therapy, barriers to treatment, and self-efficacy) affect adherence levels. Cost has also been cited as a barrier to adherence (Neugut et al., 2011; Sedjo & Devine, 2011), and this may be particularly important in developing countries (Oguntola et al., 2011).

4. INTERVENTIONS TO INCREASE ADHERENCE

Very few interventions to increase adherence to adjuvant hormonal therapies have been reported to data. Guth, Myrick, Schötzau, Kilic, and Schmid (2011) investigated whether switching endocrine therapy due to adverse effects would increase adherence to the second therapy. Of the approximately 20% of patients suffering from severe therapy-related adverse effects, 82% switched therapies. Of these women, 82% completed their therapy after the drugs were switched. The authors maintain that therapy modifications may increase adherence when severe adverse effects are observed from the primary therapy (Guth et al., 2011). In a case study report, Bryce, Bauer, and Hadji (2012) also reported that switching AIs was helpful in improving adherence.

In another study, Ell et al. (2009) randomly assigned 487 low income, mostly Hispanic women to receive written materials developed to enhance adherence alone or in combination with the services of a patient navigator who provided telephone or in person counseling for up to a year. There was no difference between the intervention conditions on the primary outcome variables. Adherence was high, at 88% or higher, in both intervention groups for adjuvant chemotherapy and radiation therapy, but adherence to hormonal therapy was not impressive, with only 59% adherent at 1 year (Ell et al., 2009). Still, the impact of patient navigators (perhaps trained cancer survivors) to provide personalized support specific to adherence might be further examined in future research.

Virtually, every paper listed in Tables 14.1 and 14.2 concluded with the suggestion that effective interventions to enhance adherence were needed. Based on the literature on adherence to medication more generally, interventions to improve adherence include educational, behavioral, pharmacological, and multidimensional approaches, such as greater involvement of oncology nurses (Miaskowski et al., 2008; Winkeljohn, 2010), counseling and education by health-care providers, particularly physicians (Chlebowski & Geller, 2006; Ruddy et al., 2009; Winkeljohn, 2010) that includes ongoing assessment and attention to psychosocial factors and side effects (Miaskowski et al., 2008) and better accessibility to health care and the dosing plan (Chlebowski & Geller, 2006; Ruddy et al., 2009).

Other specific suggestions are that oncologists and/or primary care providers should ask patients whether the regimen is causing distress or side effects, and on a regular and ongoing basis. Discussing the importance of adherence may be beneficial, as it may prompt those with poor adherence to improve, and encourage those who are already adherent to continue (Ruddy et al., 2009). Physicians may wish to recommend daily pill boxes or tricks (placing an individual pill on the bedside table) to increase adherence in those who find remembering to take their medication difficult. If possible, ongoing consultations with a pharmacist may prove beneficial, as well as providing patients with access to information about support groups and related resources, which they may not have been aware of or used. Other approaches, such as patient support groups, and online communities and blogs, remain to be explored.

Particularly important is treating any side effects, mental or physical, that may be significantly interfering with the patient's quality of life, whether by pharmacological or nonpharmacological means. Interventions specific to various side effects have been suggested, developed, and tested (Cella &

Fallowfield, 2008), but their potential impact on adherence has not yet been explored.

5. DISCUSSION

Tamoxifen and AIs are among the first examples of targeted therapies for cancer. These treatments reflect challenges associated with such approaches, including the need for prolonged and self-administered administration of treatment, and the appearance of side effects that differ from the toxicities that result from standard cancer therapies. A new paradigm for cancer treatment is needed for targeted therapies, in which monitoring for adherence is particularly important. In addition, ongoing monitoring and initiation of interventions as needed will frequently become the responsibility of the primary care provider and the well-informed patient, not only the purview of the oncologist.

In the past few years, there has been a veritable explosion in the amount of literature on nonadherence to endocrine therapies. In fact, we identified two additional reviews of this area published in 2012 subsequent to our review in 2011 (Banning, 2012; Murphy, Bartholomew, Carpenter, Bluethmann, & Vernon, 2012). This chapter updates all of these previous efforts.

Much has been learned. For example, adherence rates decrease over time are more accurately assessed by objective rather than subjective reports (which tend to produce over-estimates), are similar in men and women who receive this therapy, and are similar across the world where studies have been reported. Certain correlates such as age, cost, comorbidity, and side effects are associated with lower adherence rates. Some side effects are similar in both tamoxifen and AIs (e.g., hot flashes) and some are different (e.g., arthralgias are common with AIs but not with tamoxifen).

While these studies help us to further elucidate the myriad of factors that contribute to nonadherence, many questions remain unanswered, such as the magnitude and explanation for racial or ethnic influences on adherence, and potential biological mechanisms that may affect the experience of hormonal treatment and adherence, In particular, little is known to date as of how to effectively increase compliance to these life-saving therapies.

There are, however, a number of projects currently underway that should contribute to answering these questions. These include three studies sponsored by the pharmaceutical company, AstraZeneca (ClinicalTrials.

gov): *Compliance of Aromatase Inhibitor Assessment in Daily Practice Through an Educational Approach* (NCT00681122), *Aromatase Inhibitor Patient Compliance Program with Quality of Life Questionnaires* (NCT00523315), and *Arimidex Therapy Compliance Electronic Monitoring System* (NCT00936442). When data from these studies are published, they may provide guidance on both monitoring and improving adherence to AIs. The Southwest Oncology Group (SWOG) has launched three new protocols in this area: S0927, which tests the effectiveness of omega-3 fatty acid supplements in alleviating AI-induced joint pain; S1105 (NCT01515800), which tests the effectiveness of twice weekly text message reminders in improving oral AI adherence; and S1200, which investigates the impact of acupuncture on reducing AI-induced joint pain (SWOG, 2012). A pilot study called "adhERe" has been launched at the University of Toronto designed to enhance adherence through telephone-based motivational counseling (Jones, 2012). Finally, the Endocrine Therapy After Breast Cancer (E-ABC Study; Stanton & Partridge, 2012) is underway to collect information about the experiences of 500 American patients with tamoxifen and AIs using an Internet-based survey distributed through the national "Army of Women" Web site. There are undoubtedly other activities ongoing elsewhere that will inform this field in the future.

6. CONCLUSION

Despite the rapid expansion in the body of literature concerning adherence rates to endocrine therapies, there are still no known solutions to improve adherence rates. There is need for advancement in the therapies themselves, with new therapies needed that carry lesser side effect profiles, while simultaneously being as effective or more efficacious. It would also be advantageous if new therapies could be devised that had a longer period of action, so that daily dosage were not necessary. We expect that quality of life and symptom management issues will continue to gain prominence alongside disease-oriented outcomes in the minds of both health-care providers and the patients themselves. In addition, future interventions and those currently in progress are likely to contribute to more efficacious management of side effects and obstacles to adherence. These new developments will ensure that breast cancer survivors receiving adjuvant hormonal therapy are able to achieve the best outcomes that are possible.

REFERENCES

American Cancer Society (2012). *Cancer facts & figures 2012*. Atlanta, GA: American Cancer Society.

Banning, M. (2012). Adherence to adjuvant therapy in post-menopausal breast cancer patients: A review. *European Journal of Cancer Care, 21*(1), 10–19.

Barron, T. I., Connelly, R., Bennett, K., Feely, J., & Kennedy, M. J. (2007). Early discontinuation of tamoxifen: A lesson for oncologists. *Cancer, 109*(5), 832–839.

Bryce, J., Bauer, M., & Hadji, P. (2012). Managing arthralgia in a postmenopausal woman taking an aromatase inhibitor for hormone sensitive early breast cancer: A case study. *Cancer Management and Research, 4*, 105–111.

Burstein, H. J., Prestrud, A. A., Seidenfeld, J., Anderson, H., Buchholz, T. A., Davidson, N. E., et al. (2010). American Society of Clinical Oncology clinical practice guideline: Update on adjuvant endocrine therapy for women with hormone receptor-positive breast cancer. *Journal of Clinical Oncology, 28*(23), 3784–3796.

Carlson, R. W., Hudis, C. A., & Pritchard, K. I.National Comprehensive Cancer Network Breast Cancer Clinical Practice Guidelines in Oncology; American Society of Clinical Oncology Technology Assessment on the Use of Aromatase Inhibitors; St Gallen International Expert Consensus on the Primary Therapy of Early Breast Cancer. (2006). Adjuvant endocrine therapy in hormone receptor-positive postmenopausal breast cancer: Evolution of NCCN, ASCO, and St Gallen recommendations. *Journal of the National Comprehensive Cancer Network, 4*(10), 971–979.

Cella, D., & Fallowfield, L. J. (2008). Recognition and management for treatment-related side effects for breast cancer patients receiving adjuvant endocrine therapy. *Breast Cancer Research and Treatment, 107*, 167–180. http://dx.doi.org/10.1007/s10549-007-9548-1.

Chan, A., Speers, C., O'Reilly, S., Pickering, R., & Chia, S. (2009). Adherence of adjuvant hormonal therapies in post-menopausal hormone receptor positive (HR+) early stage breast cancer: A population based study from British Columbia. *Cancer Research, 69*(24), 36.

Chlebowski, R. T., & Geller, M. L. (2006). Adherence to endocrine therapy for breast cancer. *Oncology, 71*(1–2), 1–9.

ClinicalTrials.gov. (n.d.). *US National Institutes of Health*. Retrieved from http://www.clinicaltrials.gov. Accessed 24.05.2013.

Cluze, C., Rey, D., Huiart, L., BenDiane, M. K., Bouhnik, A. D., Berenger, C., et al. (2011). Adjuvant endocrine therapy with tamoxifen in young women with breast cancer: Determinants of interruptions vary over time. *Annals of Oncology, 23*(4), 882–890.

Davidson, B., Vogel, V., & Wickerham, L. (2007). Oncologist-patient discussion of adjuvant hormonal therapy in breast cancer: Results of a linguistic study focusing on adherence and persistence to therapy. *The Journal of Supportive Oncology, 5*(3), 139–143.

Dezentjé, V. O., van Blijderveen, N. J., Gelderblom, H., Putter, H., van Herk-Sukel, M. P., Casparie, M. K., et al. (2010). Effect of concomitant CYP2D6 inhibitor use and tamoxifen adherence on breast cancer recurrence in early-stage breast cancer. *Journal of Clinical Oncology, 28*(14), 2423–2429.

Ell, K., Vourlekis, B., Xie, B., Nedjat-Haiem, F. R., Lee, P. J., Muderspach, L., et al. (2009). Cancer treatment adherence among low-income women with breast or gynecologic cancer: A randomized controlled trial of patient navigation. *Cancer, 115*(19), 4606–4615.

Fallowfield, A. (2009). The clinical importance of patient adherence to therapy. *Advances in Breast Cancer, 6*(2), 9.

Fisher, B., Costantino, J. P., Wickerham, D. L., Redmond, C. K., Kavanah, M., Cronin, W. M., et al. (1998). Tamoxifen for prevention of breast cancer: Report of the National Surgical Adjuvant Breast and Bowel Project P-1 Study. *Journal of the National Cancer Institute, 90*(18), 1371–1388.

Fisher, B., Dignam, J., Wolmark, N., Wickerham, D. L., Fisher, E. R., Mamounas, E., et al. (1999). Tamoxifen in treatment of intraductal breast cancer: National Surgical Adjuvant Breast and Bowel Project B-24 randomised controlled trial. *Lancet, 353*(9169), 1993–2000.

Garreau, J., DeLaMelena, T., Walts, D., Karamlou, K., & Johnson, N. (2006). Side effects of aromatase inhibitors versus tamoxifen: The patients' perspective. *American Journal of Surgery, 192*(4), 496–498.

Gotay, C. C., & Dunn, J. (2011). Adherence to long-term adjuvant hormonal therapy for breast cancer. *Expert Review of Pharmacoeconomics & Outcomes Research, 11*(6), 709–715.

Guth, U., Myrick, M. E., Kilic, N., Eppenberger-Castori, S., & Schmid, S. M. (2012). Compliance and persistence of endocrine adjuvant breast cancer therapy. *Breast Cancer Research and Treatment, 131*(2), 491–499.

Guth, U., Myrick, M. E., Schötzau, A., Kilic, N., & Schmid, S. M. (2011). Drug switch because of treatment-related adverse side effects in endocrine adjuvant breast cancer therapy: How often does it work? *Breast Cancer Research and Treatment, 129*(3), 799–807.

Hackshaw, A., Roughton, M., Forsyth, S., Monson, K., Reczko, K., Sainsbury, R., et al. (2011). Long-term benefits of 5 years of tamoxifen: 10-year follow-up of a large randomized trial in women at least 50 years of age with early breast cancer. *Journal of Clinical Oncology, 29*(13), 1657–1663.

Henry, N. L., Azzouz, F., Desta, Z., Li, L., Nguyen, A. T., Lemler, S., et al. (2012). Predictors of aromatase inhibitor discontinuation as a result of treatment-emergent symptoms in early-stage breast cancer. *Journal of Clinical Oncology, 30*(9), 936–942.

Hershman, D. L., Kushi, L. H., Shao, T., Buono, D., Kershenbaum, A., Tsai, W. Y., et al. (2010). Early discontinuation and nonadherence to adjuvant hormonal therapy in a cohort of 8,769 early-stage breast cancer patients. *Journal of Clinical Oncology, 28*(27), 4120–4128.

Hershman, D. L., Shao, T., Kushi, L. H., Buono, D., Tsai, W. Y., Fehrenbacher, L., et al. (2011). Early discontinuation and non-adherence to adjuvant hormonal therapy are associated with increased mortality in women with breast cancer. *Breast Cancer Research and Treatment, 126*(2), 529–537.

Huiart, L., Dell'Aniello, S., & Suissa, S. (2011). Use of tamoxifen and aromatase inhibitors in a large population-based cohort of women with breast cancer. *British Journal of Cancer, 104*, 1558–1563.

Ishisaka, D. Y., Jukes, T., Romanelli, R. J., Wong, K. S., & Schiro, T. A. (2012). Disparities in adherence to and persistence with antihypertensive regimens: An exploratory analysis from a community-based provider network. *Journal of the American Society of Hypertension, 6*(3), 201–209.

Jones, J. (2012). *Pilot study of a brief telephone-based intervention (adhERe) to improve adherence to adjuvant hormone therapy in women with early stage breast cancer.* Toronto, ON, Canada: ELLICSR: Health, Wellness and Cancer Survivorship Centre. Retrieved July 31, 2012 from: http://www.ellicsr.ca/content/pilot-study-brief-telephone-based-intervention-adhere-improve-adherence-adjuvant-hormone.

Jordan, C. (2003). Tamoxifen: A most unlikely pioneering medicine. *Nature Reviews. Drug Discovery, 2*(3), 205–213.

Jordan, C. (2006). Tamoxifen (IC146, 474) as a targeted therapy to treat and prevent breast cancer. *British Journal of Pharmacology, 147*(S1), S269–S276.

Kahn, K. L., Schneider, E. C., Malin, J. L., Adams, J. L., & Epstein, A. M. (2007). Patient centered experiences in breast cancer: Predicting long-term adherence to tamoxifen use. *Medical Care, 4*(5), 431–439.

Kimmick, G., Anderson, R., Camacho, F., Bhosle, M., Hwang, W., & Balkrishnan, R. (2009). Adjuvant hormonal therapy use among insured, low-income women with breast cancer. *Journal of Clinical Oncology, 27*(21), 3445–3451.

Kirk, M. C., & Hudis, C. A. (2008). Insight into barriers against optimal adherence to oral hormonal therapy in women with breast cancer. *Clinical Breast Cancer, 8*(2), 155–161.

Livaudais, J. C., Hershman, D. L., Habel, L., Kushi, L., Gomez, S. L., Li, C. I., et al. (2012). Racial/ethnic differences in initiation of adjuvant hormonal therapy among women with hormone receptor-positive breast cancer. *Breast Cancer Research and Treatment, 131*(2), 607–617.

McCowan, C., Shearer, J., Donnan, P. T., Dewar, J. A., Crilly, M., Thompson, A. M., et al. (2008). Cohort study examining tamoxifen adherence and its relationship to mortality in women with breast cancer. *British Journal of Cancer, 99*(11), 1763–1768.

Miaskowski, C., Shockney, L., & Chlebowski, R. T. (2008). Adherence to endocrine therapy for breast cancer. *Clinical Journal of Oncology Nursing, 12*(2), 213–221.

Murphy, C. C., Bartholomew, L. K., Carpenter, M. Y., Bluethmann, S. M., & Vernon, S. W. (2012). Adherence to adjuvant hormonal therapy among breast cancer survivors in clinical practice: A systematic review. *Breast Cancer Research and Treatment, 134*(2), 459–478.

Myrick, M. E., Schmid, S. M., Kilic, N., & Güth, U. (2012). Eligibility, compliance and persistence of extended adjuvant endocrine therapy for breast cancer. *Acta Oncologica, 51*(2), 247–253.

Narod, S. A. (2010). Compliance with tamoxifen in women with breast cancer and a BRCA1 or BRCA2 mutation. *Journal of Clinical Oncology, 28*(33), e698–e699.

National Cancer Institute (2012). *Targeted cancer therapies fact sheet.* Retrieved from http://www.cancer.gov/cancertopics/factsheet/Therapy/targeted, December 5, 2012.

Nekhlyudov, L., Li, L., Ross-Degnan, D., & Wagner, A. K. (2011). Five-year patterns of adjuvant hormonal therapy use, persistence, and adherence among insured women with early-stage breast cancer. *Breast Cancer Research and Treatment, 130*(2), 681–689.

Neugut, A. I., Subar, M., Wilde, E. T., Stratton, S., Brouse, C. H., Hillyer, G. C., et al. (2011). Association between prescription co-payment amount and compliance with adjuvant hormonal therapy in women with early-stage breast cancer. *Journal of Clinical Oncology, 29*(18), 2534–2542.

Oguntola, A. S., Adeoti, M. I., & Akanbi, O. O. (2011). Non-adherence to the use of tamoxifen in the first year by breast cancer patients in an African population. *East and Central African Journal of Surgery, 16*(1), 52–56.

Owusu, C., Buist, D. S., Field, T. S., Lash, T. L., Thwin, S. S., Geiger, A. M., et al. (2008). Predictors of tamoxifen discontinuation among older women with estrogen receptor–positive breast cancer. *Journal of Clinical Oncology, 26*(4), 549–555.

Partridge, A. H., LaFountain, A., Mayer, E., Taylor, B. S., Winer, E., & Asnis-Alibozek, A. (2008). Adherence to initial adjuvant anastrozole therapy among women with early-stage breast cancer. *Journal of Clinical Oncology, 26*(4), 556–562.

Pellegrini, I., Sarradon-Eck, A., Soussan, P. B., Lacour, A. C., Largillier, R., Tallet, A., et al. (2010). Women's perceptions and experience of adjuvant tamoxifen therapy account for their adherence: Breast cancer patients' point of view. *Psycho-Oncology, 19*(5), 472–479.

Rae, J. M., Sikora, M. J., Henry, N. L., Li, L., Kim, S., Oesterreich, S., et al. (2009). Cytochrome P450 2D6 activity predicts discontinuation of tamoxifen therapy in breast cancer patients, *The Pharmacogenomics Journal, 9*(4), 258–264.

Ruddy, K., Mayer, E., & Partridge, A. (2009). Patient adherence and persistence with oral anticancer treatment. *CA: A Cancer Journal for Clinicians, 59*(1), 56–66.

Schmid, S. M., Eichholzer, M., Bovey, F., Myrick, M. E., Schötzau, A., & Güth, U. (2012). Impact of body mass index on compliance and persistence to adjuvant breast cancer therapy. *Breast, 21*(4), 487–492.

Sedjo, R. L., & Devine, S. (2011). Predictors of non-adherence to aromatase inhibitors among commercially insured women with breast cancer. *Breast Cancer Research and Treatment, 125*(1), 191–200.

Stanton, A., & Partridge, A. (2012). *Endocrine therapy after breast cancer (E-ABC)*. Santa Monica, CA: Army of Women. Retrieved from http://mailing.armyofwomen.org/form/armyofwomen/viewhtml/9z1zj4hvsj5qqaeth64dhimquv3mej35.

Swaby, R. F., Sharma, C. G., & Jordan, V. C. (2007). SERMs for the treatment and prevention of breast cancer. *Reviews in Endocrine & Metabolic Disorders, 8*(3), 229–239.

Southwest Oncology Group (2012). *SWOG update April 2012*. Retrieved from http://swog.org/visitors/newsletters/2012/04/index.asp?a=ai.

van de Water, W., Bastiaannet, E., Hille, E. T., Meershoek-Klein Kranenbarg, E. M., Putter, H., Seynaeve, C. M., et al. (2012). Age-specific nonpersistence of endocrine therapy in postmenopausal patients diagnosed with hormone receptor-positive breast cancer: A TEAM study analysis. *The Oncologist, 17*(1), 55–63.

van Herk-Sukel, M. P., van de Poll-Franse, L. V., Voogd, A. C., Nieuwenhuijzen, G. A., Coebergh, J. W., & Herings, R. M. (2010). Half of breast cancer patients discontinue tamoxifen and any endocrine treatment before the end of the recommended treatment period of 5 years: A population-based analysis. *Breast Cancer Research and Treatment, 122*(3), 843–851.

Visram, H., Kanji, F., & Dent, S. F. (2010). Endocrine therapy for male breast cancer: Rates of toxicity and adherence. *Current Oncology, 17*(5), 17–21.

Winkeljohn, D. (2010). Adherence to oral cancer therapies: Nursing interventions. *Clinical Journal of Oncology Nursing, 14*(4), 461–466.

Winters, L., Habin, K., Flanagan, J., & Cashavelly, B. J. (2010). "I feel like I am 100 years old!" managing arthralgias from aromatase inhibitors. *Clinical Journal of Oncology Nursing, 14*(3), 379–382.

World Health Organization, (2003). *Adherence to long-term therapies—Evidence for action*. Geneva: WHO.

World Health Organization, (2012). *Breast cancer: Prevention and control*. Retrieved from http://www.who.int/cancer/detection/breastcancer/en/. Accessed 24.05.2013.

Ziller, V., Kalder, M., Albert, U. S., Holzhauer, W., Ziller, M., Wagner, U., et al. (2009). Adherence to adjuvant endocrine therapy in postmenopausal women with breast cancer. *Annals of Oncology, 20*(3), 431–436.

INDEX

Note: Page numbers followed by "*f*" indicate figures, and "*t*" indicate tables.